M.V.H.

Clinicopathological Aspects of
# Creutzfeldt-Jakob Disease

# Clinicopathological Aspects of
# Creutzfeldt-Jakob Disease

**Edited by**

**Toshio Mizutani, M.D.**

Department of Clinical Neurcpathology,
Tokyo Metropolitan Institute for Neurosciences, Tokyo, Japan

**Hirotsugu Shiraki, M.D.**

Director, Shiraki Institute of Neuropathology,
Former Professor of Neuropathology, Institute of Brain Research,
School of Medicine, University of Tokyo, Japan

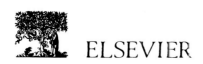 ELSEVIER    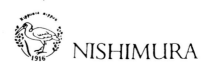 NISHIMURA

International joint publication
Publishers:

ELSEVIER SCIENCE
PUBLISHERS B.V.
P.O. Box 1126
1000 BC Amsterdam
The Netherlands

NISHIMURA Co., Ltd.
1-754-39 Asahimachi-Dori,
Niigata
951
Japan

Printed in Japan

# Preface

The history of research on Creutzfeldt-Jakob disease among the Japanese population has been conducted for a comparatively short period of time; the research of the disease actually did start mainly in the late half of 1960s, whereas a fairly large number of the papers in this field of the disease has been accumulated from the late half of 1970s to the beginning of 1980s. The verified autopsy cases of the disease in human beings, which have officially been published in different Japanese journals, on the other hand, now include 127 cases up to date and cases are still being reported. So far, Creutzfeldt-Jakob disease in the Japanese population, in fact, was fairly infrequent but never unusual or very rare.

As a consequence, almost all types of the disease, such as simple poliodystrophic (inflated neuronal) type, subacute spongiform encephalopathy, Stern-Garcin (thalamic) type and ataxic type, have been identified in the Japanese one after the other. Besides, there were also the verified autopsy cases of the familial Creutzfeldt-Jakob disease.

A new type of the disease, such as the panencephalopathic type, on the other hand, has just recently been well documented in the Japanese and published in foreign journals as well. In fact, this type of the disease in the Japanese, however, had never been identified or has quite rarely been reported in the western countries at least up to date. In addition, another new type of the disease, such as the chronic spongiform encephalopathy with plaques characterized by antecedent and long-lasting cerebellar ataxia, has been proposed by the Japanese authors, and this will be discussed in some detail in this monograph as well. Insofar as, it can be assumed that the clinicopathologic classification of Creutzfeldt-Jakob disease, particularly from a morphopathogenetic viewpoint, is still not sufficient.

One of the main purposes of this monograph is that the actual status of the disease in the Japanese should be clarified and reviewed as far as possible, since, as well known, the papers written in the Japanese language are very difficult to understand for foreign peoples.

As well known, it has been convincingly demonstrated that kuru and certain types of Creutzfeldt-Jakob disease can be transmitted from humans to animals and from animals to animals, but other types of Creutzfeldt-Jakob disease cannot. Thus, an unknown transmissible agent certainly exists, but not in all cases. For this reason and others, the term slow transmissible disease can be rationally applied here, and this classification is more scientifically sound. Without use of such a term, it is difficult to differentiate the disease in this regard because the nature of the transmissible agent, viral or otherwise, still remains unknown.

In this regard, another of the main purposes of this monograph is that there were a number of the excellent Japanese papers in this field of the disease or its allied field, some of which have internationally been accepted and evaluated; transmission experiments of the disease to small animals; experimental spongy degeneration caused by anti-folic acid agent; and biochemical aspects of Creutzfeldt-Jakob disease and allied disorders.

We particularly express our gratitude to Mr. Masanori Nishimura (President of Nishimura Co. Ltd.), who has been familiar terms with one of us (Mizutani) since medical school days. He afforded an opportunity to publish our monograph with great understanding.

The photograph was efficiently printed by Ms. Kyoko Suzuki (Department of Clinical Neuropathology, Tokyo Metropolitan Institute for Neurosciences). Mr. Nobuyuki Kobayashi at Photographic Center of Tokyo Metropolitan Institute for Neurosciences gave very useful advice for photographic technics. The manuscript was very untiringly typed by Ms. Hiroko Nemoto (Shiraki Institute of Neuropathology). We are grateful to Ms. Tomoko Shoji and Mr. Katsuaki Sakai (staffs of Nishimura Co. Ltd. ), and the staff of Elsevir Science Publisher in preparation of this book.

1985

Toshio Mizutani
Hirotsugu Shiraki

# Contents

# Contributors

AKAI, Junichiro, M. D.
Chief, Reseach Division of Pathology, National Kurihama Hospital, Lecturer, Department of Neurology, Brain Research Institute, Chiba University, 2769, Nohi, Yokosuka-City, 239, Japan.

HARIGUCHI, Shiro M. D.
Department of Neuropsychiatry, Medical School, Osaka University, Fukushima-ku, Osaka, 553, Japan.

HORITA, Naoki, M. D.
Department of Ultrastructure and Histochemistry, Psychiatric Research Institute of Tokyo, 2-1-8, Kamikitazawa, Setagaya-Ku, Tokyo, 150, Japan.

KONDO, Kiyotaro, M. D.
Professor of Public Health, Medical School, Hokkaido University, Sapporo, 060, Japan.

MIZUTANI, Toshio, M. D.
Department of Clinical Neuropathology, Tokyo Metropolitan Institute for Neurosciences, 2-6 Musashidai, Fuchu-City, Tokyo, 183, Japan.

NISHIMURA, Tsuyoshi, M. D.
Professor of Neuropsychiatry, Medical School, Osaka University, Fukushima-Ku, Osaka, 553, Japan.

SATO, Yuji, M. D.
Lecturer of Neuropathology, Neurological Institute, Faculty of Medicine, Kyushu University, Fukuoka, 812, Japan.

SATOH, Junichi, M. D.
Department of Clinical Neuropathology, Tokyo Metropolitan Institute for Neurosciences, 2-6 Musashidai, Fuchu-City, Tokyo, 183, Japan.

SHIRAKI, Hirotsugu, M. D.
Director, Shiraki Institute of Neuropathology, Former Professor of Neuropathology, Institute of Brain Research, School of Medicine, University of Tokyo, Honkomagome, Bunkyo-Ku, Tokyo, 113, Japan.

TADA, Kunitoshi, M. D.
  Department of Neuropsychiatry, Medical School, Osaka University,
  Fukushima-Ku, Osaka, 553, Japan.
TAKEDA, Masatoshi, M. D.
  Department of Neuropsychiatry, Medical School, Osaka University,
  Fukushima-Ku, Osaka, 553, Japan.
TATEISHI, Jun, M. D.
  Professor of Neuropathology, Neurological Institute, Faculty of
  Medicine, Kyushu University, Fukuoka, 812, Japan.

# Chapter I

# History of Research of Creutzfeldt-Jakob Disease

Toshio Mizutani, M. D.

The research of Creutzfeldt-Jakob disease (CJD) started with an autopsy case of a "strange disease" described by H. G. Creutzfeldt in 1920. In the next year A. Jakob reported three autopsy cases of subacute presenile dementia and identified Creutzfeldt's case as being an example of the same disorder. In his first paper he termed this disorder "spastic pseudosclerosis". Jakob's cases were reviewed in considerable detail in his second paper, which added a fourth case. In a later monograph of "Die Extrapyramidalen Erkrankungen" (1923) he added what he considered to be a fifth case. At that time, "spongy state" or "spongy degeneration" was not seriously taken into consideration, and thus, there arose no argument as to whether Creutzfeldt's case and Jakob's cases were the same disease or not. However, from the time when "subacute spongiform encephalopathy" (SSE) as a separate entity from spastic pseudosclerosis was proposed (Jacob, et al., 1958; Nevin, et al., 1960), a question as to whether the two diseases are within the same category or not occurred. The argument about this nosological problem of the disease has continued until a successful transmission of spongy degeneration to experimental animals by Gibbs, et al. in 1968. This controversy, however, is never fully settled as yet even at the present time. The delimitation of CJD remains of fundamental importance, and for this purpose clinicopathological study must still be continued at present and in the future.

## 1. Origin of the Problem of the Disease

The patient described by Creutzfeldt was a 22-year-old woman who showed psychiatric troubles since childhood. Her two sisters were mentally deficient. The total duration of illness was about 18 months. Creutzfeldt initially thought of multiple sclerosis, since nystagmus, temporal pallor of the optic discs, spastic paresis, intention tremor, scanning speech, forced laughing and a relapsing course were found. However, he set this possibility aside, since there occurred the emergence of irritative phenomena, myoclonic jerks and sensory disturbance such as hyperesthesia and hyperalgesia. The patient also exhibited mental symptoms including delirium, incoherence, incoordination, inappropriate answers, occasional states of stupor, and impaired consciousness. The postmortem examination showed laminar cortical devastation in focal and diffuse fashions, consisting of neuronal loss, swelling and homogenization, and proliferation of protoplasmic astrocytes mainly in the third layer. These changes were extensive throughout the entire cerebral cortex but more predominant in the precentral cortex. The gyral crowns were less frequently affected than the walls and depths of the sulci. In addition there were miliary lesions consisting of glial nodules and rosettes in the cortex, central nuclei and gray matter of the spinal cord. Inflated neuron (so-called "primäre Reitzung") was found in the cerebral cortex, nuclei of the brainstem, dentate nucleus and anterior horn of the spinal cord. Pyramidal tract also was involved.

Creutzfeldt summarized this case as follows: 1. unknown cause (perhaps familial predisposition); 2. relapsing course with remissions; 3. cortical symptoms referable to the motor and sensory centers (spasms and hyperalgesias); 4. mental symptoms of the type of intellectual deficit with predominance of psychomotor manifestations; 5. progressive course; 6. a noninflammatory focal disintegration of the cerebral cortex with neuronophagia and reparative glial proliferation (partly with vascular proliferation); 7. a noninflammatory diffuse cell disease with cell outfall throughout almost the entire gray substance.

Jakob, on the other hand, summarized the clinical and pathological features of this disease based on the observations of his five cases, and considered that "this disease occupies a place between the spastic system diseases, particularly amyotrophic lateral sclerosis (ALS), and the disease primarily localized to the striatum, particularly Westphal and Strümpell's pseudosclerosis, Wilson's disease, and chorea" (1921). This idea lead to propose "spastic pseudosclerosis" for this disease. Its neuropathology was a severe, purely parenchymatous degeneration consisting of the occurrence of numerous neuronophagic foci, the development of glial rosettes, the presence of diffuse and circumscribed foci of devastation with a preferential localization in particular regions (precentral gyrus, anterior part of the striatal system, the posterior frontal region, and the temporal region, medial nucleus of the thalamus, the motor nuclei of the medulla oblongata and spinal cord) with neuronal inflation, and generalized proliferation of protoplasmic astrocytes. Pyramidal tract degeneration in variable degrees was found in all cases.

When Jakob emphasized a close relationship of Creutzfeldt's pathological findings to those of his patients, a question proposed by other authors about the linking of the disease of Creutzfeldt's 22-year-old patient to Jakob's middle-aged group (Heidenhain, 1928). Furthermore, it has been pointed that Jakob's own case group was far from being uniform. Clinically his first case had temporarily positive Wassermann reaction and had attempted suicide with carbon monoxide gas; the second and fourth cases indulged in alcohol and had malnutrition; and as to the third and fifth patients a relationship to infectious and postencephalitic states was speculated. Pathologically, status spongiosus was found in only the fifth case, while in the early four cases there was no description of status spongiosus. Moreover, Van Rossum (1965) considered Jakob's fourth case as ALS, while Kirschbaum stated that this case was clearly distinguishable from ALS (1968). Recently, reviewing the original sections used by Jakob, Masters and Gajdusek concluded that his third and fifth cases fell within the category of spongiform encephalopathy from the conception of CJD at the present time, while his second and fourth cases were considered as acquired toxic-metabolic encephalopathies and his first case could be classified as an amyotrophic form of CJD (1982).

Nevertheless, it should be recognized that Jakob separated his spastic pseudosclerosis from ALS and various striatal degenerations, based on the striking similarities of the histopathological findings conjoined the five clinical observations.


## 2. Extended Concept of the Disease

### 1) Description of the representative cases

It seems certain that Jakob's wider concept permitted the collection and differentiation of the many more observations which afterward accumulated, as discussed below.

Heidenhain reported three cases of presenile corticostriatal degeneration (1928). The patients disclosed prodromal sensory disturbances, minor pyramidal and extrapyramidal signs, and prominent visual-agnostic symptoms. In his cases the occipital lobe, particulalry the visual cortex, was preferentially damaged and small neurons were selectively affected. Status spongiosus was found in two of them. He differentiated his cases from the Jakob's spastic pseudosclerosis on account of the main localization in the occipito-parietal cortex and relative sparing of the frontal and central gyri, although his second and third cases showed widespread degeneration including anterior sector, basal ganglia and cerebellum. He linked his cases to Kirschbaum's two cases (1924) in which comparable clinical features and notably topographical change were not fully comforming with the Jakob's original reports. He also stated that the Creutzfeldt's case should be excluded from the disease since the disease onset was of the early age, and the patient became psychotic and his extrapyramidal signs were not conspicuous, and that the histological picture also differed. In later years Heidenhain's cases qualified "Heidenhain's syndrome" as a subgroup with prevalent occipitoparietal clinical and anatomical disturbances (Meyer, 1954).

Familial cases of CJD were reported. The first, Baker's family pedigree was compiled firstly by Meggendorfer (1930) and followed by Stender (1930) and Jakob (1950), although the first case of this family was reported by Kirschbaum (1924). The similarities of clinicopathological process among the members of this family were obvious. The second family "R" was observed by Davison (1932) and followed by Davison and Rabiner (1940). Thereafter, five families were added. In 1979 Akai reported the first family of CJD in Japan (see Chapters II & IV).

In 1939 Stern published a case of 51-year-old man in whom dementia, sensory aphasia and apraxia developed. The neuropathology comprized an extensive degeneration of the cerebral cortex and thalamus. Similar cases of combined degeneration of the cerebral cortex and thalamus were reported (Schulman, 1956; Jacob, et al., 1950; Poursines, et al., 1953; Khochneviss, 1960; Garcin, et al., 1962). The lesions of the corticothalamic projections were associated with the secondary degenerations from the cortical devastation into the alterations of the medial and dorsolateral thalamic association nuclei. Martin, on the other hand, showed that essentially primary thalamic degeneration became manifested even when the related cortical fields were spared, and the form consisted of an independent degeneration of the intralaminary relay nuclei centralis medialis and lateralis of the thalamus (1966). Martin's findings supported the occurrence of pronounced primary involvement of thalamic nuclei in special cases of CJD (Forme thalamique, Garcin, et al., 1962, 1963; Stern-Garcin syndrome, McMenemy, et al., 1965; Thalamic type, Kirschbaum, 1968). Shiraki also categorized this type into a subtype of CJD with emphasis on combined system degeneration (1973), but later, he set this type aside, from clinicopathological point of view (Mizutani, 1981b; Shiraki & Mizutani, 1983, see Chapter III-4).

Alajouanine and Van Bogart in 1950 published two cases characterized by dementia, hyperkinesias and attacks of tetanus-like spasms. The patients died within a few months. There was neuronal degeneration and glial cell proliferation in the cortex, putamen, pallidum, thalamus, pontine nuclei and inferior olives. The authors did not diagnose these cases as spastic pseudosclerosis. Whereas, Jacob, et al. (1958), Alema, et al. (1959) and Khochneviss (1960) considered them to belong to the category of CJD.

Prominent neuronal degeneration and astrocytic proliferation in the cerebellum were emphasized by Foley and Denny-Brown (1955), and Brownell and Oppenheimer (1965). Schwarz and Barrows described a case limited to cerebellum, brainstem and anterior horn of the spinal cord (1958).

Mirianthopoulos, et al. reported an autopsy case of a 67-year-old man with the total duration of 60 months (1962). In this case there occurred severe neuronal depletion of the anterior horns of the spinal cord and corticospinal tract degeneration, while the cerebral cortex showed a laminar neuronal degeneration, status spongiosus and astrocytic proliferation, particularly predominant in the temporal cortex. The authors considered it as ALS with CJD. The clinical features comparable with those of ALS have been recognized in the CJD, while the pathological findings of motor neuron system usually were mild in contrast with those of ALS. However, this syndrome of motor neuron disease with dementia has been grouped together under the heading of amyotrophic form of CJD.

Brownell and Oppenheimer (1965) described "an ataxic form of CJD" which has been widely accepted. The point they stressed was that the cerebellar cortex is one of the structures at risk. The common clinical feature of this type was that cerebellar ataxia was predominant at the early stage and even at the later stage. The neuropathology of the cerebellum showed a selective degeneration of the granule cells with the comparatively well-preserved Purkinje cells which occurred in the entire cortex symmetrically and bilaterally, irrespective of neo- and paleocerebellum. Furthermore, Mizutani pointed out in the Brownell and Oppenheimer's cases that cerebellar degeneration far exceeded cerebral involvement (1977, 1981a). It is remarked that the fourth case reported by Brownell and Oppenheimer was first diagnosed as cerebellar degeneration both clinically and pathologically. On the other hand, the cases cited by Brownell and Oppenheimer (Foley & Denny-Brown, 1955; Lesse, et al., 1957; Katzman, et al., 1961; Silberman, et al., 1961) showed severe cortical lesion of the cerebrum in comparison with the Brownell and

Oppenheimer's cases.

Among the Japanese autopsy cases of CJD about a half of them had this cerebello-cortical degeneration mostly combined with primary involvement of both the cerebral and cerebellar white matter (Panencephalopathic type of CJD, see Chapter III- 6 & Appendix).

## 2) Spastic pseudosclerosis and subacute spongiform encephalopathy

In 1954 Jones and Nevin published the paper entitled "rapidly progressive cerebral degeneration (subacute vascular encephalopathy) with mental disorder, focal disturbances and myoclonic epilepsy". They implicated primary vascular disturbances but their view was not fully substantiated and not commonly shared by other authors who considered vascular disturbances as merely obligatory to the pathogenesis in certain cases. They considered spastic pseudosclerosis strictly unrelated to their group of patients which they included in a discussion of previously published cases (Nevin, et al., 1960). According to them, Heidenhain appeared to have confused the issue by suggesting that the Kirschbaum's two cases of Jakob's spastic pseudosclerosis should be grouped along with his own cases, despite that he distinguished his cases from the Jakob's spastic pseudosclerosis. They listed several pathological differences between SSE and spastic pseudosclerosis: 1) distribution of the cortical lesions; 2) cytological differences; 3) pathological changes in focal fashion; 4) behavior of astrocytes such as glial rosettes and neuronophagias; 5) status spongiosus. The authors considered status spongiosus as a non-specific change in SSE and it could commonly be found in other pathogenetic influences of metabolic-toxic, infectious, traumatic, or purely degenerative factors singly or combined.

Coupled with Nevin's paper, Jacob's report of "subacute presenile spongiform cerebral atrophy" raised the question regarding the relationship to CJD (1958). However, Jacob, et al. discussed on a separate entity of spongiform cerebral atrophy independently. They considered that the disease was characterized by degeneration of interstitial tissue and by a reaction of fibrillary glia, while in CJD there was degeneration of neurons and in particular there was a reaction of protoplasmic astrocytes. They considered the histological difference between the two diseases more pronounced than the clinical one. They, therefore, suggested that spongy encephalopathy and spastic pseudosclerosis could be grouped together clinically along with other subacute encephalopathies described by the French school (Garcin, et al., 1950; Poursiness, et al., 1953).

Kirschbaum's monograph of "Jakob-Creutzfeldt Disease" has a great influence on clinicopathological delimitation of CJD (1968). He summarized the neuropathology of CJD and stated that the neuronal and glial changes occurred either side by side or alternatively; status spongiosus appeared independently. Neuronal and glial changes may be less conspicuous and relatively minor, and status spongiosus may be prominent. Such conditions have promoted the use of such terms as "subacute spongious atrophy" (Jacob, et al., 1958) and "spongiform encephalopathy" (Nevin, et al., 1960). It was worthy of note that status spongiosus is not more frequent in the occipital (Heidenhain) type. Status spongiosus varied greatly in intensity and distribution in the gray and potentially also in the white matter and appeared separate and distinct from the general histopathological picture. That is his concept of CJD. Therefore, he did not consider SSE as a separate entity from spastic pseudosclerosis. Apart from whether SSE and spastic pseudosclerosis are the same disease or not, however, Kirschbaum's conclusion appeared to be incomplete in our opinion because he did not fully discuss a pathogenetical interrelationship among the three elementary changes, i.e., status spongiosus, astrocytic reaction and neuronal change. The problems, such as what kind of combination of these factors occurred and which of them was or were predominant, seemed to be explained by accidental occurrence.

In this connection, there has been an argument as to whether the change of neuron or astrocyte should be cosidered as primary. Meyer thought the neuronal degeneration to be primary and the glial proliferation secondary (1929). On the contrary, Zimmermann pointed that there was frequent disproportion between the extent and degree of neuronal and glial changes and sometimes marked astrocytic hypertrophy in the area of minor loss of neurons (1928). This was interpreted as a primary astroglial disturbance, and thus, induced that astrocytic hypertrophy migth occur not only as a sequel to neuronal degeneration, but also simultaneously as a primary response to unknown noxious agents. Since then, it has been repeatedly observed and similarly commented upon by Foley and Denny-Brown (1955), Jacob, et al. (1958), Silberman, et al. (1961), Shiraki (1974), and Mizutani, et al. (1981a, 1981b). Among them, Jacob's idea was remarked in that the pathological change of interstitial tissue of the cerebral cortex could play an important role in morphopathogenesis of SSE. This was further strengthened by electron microscopical studies. Gonatas, et al. reported the most reliable findings (1965). They observed about 40 sectioned blocks taken from the biopsy materials of two cases of CJD electron microscopically and concluded that status spongiosus probably was not related to cortical edema, but was rather a focal, intracytoplasmic process affecting only astrocytes and, less frequently, neurons. Shiraki pointed out that some glial dysfunction existed in CJD based on the observations that there occurred no obvious fibrillary gliosis, in spite of conspicuous proliferation of astrocytes, and there was no tendency of fat granule cells to accumulate around the vessels. On the contrary, since Lampert, et al. observed vacuolation in the neuronal processes (1971, 1972), the idea that status spongiosus is due to neuronal vacuolation is gaining ground. Recently, using a Golgi impregnation technique, a prominent and selective loss of dendritic spines, and focal swelling of dendrites were demonstrated (Landis, et al., 1981; Ferrer, et al., 1981).

Pellagra, on the other hand, was suggested as playing a part in the etiology of CJD (Josephy, 1936; Stadler, 1939; Jervis, et al., 1942; Stengel & Wilson, 1946). McMenemy stated that some of the earlier described cases of CJD should be considered as pellagra, and intoxication, particularly of lead, barbiturates and alcohol, should also be considered in the differential diagnosis (1958). This problem was taken up again by Jacob (1960), Matsuoka and Miyoshi (1964) and Shiraki (1974).

## 3) Clinicopathological aspects

There have been published many papers on the clinical and clinicopathological features of CJD. In 1938 Jansen and Monrad-Krohn divided the clinical course of CJD into three stages and this is still useful. The main clinical features of CJD, such as akinetic mutism, myoclonus, flexion posture and EEG changes, were emphasized by Foley and Denny-Brown (1955), by Pallis and Spallane (1957), by Nevin, et al. (1960) and by Katzman, et al. (1961).    The term "akinetic mutism" first described by Cairns was used to describe a patient who lay quietly and did not speak or respond to stimuli except that their eyes followed movements or objects (1953).    A state, reminiscent of akinetic mutism, was described in CJD (Pallis & Spillane, 1957; Nevin, et al., 1060; Katzman, et al., 1961). Cairns ascribed this state as interference with the upper portion of the reticular formation and its connections with the thalamus and hypothalamus.    Pallis and Spillane, on the other hand, noted the paucity of pathological findings in the region of the upper reticular formation, thalamus and hypothalamus.    They postulated that akinetic mutism resulted from a functional rather than a pathologically demonstrable lesion.    Katzman, on the other hand, speculated that akinetic mutism was a consequence not of involvement of the activating system itself but of the almost total involvement of the end organ of the activating system, the cerebral cortex.    Our observations showed that there occurred degeneration of both the ascending and descending pathways through, into and from the brainstem reticular formation as well as of the cerebrum in the panencephalopathic type of CJD, and thus, this finding should be remarked in development of akinetic mutism.

In 1958 Lesse and Hoeffer published the results of EEG examinations of eleven cases of diffuse encephalopathy, who all showed a similar type of EEG, i.e., periodical discharges consisting of synchronous slow waves and spike-wave activity (PSD, periodic synchronous discharge).    One of their cases showed CJD on postmortem examination.    Jacob, et al. described this EEG change as epilepsia partialis continuans in one patient (1958).    It has been suggested that myoclonus and PSD were the common manifestations of the same underlying disturbance.    Foley and Denny-Brown regarded it as a cerebellar type of myoclonus released or conditioned by cerebellar and cortical damage (1955).    Katzman stated that the subcortical centers from which the discharges arise were more likely to fire when they are released from cortical inhibition and, in addition, received impulses from degenerating neurons.    Finally Katzman, et al. defined akinetic mutism, myoclonus and PSD as the clinical triad of CJD (1961).

## 4) Different classifications of CJD

By the early 1970s, several outstanding classifications had been proposed from different standpoints.    For a long time CJD was considered a rare form of presenile dementia usually diagnosed only by postmortem examination, but nearly 200 autopsy cases had been accumulated by the end of the 1960s.    Siedler and Malamud (1963) stated that the disease was actually uncommon but not rare.    The problem as to whether spastic pseudosclerosis and SSE were within the same category arose, as mentioned above.    This included pathogenesis of status spongiosus, variable pathological relationships among the changes of neurons, glias and neuropil, and a variety of the anatomical distribution of lesions from case to case.    Besides, no evidence of cause has been identified.    However, none of the classifications did much take account of histopathogenetic aspects.    Such a broad spectrum of both clinical and pathological features induced many authors to make an attempt to classify into subtypes based on either clinical features or anatomical distribution of lesions. As a result, the concept of CJD tended to become extended.

Meyer (1929) proposed to classify CJD into two clinical types, one resembling presenile dementia and the other resembling amyotrophic lateral sclerosis (ALS). This was probably the first classification of CJD but it has not been generally accepted, since his classification did not refer to the presence of extrapyramidal signs.

Alema and Bignami defined CJD as the general heading of "polioencephalopathia degenerativa". They distinguished five types as follows: 1) the myoclonus type (Myoclonus, a specific EEG pattern and a rather rapid course were characteristics, but the pathology was not uniform and marked status spongiosus was found in a half of the cases.); 2) the amaurotic type (Heidenhain's sydrome); 3) the so-called intermediate type which was identical to the clinical picture originally described by Creutzfeldt and Jakob; 4) the dyskinetic type (Tremor, chorea, athetosis and ballismus, and sometimes parkinsonism occur. In the terminal stage epileptic seizures occur and dysarthria and dementia become pronounced. Neuronal shrinkage and inflation with proliferation of astrocytes are predominant in the posterior frontal and temporal lobes, and striatum, thalamus, motor nuclei in the brainstem and anterior horn of the spinal cord.); 5) the amyotrophic type (Pyramidal signs and lower motor neuron signs with tremor and rigidity are predominant. Neuropathology bears a strong resemblance to the dyskinetic type). The kernel of Alema and Bignami's monograph is the introduction of a new classification of the clinical pictures under polioencephalopathy. This classification was based preferentially on the clinical pictures, while pathological features were unsatisfactory. A similar classification proposed by Khochneviss (1960) and Garcin, et al. (1963) consisted of five types: 1) the classical type; 2) the amyotrophic type; 3) the thalamic type; 4) Heidenhain's type; 5) the spongious type. They introduced the thalamic type and used the term subacute spongious encephalopathy following Jacob et al. (1958).

Van Rossum (1962, 1965, 1968) proposed a classification of CJD based mainly on the histological findings; 1) the spongious (cortical) type (This type is almost identical to SSE in a modern criteria. The author stressed spongy degeneration in the striatum as well as the cortex); 2) the optic type (This type is so-called Heidenhain's type); 3) the striatal type (The author stated that this was the most common type in which hyperkinesias, especially chorea and myoclonus, pyramidal sign, focal signs including aphasia and apraxia, muscle atrophy, dysarthria, and dementia occurred. There occurred neuronal degeneration in cortex, subcortical gray, cranial motor nuclei and anterior horn of the spinal cord. No spongy degeneration was found.); 4) the thalamic type; 5) the niger type (This was the new type introduced by Van Rossum. Three cases were included. The clinical course was exceedingly protracted. The main feature was hypokinesia-rigidity syndrome as well as hyperkinesia (tremor, myoclonus, and athetosis) and organic mental syndrome. The substantia nigra disclosed conspicuous degeneration. Neuronal degeneration also occurred in the cerebral and cerebellar cortex, thalamus, and pontine and inferior olivary nuclei. No spongy degeneration was described.); 6) the anterior horn (amyotrophic) type. It was of an interest that nigral involvement was taken up as one of the main features of CJD. However, the significance of spongy degeneration was obscure in his classification.

A classification based on the anatomical distribution of lesions was also proposed by Kirschbaum (1968). He divided into three types which are frequently used even at the present time: 1) the frontopyramidal, spastic pseudosclerosis type (A. Jakob); 2) the occipitoparietal, agnostic-visual, and dyskinetic syndrome (Heidenhain); 3) the diffuse cerebral and cortical and basal ganglia type with (as also in types 1 and 2) thalamic, midbrain, cerebellar, spinal participation.

May stated that although many authors considered only the anatomical distribution of the lesions, the variable distribution of lesion in this disease made subdivision by strictly anatomical criteria problematic and that the classifications by Meyer, et al.(1954), by Alema and Bignami (1959), and by Garcin, et al. (1963) seemed to be more useful (1968). He divided into the four types based mainly on the different durations of the total illness; 1) the amyotrophic type; 2) the classical type; 3) the transitional type; 4) SSE.

Finally it is noteworthy to refer the paper by Siedler and Malamud because a similar classification based on the findings of experimental transmission of spongy state appeared, as mentioned below (Roos, et al., 1973). Siedler and Malamud examined their 15 cases of CJD and reviewed the literatures (1963), and concluded that a separate entity of SSE existed apart from CJD was not warranted, rather the disease had broad clinical and pathological spectra. The authors proposed two subtypes: 1) the cases with fronto-centro-temporal accentuated cortical atrophy, lower motor neuron disease and a longer duration of illness and 2) the cases with more generalized atrophy of the cerebral cortex, absence of motor neuron changes and more subacute course. On the other hand, Roos and his associates analysed the clinical features of the cases with and without successful transmission of spongy state to the animals. Thus, the cases with successful transmission showed a rather short duration and no lower motor neuron signs, while the cases with failure of transmission disclosed a long duration of illness and lower motor neuron signs.

In the period before 1968 when status spongiosus in human brain of CJD was successful in experimental transmission by Gibbs, et al., most investigators already regarded the disease as a single nosological entity, although Nevin had asserted SSE as a distinct entity different from CJD as mentioned before. Each histological change in neuron, astrocyte and neuropil of CJD was nonspecific and combinations of the three elements were variable from case to case, as pointed out by Kirschbaum. Furthermore, the problem as to which change or changes were the most essential feature in CJD has not yet been well established. The morphopathogenesis of status spongiosus seems to be one of the critical problems, at least. This neccesiates the comparative study of the status spongiosus in CJD with the presenile dementia, such as Pick's disease, Alzheimer's disease and other dementias, and normal senile brain. Unfortunately, such comparative studies have never been well documented as yet. These resulted into widening of the spectrum of CJD and reflected on the various classifications of CJD. Thus, almost all classifications were based not on the histopathogenetical aspects but on the clinical features and/or the anatomical distribution of the lesions. It is certain that Jakob's idea in which he put heterogenous cases of presenile neuropsychiatric disorders and Creutzfeldt's case into a distinct entity, played a role in widening of the concept of the disease. Nevertheless, it should be remarked that a presenile degenerative disorder separated by Jakob from various cortical, pyramidal and extrapyramidal degenerations certainly existed, apart from whether his cases were CJD or not in modern knowledge. Masters and Gajdusek stated that two of Jakob's original cases could be considered to be etiologically some toxic-metabolic encephalopathies. If it is true, CJD may be a syndrome caused by different etiologies.

# 3. Modern Concept and Problems of the Disease

In 1965, Gajdusek discussed the possibility that CJD is a slow virus infection. In the next year he demonstrated that a brain specimen of patients with Kuru was inoculated into the brain of chimpanzee, and a spongy degeneration developed in the chimpanzee's brain after a long latent interval (1966). Finally both spongy degeneration and astrocytosis of CJD were similarly transmitted from a patient to a chimpanzee (Gibbs, et al., 1968). Thereafter, the disease has been transmitted in second passage from chimpanzee to chimpanzee (Gibbs & Gajdusek, 1969). These epoch-making results compelled an interest to demonstration of causative agent of CJD, despite that the clinicopathological delimitation of CJD has not been fully clarified. Transmission of the disease to experimental animals has been performed in the numerous laboratories of the world, and thus, spongy degeneration can be transmitted to small rodents. Beck, et al. reported the detailed neuropathological findings of the chimpanzee in comparison with those in human CJD, and they pointed out surprisingly great similarities between the two conditions (1969). According to the authors, in both conditions the primary degeneration was entirely confined to gray matter, while the white matter lesions were considered to be secondarily originated from the destruction of cortical neurons. The topographical distribution of the lesion was also similar in both conditions. The histological changes consisted of neuronal loss, status spongiosus and proliferation of astrocytes with many reactive microglial cells. It also was remarked that both specimens showed inflated neurons. They also stressed that the degeneration in the hypothalamo-neurohypophysial system was found in both conditions. On the contrary, there were some differences between the two. In CJD of humans the dorsomedial nucleus and pulvinar of the thalamus were severely damaged, while in the chimpanzee the ventrolateral group showed the severest changes. Further differences lay in the severe degeneration with almost complete neuronal loss in the rostral part of the pontine nuclei of the experimental case. They considered that such differences may represent another variant in CJD in humans or may be due to differences in the susceptibility to the pathogenetic agent of certain gray matters. In our opinion, neuronal loss in the rostral pontine nuclei of the chimpanzee, however, may be comparable with the findings in which this could be regarded as a part of multisystem degeneration in CJD, but this will be discussed more in detail later on. Finally they discussed the view that a primary degeneration of the astrocytes leads to secondary degeneration of the neurons. They carefully assessed the pathological findings and thought that the question as to which cell is primarily affected by the agent and which cell reacts secondarily must remain open. However, since Lampert, et al. stressed that status spongiosus occurred exclusively in neuron (1969, 1971), the concept of neuronal disease in CJD has been widely accepted, rather than Gonatas' view in which vacuoles occurred mainly in the astrocytic processes.

Roos, et al. stated that they have successfully transmitted the disease to animals and named this as "the CJD type of subacute spongiform virus encephalopathy" (1973). Against Nevin's opinion they stated that the successful transmission of a case that satisfied the Nevin's clinical and pathological criteria for CJD (1960) would serve as a unifying factor in attempting to classify SSE and CJD. Virus-like particles have been described repeatedly in the brains of both natural and experimental spongiform encephalopathies (Roth, et al., 1979; Chou, et al., 1980, Narang, et al., 1980; Baringer, et al., 1981), but none of these observations have been consistently confirmed up to date. Thus, it remains open whether the causal agent of spongy degeneration is a virus or not. This is a weak point of the viral infection theory. The view, therefore, seems to be premature that CJD is a slow virus infection. Recently, there is a tendency in which the term "subacute spongiform virus encephalopathy" has been replaced by the term "transmissible dementia", although the term "transmissible dementia" seems to reflect the extension of the concept of CJD.

Roos, et al. divided 47 cases into two groups on the basis of whether or not inoculation of their frozen brain tissues successfully transmitted the disease to primates, and compared two groups clinically (1973). According to them, the most statistically significant features were based upon a variety of a total duration of illness and a presence of lower motor neuron signs. As a consequence, they stated that the group with failure of transmission showed a longer duration and prominent signs of lower motor neuron involvement. As mentioned above, the similar differences were pointed out by Siedler and Malamud from a different point of view (1963). Furthermore, Traub, et al. reported that the patients with the amyotrophic form of CJD have not yet been shown to have experimentally transmissible disease (1977).

The neuropathology of spongy degeneration in CJD was reviewed by Masters and Richardson (1978). According to them, a distinction was drawn between the vacuolation of the neuropil which was characteristic of the disease (spongiform change) and the rather coarse loosening of the brain parenchyma associated with severe gliosis which was a non-specific change (status spongiosus). Spongiform change was most severe and readily apparent in the cases of relatively short duration (6 months or less), while status spongiosus with concomitant gliosis was seen in those cases of longer duration.

In Japan several critical papers to the theory of slow virus infection were reported in "Symposium on Creutzfeldt-Jakob Disease" held in the 14th Annual Meeting of Japanese Society of Neuropathology. Shiraki discussed that transmissible agent did not always suggest only a virus (1974). He proposed a classification with emphasis on the histopathogenetic aspects: Simple poliodystrophic type; SSE; Stern-Garcin type. He stressed that simple poliodystrophic type has an aspect of toxic-metabolic disorders including pellagra, while in SSE glial dysfunction could play a part of histopathogenesis. He also emphasized that the pathological aging and system degeneration in CJD were not coincidental but closely interrelated (see Chapter III- 9). Matsuoka, on the other hand, regarded CJD as a representative of glioneuronal dystrophies, since astrocytic reaction appeared to be primary in CJD (1974). Moreover, he referred to a group of "dissociation anatomo-clinique". This has been proposed for SSE (Jacob & van Bogart, 1967; Macchi & Lechi, 1967; Terzian, et al., 1967), while he stated anatomo-clinical dissociation in spastic pseudosclerosis. Ikuta demonstrated cholesterol-ester in the spongy cavities of the cortex in SSE, and he discussed a metabolic disorder as a cause of SSE (1974).

It is well-known that CJD has been regarded as a disease of the gray matter (polioencephalopathy). Mizutani, et al., on the other hand, proposed "panencephalopathic type" as a subtype of CJD and emphasized the primary involvement of the white matter combined with system degeneration in this subtype (1977, 1981a, 1981b, 1983). In this regard, the first case reported by Jacob, et al. showed a diffuse loss of myelin in the cerebral and cerebellar white matter, and pyramidal tract and posterior column of the spinal cord (1958). Jacob suggested a possibility in that a more widespread involvement of the white matter may be found in the future. The panencephalopathic type of CJD was marked not only by the primary invovlement of the white matter but also by the systematized degeneration in the cerebellum, brainstem and spinal cord. The latter change was confined precisely to the anatomically-interrelated nuclei and fiber tracts, accompanied by fibrillary gliosis. Thus, many of these lesions could be compatible with the previously well-known system degenerations, such as Friedreich's ataxia, olivopontocerebellar atrophy and dentatorubro-pallidoluysian atrophy (see Chapter III-6). Furthermore, these findings were also found in the other subtypes of CJD. Mizutani, et al. stressed that system degeneration could be no more than coincidental but one of the essential features of CJD. The panencephalopathic type of CJD, on the other hand, appeared to be prevailing in Japanese, but several sporadic or familial cases have been reported in other countries (see Chapter III-6 & Appendix).

In 1979 Tateishi and his associates succeeded in experimental transmission of spongy degeneration to the white matter of small rodents (Tateishi, et al., 1979; Tateishi, et al., 1980; Tateishi, et al., 1980) (see Chapter V). In 1983 they also succeeded in the reproduction of kuru plaques in small animals (Tateishi, et al., 1984).

The experimental spongy degeneration suggested a possibility that other dementing diseases would be found to be transmissible and would eventually be included into the category of transmissible dementia. This extension of concept is apparently different from that in the time before 1968. Alzheimer's disease now becomes a candidate for transmissible dementia. Masters, et al. emphasized the possibility that Alzheimer's disease shares a common pathogenesis with CJD, based on epidemiological, clinical and experimental studies of familial Alzheimer's disease and familial CJD (1981). They also discussed the relation of CJD with kuru or kuru-like plaques and Gerstmann-Sträussler-Scheinker disease (GSSD) and proposed the term Gerstmann-Sträussler syndrome to include the cases with ataxia, dementia and co-existence of multiform plaques (1981). This hypothesis appears to be supported further by Tateishi's excellent experiment of kuru plaque. In Japan the cases with long prodromal stage characterized by severe cerebellar and/or ataxic symptoms simulated to spinocerebeller degeneration and GSSD, and by kuru or kuru-like plaques have been accumulated (Mizutani, 1981b, see Chapter III-7). Thus, amyloid plaques are common in CJD with plaques, Kuru, Alzheimer's disease and GSSD. However, the problem whether amyloid plaque are related causally to the essential process of CJD or not, remains still unsolved. Furthermore, system degeneration in these disease groups has not been fully considered. Prior to discuss this the detailed and careful clinicopathological observation in those human cases should be performed.

It now becomes obvious that spongy degeneration and amyloid plaque have become the most reliable target as the transmissible change in CJD research. This certainly made clear some aspects of so-called "status spongiosus", and appears to define the spectrum of CJD, since the experimental studies have showed that some cases of CJD were transmissible, while the others not. This was a marked progress in an etiological aspect of CJD research. However, it should be pointed out that since the aspects based on the experimental results were emphasized to excess, the other clinicopathological features including system degeneration, pathological aging and cytological changes in neuron and astrocyte tended to be neglected.

Modern knowledge suggests that CJD as a clinicopathological entity may be a syndrome due to different causes.   This possibility forces us to clarify the clinicopathological similarities and dissimilarities among the subtypes of CJD in relation to the results of experimental studies.   At least at present, however, one should keep in mind that only spongy degeneration, inflation of neuron and plaques can be transmitted to experimental animals, but as far as another important criteria of CJD, i,e., system degenerations, are concerned, they have never been transmitted to animals at least up to date.

# REFERENCES

**Alajouanine, T. and van Bogart, L.**:   Sur une affection caractérisée par une contracture téta-noïde diffuse avec hypercinésies variab es et à évolution subaiguë mortelle, Rev. Neurol., 82: 21-34, 1950.

**Alema, G. and Bignami, A.**:   Polio encefalopatia degenerativa subacuta del presenio con stupore acinetico e rigidita decorticata con mi clonie, Riv. sper. Freniat., 83, Suppl. IV, 1485-1622, 1959.

**Baringer, J. R., Prusiner, S. B. and Wong, J. S.**:   Scrapie-associated particles in postsynaptic processes.   Further ultrastructural studies, J. Neuropathol. exp. Neurol., 40: 281-288, 1981.

**Beck, E., Daniel, P. M., Matthews, W. B., Stevens, D. L., Alpers, M. P., Asher, D. M., Gajdusek, D. C. and Gibbs, C. J. Jr.**:   Creutzfeldt-Jakob disease.   The neuropathology of a transmission experiment, Brain, 92: 699-716, 1969.

**Brownell, B. and Oppenheimer, D. R.**:   An ataxic form of subacute presenile polioence-phalopathy (Creutzfeldt-Jakob disease), J. Neurol. Neurosurg. Psychiat., 28: 350-361, 1965.

**Chou, S. M., Payne, W. N., Gibbs, C. J. Jr. and Gajdusek, D. C.**:   Transmission and scanning electron microscopy of spongiform change in Creutzfeldt-Jakob disease, Brain, 103: 885-904, 1980.

**Creutzfeldt, H. G.**:   Über eine eigenartige herdförmige Erkrankung des Zentralnervensystems, Z. ges. Neurol. Psychiat., 57: 1-19, 1920.

**Davison, C.**:   Spastic pseudosclerosis, Brain, 55: 247-264, 1932.

**Davison, C. and Rabiner, A. M.**:   Spastic pseudosclerosis, Arch. Neurol. Psychiat., 44: 573-598, 1940.

**Ferrer, I., Costa, F. and Grau Veciana, J. M.**:   Creutzfeldt-Jakob disease: a Golgi study, Neuropathol. Appl. Neurobiol., 7: 237-242, 1981.

**Foley, J. M. and Denny-Brown, D.**:   Subacute progressive encephalopathy with bulbar myo-clonus, Excerpta med., Sect. VIII, 3: 782-784, 1955.

**Gajdusek, D. C., Gibbs, C. J. Jr. and Alpers, M.**:   Experimental transmission of a kuru-like syndrome to chimpanzees, Nature, 209: 794-796, 1966.

**Gajdusek, D. C., Gibbs, C. J. Jr. and Alpers, M.**:   Transmission and passage of experimental "kuru" to chimpanzees, Science, 155: 212-214, 1967.

**Garcin, R., Brion, S. and Khochneviss, A.**:   Le syndrome de Creutzfeldt-Jakob, Rev. Neurol.,

106: 506-508, 1962.

**Garcin, R., Brion, S. and Khochneviss, A.:** Le syndrome de Creutzfeldt-Jakob et les syndromes cortico-striés du presenium, Rev. Neurol., 109: 419-441, 1963.

**Gibbs, C. J. Jr., Gajdusek, D. C., Asher., D. M., Beck, E., Danniel, P. M. and Matthews, W. B.:** Creutzfeldt-Jakob disease (Spongiform encephalopathy); Transmission to the chimpanzee, Science, 161: 388-389, 1968.

**Gibbs, C. J. Jr. and Gajdusek, D. C.:** Infection as the etiology of spongiform encephalopathy (Creutzfeldt-Jakob disease), Science, 165: 1023-1025, 1969.

**Gonatas, N. K.:** Electron microscopic study in two cases of Creutzfeldt-Jakob disease, J. Neuropathol. exp. Neurol., 24: 575-598, 1965.

**Heidenhain, A.:** Klinische und anatomische Untersuchungen über eine eigenartige organische Erkrankung des Zentralnervensystems im Presenium, Z. ges. Neurol. Psychiat., 118: 49-114, 1928.

**Ikuta, F., Kumanishi, T., Ohashi, T. and Koga, M.:** Studies on Creutzfeldt-Jakob disease - Is this disease a metabolic disorder ?, Adv. Neurol. Sci. (Japan), 18: 46-61, 1974.

**Jacob, H., Pyrkosch, W. and Strube, H.:** Die erbliche Form der Creutzfeldt-Jakoben Krankheit, Arch. Psychiat. Nervenkr., 184: 653-674, 1950.

**Jacob, H., Eicke, W. and Orthner, H.:** Zur Klinik und Neuropathologie der subakuten praesenilen spongiösen Atrophien mit dyskinetischem Endstadium, Dtsch. Z. Nervenheilk., 178: 330-357, 1958.

**Jakob, A.:** Über eigenartige Erkrankungen des Zentralnervensystems mit bemerkenswertem anatomische Befunde, Z. ges. Neurol. Psychiat., 64: 147-228, 1921.

**Jakob, A.:** Über eine der multiplen Sklerose klinisch nahestehende Erkrankung des Zentralnervensystems (spastische Pseudosklerose) mit bemerkenswertem anatomische Befunde, Med. Klin., 17: 372-376, 1921.

**Jakob, A.:** "Die Extrapyramidalen Erkrankungen", Springer, Berlin, 1923.

**Jansen, J. and Monrad-Krohn, G. H.:** Über die Creutzfeldt-Jakobsche Krankheit, Z. ges. Neurol. Psychiat., 163: 670-704, 1938.

**Jervis, G. A., Hurdum, H. M. and O'Neill, F. J.:** Presenile psychosis of the Jakob type, Amer. J. Psychiat., 99: 101-109, 1942.

**Jones, P. and Nevin, S.:** Rapidly progressive cerebral degeneration (subacute vascular encephalopathy) with mental disorder, focal disturbances and myoclonic epilepsy, J. Neurol. Neurosurg. Psychiat., 17: 148-151, 1954.

**Josephy, H.:** Jakob-Creutzfeldtsche Krankheit. In: Handbuch der Neurologie, eds. Bumke, F. and Foerster, O., Vol. XVI, Berlin, Springer-Verlag, 1936, p.882.

**Katzman, R., Kagan, E. H. and Zimmerman, H. M.:** A case of Jakob-Creutzfeldt disease, J. Neuropathol. exp. Neurol., 20: 78-94, 1961.

**Khochneviss, A.:** Contribution à l'étude du syndorme de Creutzfeldt-Jakob, et des syndromes cortico-striés du présénium, Thèse Paris, 1960.

**Kirschbaum, W. R.:** Zwei eigenartige Erkrankungen des Zentralnervensystems nach Art der spastischen Pseudosklerose (Jakob), Z. ges. Neurol. Psychiat., 92: 175-220, 1924.

**Kirschbaum, W. R.:** Jakob-Creutzfeldt Disease, American Elsevier, 1968.

**Lampert, P. W., Gajdusek, D. C. and Gibbs, C. J. Jr.:** Experimental spongiform encephalopathy (Creutzfeldt-Jakob disease) in chimpanzees: electronmicroscopic studies, J. Neuropathol. exp. Neurol., 30: 20-32, 1971.

**Lampert, P. W., Gajdusek, D. C. and Gibbs, C. J. Jr.:** Subacute spongiform virus encephalopathies. Scrapie, Kuru and Creutzfeldt-Jakob disease, Am. J. Pathol., 68: 626-646, 1972.

**Landis, D. M., Willams, R. S. and Masters, C. L.:** Golgi and electronmicroscopic studies of spongiform encepehalopathy, Neurology, 31: 538-549, 1981.

**Lesse, S., Hoefer. P. F. A. and Austin, J. H.:**  The electroencephalogram in diffuse encephalopathies, Arch. Neurol. Psychiat., 79: 350-357, 1958.

**Martin, J. J.:**  Topographie et signification des lésions thalamiques dans la maladie de Creutzfeldt-Jakob et les formes apparentées, J. Hirnforsch., 8: 137-159, 1966.

**Masters, C. L. and Richardson, E. P. Jr.:**  Subacute spongiform encephalopathy (Creutzfeldt-Jakob disease).  The nature and progression of spongiform change, Brain, 101: 333-344, 1978.

**Masters, C. L., Gibbs, C. J. Jr. and Gajdusek, D. C.:**  The familial occurrence of Creutzfeldt-Jakob disease and Alzheimer's disease, Brain, 104: 535-558, 1981a.

**Masters, C. L., Gajdusek, D. C. and Gibbs, C. J. Jr.:**  Creutzfeldt-Jakob disease virus isolation from the Gerstmann-Sträussler syndrome: With an analysis of the various forms of amyloid plaque deposition in the virus-induced spongiform encephalopathies, Brain, 104: 559-588, 1981b.

**Masters, C. L. and Gajdusek, D. C.:**  The spectrum of Creutzfeldt-Jakob disease and the virus-induced subacute spongiform encephalopathies, In: Recent Advances in Neuropathology, eds., Smith, W. T. and Cavanagh, J. B., Churchill Livingstone, Edinburgh, 1982, pp. 137-163.

**Matsuoka, T. and Miyoshi, K.:**  An autopsy case of Creutzfeldt-Jakob disease - A contribution to the understanding of presenile-involutive encephalopathies, Adv. Neurol. Sci. (Japan), 8: 427-438, 1964.

**Matsuoka, T.:**  Creutzfeldt-Jakob disease - Clinical manifestations and pathological features, Adv. Neurol. Sci. (Japan), 18: 33-45, 1974.

**May, W. W.:**  Creutzfeldt-Jakob disease. 1. Survey of the literature and clinical diagnosis, Acta Neurol. Scandinav., 44: 1-32, 1968.

**McMenemy, W. H.:**  The dementias and progressive diseases of the basal ganglia. In: Greenfield's Neuropathology, 1st edition. London, Edward Arnold (1958), pp. 475-521, 2nd edition, 1963.

**Meggendorfer, F.:**  Klinische und genealogische Beobachtungen bei einem Fall von spastischen Pseudosklerose Jakobs, Z. ges. Neurol. Psychiat., 128: 337-341, 1930.

**Meyer, A.:**  Über eine der amyotrophischen Lateralsklerose nahestehende Erkrankung mit psychischen Störungen, Z. ges. Neurol. Psychiat., 121: 107-138, 1929.

**Meyer, A., Leigh, D. and Bagg, C. E.:**  A rare presenile dementia associated with cortical blindness, J. Neurol. Neurosurg. Psychiat., 17: 129-133, 1954.

**Mizutani, T.:**  Creutzfeldt-Jakob disease with cerebellar cortical degeneration - Special reference to a subtype of Creutzfeldt-Jakob disease with severe cerebrocerebellar atrophy, Adv. Neurol. Sci. (Japan), 21: 135-143, 1977.

**Mizutani, T., Okumura, A., Oda, M. and Shiraki, H.:**  Panencephalopathic type of Creutzfeldt-Jakob disease: Primary involvement of the cerebral white matter, J. Neurol. Neurosurg. Psychiat., 44: 103-115, 1981a.

**Mizutani, T.:**  Neuropathology of Creutzfeldt-Jakob disease in Japan.  With special reference to the panencephalopathic type, Acta Path. Jpn., 31: 903-922, 1981b.

**Narang, H. K., Chandler, R. L. and Anger, H. S.:**  Further observations on particulate structures in scrapie affected brain, Neuropathol. Appl. Neurobiol., 6: 23-28, 1980.

**Nevin, S., McMenemy, W. H., Behrman, S. and Jones, D.P.:**  Subacute spongiform encephalopathy - A subacute form of encephalopathy attributable to vascular dysfunction (Spongiform cerebral atrophy), Brain, 83: 519-564, 1960.

**Nevin, S., Barnard, R. O. and McMenemey, W. H.:**  Different types of Creutzfeldt-Jakob disease, Acta Neuropathol., Suppl. III, 7-13, 1967.

**Pallis, C. A. and Spillane, J. D.:**  A subacute progressive encephalopathy with mutism, hypokinesia, rigidity and myoclonus, Quart. J. Med., 26: 349-373, 1957.

**Poursines, Y., Boudouresques, J. and Roger, R.:**  Processus dégénératif atrophique diffus à prédominance thalamo-striée, Rev. Neurol., 89: 266-271, 1953.

**Roos, R., Gajdusek, D. C. and Gibbs, C. J. Jr.:** The clinical characteristics of transmissible Creutzfeldt-Jakob disease, Brain, 96: 1-20, 1973.

**Schulman, S.:** Bilateral symmetrical degeneration of the thalamus, J. Neuropathol. exp. Neurol., 15: 208-209, 1956.

**Schwarz, G. A. and Barrows, L. J.:** Polioencephalopathy reminiscent of Creutzfeldt-Jakob syndrome, J. Neuropathol. exp. Neurol., 17: 352-366, 1958.

**Shiraki, H.:** The neuropathological background for Creutzfeldt-Jakob disease (Creutzfeldt-Jakob sydrome), Adv. Neurol. Sci. (Japan), 18: 4-30, 1974.

**Shiraki, H. and Mizutani, T.:** Neuropathologic characteristics of types of Creutzfeldt-Jakob disease with special reference to the panencephalopathic type prevalent among Japanese, In: Neuropsychiatric Disorders in the Elderly, eds. Hirano, A. and Miyoshi, K., Igaku-Shoin, Tokyo, New York, 1983, pp. 139-188.

**Siedler, K. and Malamud, N.:** Creutzfeldt-Jakob's disease, Clinicopathologic report of 15 cases and review of the literature (with special reference to a related disorder designated as subacute spongiform encephalopathy), J. Neuropathol. exp. Neurol., 22: 381-402, 1963.

**Silberman, J., Cravioto, H. and Feigin, J.:** Corticostriatal degeneration of Creutzfeldt-Jakob type, J. Neuropathol. exp. Neurol., 20: 105-118, 1961.

**Stadler, H.:** Über Beziehungen zwischen Creutzfeldt-Jakobscher Krankheit und Pellagra, Z. ges. Neurol. Psychiat., 165: 326-332, 1939.

**Stender, A.:** Weitere Beitrage zum Kapitel "spastische Pseudosklerose Jakobs", Z. ges. Neurol. Psychiat., 128: 528, 1930.

**Stengel, E. and Wilson, W. E. J.:** Jakob-Creutzfeldt disease, J. Ment. Sci., 92: 370-378, 1946.

**Stern, K.:** Severe dementia associated with bilateral symmetrical degeneration of thalamus, Brain, 62: 157-171, 1939.

**Tateishi, J., Ohta, M., Koga, M., Sato, Y. and Kuroiwa, Y.:** Transmission of chronic spongiform encephalopathy with kuru plaques from humans to small rodents, Ann. Neurol., 5: 581-584, 1979.

**Tateishi, J., Koga, M., Sato, Y. and Mori, R.:** Properties of the transmissible agent derived from chronic spongiform encepehalopathy, Ann. Neurol., 7: 390-391, 1980.

**Tateishi, J., Sato, Y., Nagara, H. and Boellaard, J. W.:** Experimental transmission of human subacute spongiform encephalopathy to small rodents. IV. Positive transmission from a typical case of Gerstmann - Sträussler - Scheinker's disease, Acta Neuropathol., 64: 85-88, 1984.

**Traub, R., Gajdusek, D. C. and Gibbs, C. J. Jr.:** Transmissible virus dementia: The relation of transmissible spongiform encephalopathy to Creutzfeldt-Jakob disease, In: Aging and Demenia, eds. Kinsbourne, M. and Smith, L., Spectrum, New York, 1977, pp. 91-127.

**Van Rossum, A.:** Die spastische pseudosklerose (Creutzfeldt-Jakob), Proceedings of the 4th International Congress of Neuropathology, München, Stuttgart, Vol. 3, p. 349, 1962.

**Van Rossum, A.:** De spastische pseudosclerose (Ziekte van Creutzfeldt-Jakob), Utrecht, Schotanus en Jens, 1965.

**Van Rossum, A.:** Spastic pseudosclerosis (Creutzfeldt-Jakob disease), In: Handbook of Clinical Neurology, eds. Vinken, P. J. and Bruyn, G. W., Vol. 6., North-Holland Pub. Comp., Amsterdam, 1968, pp 726-760.

**Zimmermann, R.:** Ein weiterer Fall von Pseudosklerosis spastica, Z. ges. Neurol. Psychiat., 116: 1-15, 1928.

# Chapter II

# Epidemiology of Creutzfeldt-Jakob Disease in Japan

Kiyotaro Kondo, M.D.

Epidemiology is concerned with the frequency of a disease and its determinants. It evaluates etiological hypotheses and often gives clues on the cause. Creutzfeldt-Jakob disease (CJD) still remains an enigma in neurosciences, particularly regarding its agent and the mechanism of its natural spread (Brown,1980; Kondo, 1982; Malmgren, et al., 1979). This report describes current epidemiological data of CJD with emphasis on the findings from Japan.

## 1. Diagnosis and Classification

CJD is one of the subacute spongiform encephalopathies (SSE) caused by an unconventional subviral agent. The group includes, besides CJD, Gerstmann-Sträussler-Scheinker disease, some cases with familial Alzheimer disease in humans, along with animal diseases such as scrapie and transmissible mink encephalopathy.

Following the first reports by Creutzfeldt (1920) and Jakob (1921), a total of 150 cases were reviewed by Kirschbaum (1963), but an increasing number of cases have been reported since Gibbs, et al. (1968) transmitted CJD to chimpanzees. Masters, et al. (1979) reviewed 1,435 reported cases, in which transmission experiments were successful in 111. In Japan, Omaru (1961) described the first case. Shinpuku, et al. (1978) summarized 88 cases of his own and from the literature. The Japan Ministry of Health and Welfare since 1976 supported a Research Group for Slow Virus Infections. The group identified 72 and 66 cases from departments of neurology and psychiatry, respectively, with few overlappings. Clinical and other patterns in these cases were analyzed by Tsuji, et al. (1980), disclosing no difference from the western cases.

Diagnosis of CJD has long been dependent on autopsy findings, but recently rather characteristic patterns in EEG and the CAT scans provided reasonably convincing basis for antemortem diagnosis, thus making CJD a target of epidemiological studies. Clinical-pathological subdivision, which will be discussed by other contributors, is of little epidemiological importance. For such studies, the following classification proposed by Masters, et al. (1979) is more useful which classifies the available diagnostic evidence;

    (1) Transmissible. cases whose brain material successfully transmitted SSE to an experimental animal

    (2) Definite. cases verified pathologically

    (3) Probable. cases showing typical clinical pictures

    (4) Possible. clinical cases atypical to accept as probables, but CJD cannot be excluded.

In the absence of pathognomonic laboratory findings, this classification is useful for statistical and epidemiological studies. The first three groups can be accepted as CJD, but the last group should be treated with proper care.

# 2. Frequency and Distribution

CJD is known in 47 countries of the world (Masters, et al., 1979) including a case from Papua New Guinea where kuru occurs in the Eastern Highland Province. Subsequent cases have been reported from a few more countries.

## 1). Reported frequencies

Available data on the frequency of CJD are summarized in Table 1, which includes Japanese data. Methods of the survey are varied, but relatively uniform figures have been reported from the countries with grossly varying latitudes, natural environments, races, socioeconomic conditions, being rather unusual for an infectious disease. Roughly, prevalence rates, annual incidence and mortality rates are less than 1 per 1,000,000, except for the Libyan Jews in Israel. CJD among the Libyan immigrants to Israel are mostly familial cases (Neugut, et al., 1979), and no information is available for their motherland.

## 2). Age and other determinants of frequency

Reported cases include one patient who died of CJD at 17, and a few manifesting at elderly ages of 90s. Both sexes are equally affected in all surveys. According to Tsuji, et al. (1980), Japanese cases were 25-77 years old at onset, the average being 56. Age-specific incidence rate is reported only in France by Brown, et al. (1979), disclosing a unimodal curve rising around 35 years, steeply increasing around 50 to a peak at 65-69, then dropping drastically.

Long-term change of the frequency is not likely although more cases are reported more recently, obviously due to increasing interest in this disease. Bobowick, et al.(1973)

**Table 1.** Frequency of Creutzfeldt-Jakob Disease in Various Areas of the World

| Reports | Survey areas | Periods | Population (1,000) | Methods of case finding | Number of case | Frequency per million | | |
|---|---|---|---|---|---|---|---|---|
| | | | | | | Prevalence rate | Annual incidence rate | Annual mortality rate |
| Tsuji et al., 1980 | Japan-All | 1975-77 | ? | Cases of CJD and ALS, 3 years, 6 departments of neurology | 7 | 1.1 | | |
| | -Fukuoka | ? | 4,440 | Cases reported from local hospitals for June, 1978 | 5 | 1.1 | 0.12-0.19 | 0.15 |
| Kahana et al., 1973 | Israel-Non-Lybian -Lybian | 1963-72 ditto | 2,122 31 | Nationwide discharge summaries, Autopsy reports, etc | 16 13 | | 0.4-1.9 31.3 | |
| Palsson, 1979 | Iceland | Past 20 years | 200 | Cases of the only neurologist in country | 2 | | 0.5 | |
| Matthews, 1975 | England-Wales | 1964-73 | | Own cases, those reported by colleagues | 46 | | 0.09 | |
| Brown et al., 1979 | France-All -Paris | 1968-77 ditto | | Cases in major neuro-clinics in 94 areas of 21 prefectures | 170 59 | | | 0.32 1.33 |
| Alema, 1973 | Italy-All -Rome | 1958-71 ditto | | Hospital records and referrals to neurologists | 32 | | | 0.05 0.38 |
| Majtényi, 1978 | Hungary-All -Budapest | 1955-77 ditto | | Hospital and autopsy records | 37 16 | | | 0.18 0.41 |
| Masters et al., 1979 | USA-All -Boston, MA | 1973-77 1957-76 | 2,533 | Cases reports and NIH referrals Hospital records | 265 22 | | | 0.26 0.43 |
| Malmgren et al., 1979 Farmer et al., 1978 | -Rochester, MN -New York, NY | 1960-74 1959-75 | 50 | Cases in Mayo Clinic Autopsy records | 0 11 | 0 | 0 0.24 | 0 |
| Galves et al., 1980 | Chile-All -San Tiago | 1973-77 ditto | 10,400 29% of citizen | Hospital records and referrals to neurologists | 16 11 | | | 0.31 0.73 |

suspected a seasonal variation of the incidence, but this is rejected in most other reports.

Racial difference is unlikely. Elevated occurrence among Libyan Jews was ascribed to their eating behavior of sheep eyes but this delicacy is not unique to the Libyans, but rather widely enjoyed in the Middle-east.

Urban-rural difference in the frequency was noted in a few reports as seen in Table 1, but is probably due to better case finding in the urban centers. Applying the Knox method, Masters, et al. (1979) rejected a time-space clustering in Boston. Brown (1983), however, found a significant correlation of the incidence rate of the cases of CJD with the population density in France and suggested that a role for random inter-human spread, either direct or indirect, in natural disease transmission.

Fig. 1 represents an area-adjusted map of Japan in which cases of CJD are plotted which include those identified by the stated Research Group as well as death certificates for 1977-1981. A small square with 5 cases west to the large square for Tokyo containing 43 cases represents the prefecture of Yamanashi. Akai, in this volume, describes a pedigree from this prefecture. Three adjacent squares northwest of Yamanashi are Toyama, Ishikawa and Fukui, which appear to contain numerous cases relative to their population. Neurology is still evolving in this area, and this clustering may be significant.

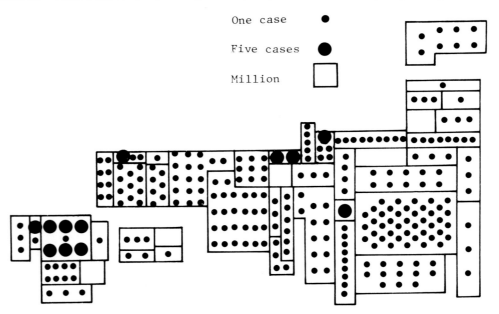

**Fig. 1.** Area-adjusted mapping of Creutzfeldt-Jakob Disease in Japan

Squares represent 47 prefectures in the country without changing their geographical interrelations. The area of a square is proportional to the population of the prefecture it represents. A small dot represents a case, and a large dot represents five cases. Cases appear to aggregate in few regions, but their significance is debatable.

## 3). Local clustering

This was observed in a few relatively isolated villages in various countries.    Matthews (1975) observed three cases during 1964-71 in small villages in Midlands, England, and five in another less documented focus in the eastern part of the country.    Suspected clustering in Slovakia motivated a nationwide survey in Czekoslovakia for 1972-79.    As summarized by Mitrova (1980), six cases were accumulated in rural area in the south-eastern Slovakia, along with three cases in the adjacent part of Hungary.    In this country, Majtényi (1978) reported that 1/3 of the cases outside Budapest, five cases in two years, occurred in a small area along the river Tisza.    Two more episodes were communicated to Masters, et al. (1979).    In Italy, rural concentration of six cases in the Parma-Mantova area was seen during 1975-77.    Five cases were observed over five years' period in the area of Burlington, Vermont, USA.

A small, but striking clustering was observed in two small adjacent cities in Hokkai-

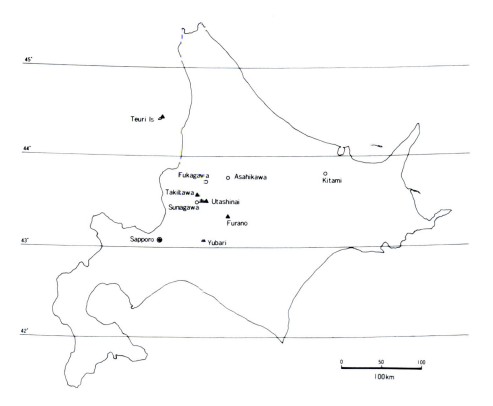

**Fig. 2.**   Hokkaido, Japan with Cases of Creutzfeldt-Jakob Disease
Each case of CJD is represented by a triangle.   Cities inhabited by the three cases in the Takikawa-Utashinai cluster are shown by open circles, along with Sapporo, the capital of Hokkaido, where about 1/2 of residents of Hokkaido live but no case is found.

do island in the northern Japan, as seen in Fig.2, during a period of five years.   All cases were females.

**Case 1.**   Aged 58, lived in Takikawa city, manifested the first symptoms in July, 1973, became progressively demented, exhibited myoclonus and convulsions.   Brain atrophy evident in CAT scans, and periodic synchronous discharges in EEGs.

**Case 2.**   Aged 43, lived in Monju, Utashinai city, first abnormalities observed in the fall, 1977, typical picture, course, CAT and EEG patterns.   Death in 1983.   Autopsy disclosed a typical SSE.

**Case 3.**   Aged 42, lived in Kamoi, Utashinai city, abulia in June, 1978.   Typical picture, course and EEG patterns.   CAT disclosed moderate brain atrophy.

Three cases were not related or acquainted, and had no opportunity of physical contacts among themselves.   However, all three lived in Kamoi, Utashinai, a small coal miners' village, in different years during 1943 through 1979.   There were three more cases in the surrounding areas in Hokkaido, but they had no relation with the stated three cases. Two more cases reportedly manifested CJD recently in the same area.

While such observations may give clues to the pathogenesis of the disease, it is predictable that instances of clustering of any given rare disease may be encountered in few places in the world because the probability of observing 0,1,2,⋯ cases in a small community obeys the Poisson distribution, and there are, theoretically, few places involving unusual numbers of cases.

# 3. Histories of Exposures, Risk Factors and Associated Disease

An event predating clinical onset is referred to as risk factor of a given disease, when individuals having the factor have increased probability of being affected.   Risk factors give useful clues for further etiological studies, identification of high-risk group, or prevention of the disease by means of environmental prophylaxis.   If a disease occurs dependently with other disorders with known on conjectured etiologies, the association may also give clues on its cause, because both diseases may have the same or related etiology, or share common precipitating factors, or associated disorder may predispose to the disease or vice versa.   Alert clinicians are often first runners to suspect risk factors or associated disease which must be established by statistically adequate methods, including case-control observations.

## 1). Occupation

There are claims that workers in some occupations are liable to CJD.   In a summary of Masters, et al. (1979), occupational analysis in 308 patients showed 19 in the health professions, including 2 physicians, one neurosurgeon and 4 dentists.   They concluded that, although the natural mechanism of the spread and reservoir or the CJD agent remain unknown, the possibility of iatrogenic or occupational spread in a significant proportion of cases deserves careful consideration.  In our case-control study stated in the follows, this claim has not been supported, however.

## 2). Associated disease and physical injuries

Various authors suggested that CJD is associated with a few other disorders.

Review of cases.  Masters, et al. (1979) reviewed 1,435 cases which represent the majority of the world cases.  In 337 patients in whom past medical or surgical histories were known, there were 53 (16%) with a history of surgery and 13 (4%) with a history of cranial or ocular surgery in the 6 months to 3 year interval before the onset.  286 (85%) had a history of major medical illnesses more than 6 months before onset.  A high proportion, 27%, of these medical illnesses were neurologic or psychiatric, a finding

**Table 2.** Surgical Operations, Mechanical Injuries, Tooth Extractions, Blood Transfusions, and Lumber Puncture during the Five-Year Period prior to Onset of Creutzfeldt-Jakob Disease (Kondo and Kuroiwa, 1982)

| Interventions or Injuries | Male | | | Female | | |
|---|---|---|---|---|---|---|
| | Cases | Spouses | Neighbors | Cases | Spouses | Neighbors |
| Total individuals | 27 | 25 | 26 | 33 | 22 | 30 |
| Surgical operations | | | | | | |
| Eye | | | | | 1 | |
| Ear | | | | | | |
| Nose | | | | | | |
| Neurosurgical | | | | | | |
| Neck | 2 | 1 | | 1 | | |
| Chest | 1 | | | | | |
| Abdomen | 2 | | 1 | 3 | | 2 |
| Pelvis | 1 | | | 2 | 1 | |
| Extremities | 1 | | 2 | 2 | | 1 |
| Mechanical injuries | | | | | | |
| Eye | 1 | | 3 | 3 | | |
| Head and face | 1 | | | | 1 | 2 |
| Neck | 1 | 1 | | | | 1 |
| Chest | 2 | | | | | 1 |
| Abdomen | | | | 1 | | |
| Pelvis | | | | | | |
| Extremities | 4 | | 1 | 2 | | 2 |
| Tooth extractions | | | | | | |
| Maxillary | 10 | 9 | 13 | 10 | 5 | 15 |
| Mandibular | 10 | 6 | 14 | 11 | 7 | 14 |
| Blood transfusions | | | 2 | 1 | 1 | |
| Lumbar punctures | 2 | | 1 | | | 2 |

emphasized since the most likely place for a patient to encounter a CJD patient is on a neurologic or psychiatric service. These are provocative suggestions, but require statistical confirmation, because they are unilateral observations devoid of controls.

Case-control studies. Kondo and Kuroiwa (1982) made a case-control study in Japan. Histories in 60 cases reported by 902 neurological clinics were compared by sex among the cases, the neighbors as well as spouses of the cases of the opposite sex. No association was observed in the both sexes with 5 socioeconomic variables; occupation; exposures to 9 species of animals; ingestion of raw meat or quadruped brains; 18 diseases, allergies or immunizations, tooth extraction, blood transfusion and lumber puncture. On the other hand, surgical operations were encountered in 25.9% and 7.8% of male cases and pooled controls, whilst in 24.2% and 9.6% of female cases and controls. Mechanical injuries were observed in 33.3% and 9.8% of male cases and controls, and in 18.2% and 13.5% of female cases and controls. The operations and mechanical injuries were varied in nature and clustered in no particular region of the body, as described in Table 2.

In a study involving 38 cases of CJD, Bobowick, et al. (1973) observed that 1) upper respiratory infections were recalled in 1/3 of the cases for the year prior to onset, 2) 1/3 of the cases and the controls ate brains with greater preference of the cases for hog brains, whereas 3) no difference was observed in the marital status, years of schooling, socioeconomic status, occupation, residence pattern, 16 selected diseases, 5 selected immunologic histories as well as in exposures to various animals. Surgical operations and mechanical injuries were not specifically inquired in their study.

Analysis of autopsy. The present author, in an unpublished study, compared pathological complications in 88 autopsies of CJD with those of control diseases; 550 craniocervical injuries, 403 myocardial infarction and 440 pulmonary tuberculosis retrieved from the "Annual or Pathological Autopsies in Japan" for 1964-1978. Recorded pathological findings excluding those of the stated diseases, their treatments, agonal and other irrelevant changes, were classified and compared by age and sex. No excess was observed over control disease, in the frequencies of non-neoplastic complications in CJD, regardless of the classification made from etiological, functional, topographical or morphological points of view. Numbers of neoplasms were also comparable among these diseases. However, frequency of organ resections were higher, as shown in Table 3. CJD was associated with no other disorders recognizable in antopsy, excluding organ resections.

## 3). Contacts with other patients

It is remarkable, that aside from a few iatrogenic cases, cases with CJD have no history at all of exposure to the other cases prior to the onset. No case used in our case-control study had this history. In 170 French cases, extensive inquiry identified no contact with other cases (Brown, et al., 1979). Such contact does not increase the risk to CJD, unlike scrapie which often causes satellite cases to happen. Only two examples of conjugal cases of CJD have been reported.

**Table 3.** Organ Resections in Autopsies of Creutzfeldt-Jakob Disease and Three Control Diseases

| Organ resections | Creutzfeldt-Jakob disease | | Craniocervical injuries | | Myocardial infarction | | Pulmonary tuberculosis | |
|---|---|---|---|---|---|---|---|---|
| | Male | Female | Male | Female | Male | Female | Male | Female |
| Number of autopsied cases | 47 | 41 | 452 | 98 | 269 | 134 | 326 | 114 |
| Cases with resective surgery | 4 | 3 | 15 | 3 | 8 | 2 | 7 | 4 |
| % resected cases | 8.5 | 7.3 | 3.3 | 3.1 | 3.0 | 1.5 | 2.1 | 4.4 |
| Number of organ resected | 4 | 3 | 15 | 3 | 10 | 2 | 7 | 5 |
| Tongue | | | | | 1 | | | |
| Stomach | 1 | 1 | 9 | 1 | 4 | 1 | 3 | 1 |
| Intestine | 1 | 1 | 4 | | 1 | | 3 | 1 |
| Pancreas | | | | | 1 | | | |
| Gall bladder | | | | | 1 | | | |
| Lung | | | 1 | | | | | |
| Kidney | 1 | | | 1 | 1 | | | |
| Urinary bladder | 1 | | | | | | | |
| Prostate | | | 1 | | | | 1 | |
| Uterus | | 1 | | 1 | | | | 2 |
| Mammary gland | | | | | | | | 1 |
| Artery | | | | | | 1 | | |
| Extremities | | | | | 1 | | | |

1) Numbers of cases with recorded resective surgery are shown along with numbers of organs resected including those partially or unilaterally resected. Incisions, sutures or simple anastomoses are excluded.

2) Proportion of cases with resective surgery significantly differed in male from pulmonary tuberculosis only (p < 0.05).

**Table 4.** Selected Case Reports of Creutzfeldt-Jakob Disease with Suggestive Exposure Histories

| Authors | Cases | Histories prior to CJD | Months from the history to CJD | Original authors' comments |
|---|---|---|---|---|
| Packer et al. (1980) | Female, 20 | Dissected a rhesus monkey | 3-4 | |
| Matthews et al. (1979) | Male, 63 | Kept ferrets until 1939, bitten in 1971 | About 2 years after the bite | Ferrets are animal reservoir of CJD? |
| Alter et al. (1975) | | Habitual eating of sheep brains, 1944-65 | ? | Acquired the agent during a gourmet for 20 years? |
| Nevin et al. (1960) | Male, 58; male, 68; female, 47 | Craniotomy for meningioma, abscess and "neurosis" by one surgeon | 15, 27, 17 | Might be regarded as a possible mode of entry, rather than as precipitating CJD |
| Duffy et al. (1974) | Female, 55 | Corneal transplantation from a CJD patient | 18 | Example of person-to-person transmission? |
| Bernoulli et al. (1977) | Female, 23; male, 17 | Intracerebral electrode formerly used in a CJD patient | 20, 18 | Infected from the contaminated electrode, conventional sterilisation inadequate? |
| Quoted by Traub et al. (1977) | Male, 54* | Neurosurgeon | ? | Self-inoculated in operation room? |

*Complicated with papulosis atrophicans maligna.

### 4). Contacts with animals

In view of the transmission experiments, exposures to animals appeared significant. A few interesting cases are quoted in Table 4 with the original authors' comments. In two case-control studies stated exposures to various animals were not excessive in the cases than in the controls, however. Worldwide distribution of CJD is rather uniform, being totally incompatible with that of scrapie. In an extensive study in France, Chatelain, et al.(1981) rejected a regional correlation of the incidence patterns between CJD and scrapie.

### 5). Iatrogenic cases

A few instances of so-called iatrogenic transmission of CJD are included in Table 4. Two cases of Bernoulli, et al. (1977) deserve a special notice in their younger age for this disease and in the fact they manifested CJD 18-20 months after the intracerebral EEG recording with the same electrode which has been likewise used in a CJD patient. These "iatrogenic" cases contracted CJD in a situation comparable to the transmission experiments, after incubation periods similar to those observed in the experimentally affected animals.

### 6). Risk factors to Creutzfeldt-Jakob disease, a tentative view

Sofar known, following factors can be accepted as associated with an increased development of CJD: 1) age, 2) mechanical injuries and surgical operations, 3) intracorporeal contacts with the polluted material and 4) CJD in the other family members. No single or unitarian interpretation explains these associations, but definitely, they give clues to test hypotheses regarding pathogenesis and the natural spread of CJD.

## 4. Familial Aggregation

The familial nature of CJD was first noted by Jakob himself. May, et al. (1968) suspected autosomal-dominant heredity based on a few pedigrees including the famous Backer family. The largest family was reported by Cathala, et al. (1980), which included 14 cases in three generations. Haltia, et al. (1979) observed a family involving 9 cases. In these and other families, CJD is transmitted regardless of the affected sex always through one of the parents.

Masters, et al. (1979) observed a positive family history in 15% of 1,435 cases they reviewed, and concluded that 1) transmission is "dominant" equally through the paternal and the maternal lines, 2) familial cases are younger at onset but otherwise identical to the sporadic cases, and 3) the incubation time extends over 40 years, if the cases in the same family are due to single exposures. Several instances of familial CJD are known in Japan, which will be reviewed by Akai in this volume (see Chapter IV). The proportion of the Japanese cases with positive family history in 2 of 72 in the material reported by Tsuji, et al. (1980).

Mechanisms of the familial aggregation include; 1) person-to-person transmission, 2) inherited predisposition, 3) genomic incorporation of the genetic material of the agent. In view of the lack of histories of exposure to other patients with CJD in all large case series, and that only two instances of the conjugal CJD have ever been reported, 1) is unlikely. Even in large pedigrees with CJD, contacts do not adequately explain the family patterns. "Horizontal" transmission can be suspected only in the pedigrees of Brown, et al. (1979) and Galves, et al. (1980). That the paternal and maternal ancestors are equally affected denounces infection through placentae, deliveries or lactation. Two examples of CJD twins with unknown zygosity are reported, one discordant, the other concordant. Inherited predisposition is known in scrapie in some susceptible animals, but it is unlikely in kuru and probably in CJD as well.

In summary, although CJD runs in families, no convincing evidence supported a familial exposure to a single source of infection or an intrafamilial contagion. No formal-genetic analysis has been attempted to test an "autosomal-dominant" hypothesis of the transmission. Incorporation of the agent's genetic material in the host's germ cells may cause a seemingly Mendelian pattern, but this possibility is yet to be evaluated.

## 5. Agent and the Natural Spread

Enormous information has been accumulated regarding the nature of the agent. Although genetic information is contained in nucleic acids in microorganisms including viruses, even this point has been debated with respect to the scrapie agent. Prusiner (1982) proposed a term "prion" to denote the small *proteinaceous infectious* agent, which is resistant to inactivation by most procedures that modify nucleic acids. Possible mechanisms of its replication include, 1) prions, if they contain undetectable nucleic acids, code for prion protein(s) or activate transcriptions of host genes coded for prion protein, or 2) prions, if devoid of nucleic acids, activate transcription of host coding for prion protein or code for their own replication by a reverse translation or protein-directed protein synthesis. The origin of such agents is totally enigmatic, however.

Aside from few case reports of presumed iatrogenic transmission, in which deep tissue of the victims came in direct contact with infected materials, mechanisms of the natural spread remains obscure. Such cases are rare and special, and do not straightforwardly provide hypothesis for the natural spread in the majority of cases.

Other possibilities of the natural spread include, 1) natural person-to-person transmission, 2) transmission via environmental sources, 3) familial transmission, 4) zoonotic transmission. Brown (1980) quoted extensive circumstantial data against all of these hypotheses, for which there is no direct evidence.

One more hypothesis, which is currently totally devoid of a direct support, but perfectly compatible with known epidemiological characteristics of CJD, is that the agent(s) is created *de novo* in each patient individually through unknown mechanism(s) in which the DNA-RNA-oligopeptides sequence is troubled. Most patients therefore, contracted CJD absolutely independently from the other patients due to an endogenous agent, although such agent(s) is capable of producing the disease in other hosts under special iatrogenic situations and is capable of inheriting when the agent is incorporated in germ cells.

# 6. Summary

CJD occurs uniformly at an incidence rate of 1 per million per year throughout the world, but a few instances of regional clustering have been reported. Both sexes are equally affected. Known risk factors include age, physical injuries, intracorporeal contacts with an infected material and CJD in family. Japanese cases showed no special characteristics in these regards.

This study was supported by a grant for the Research Group for Slow Virus Infection, from the Japan Ministry of Health and Welfare. Cordial thanks are due to Ms. Kyoko Kato for technical assistance.

# REFERENCES

**Alema, G.**: Quoted from Brown (1980).

**Alter, M., Yitzak, F., Holly, D. and Webster, D. D.**: Creutzfeldt-Jakob disease after eating ovine brains? N. Engl. J. Med., 292 : 927, 1975.

**Bernoulli, C., Siegfried, J., Baumgartner, G., Regli, F., Rabinowicz, T., Gadjusek, D. C. and Gibbs, Jr. C. J.**: Danger of accidental person-to-person transmission of Creutzfeldt-Jakob disease by surgery, Lancet, 1: 478-479, 1977

**Bobowick, A. R., Brody, J. A., Matthews, M. R., Roos, R. and Gajdusek, D. C.**: Creutzfeldt-Jakob disease; a case-control study, Am. J. Epidemiol., 98 : 381-394, 1973.

**Brown, P.** : An epidemiologic critique of Creutzfeldt-Jakob disease, Epidemiol. Rev, 2 : 113-135, 1980.

**Brown, P., and Cathala, F.** : Creutzfeldt-Jakob disease in France, 1. Retrospective study of the Paris area during the ten-year period 1968-1977, Ann. Neurol., 5 : 189-192, 1979.

**Brown, P., Cathala, F. and Gajdusek, D. C.**: Creutzfeldt-Jakob disease in France, 3. Epidemiological study of 170 patients dying during the decade 1968-1977. Ann Neurol 6 ; 438-446, 1979.

**Brown, P., Cathala, F. and Sadowsky, D.**: Correlation between population density and the frequency of Creutzfeldt-Jakob disease in France, J. neurol. Sci., 60 : 169-176, 1983.

**Cathala, F., Chatelain, J., Brown, P., Dumas, M. and Gajdusek, D. C.** : Familial Creutzfeldt-

Jakob disease, autosomal dominance in 14 members over 3 generations,    J. Neurol. Sci., 47 : 343-351, 1980.

**Chatelain, J., Cathala, F., Brown, P., Raharison, S., Court, L. and Gajdusek, D. C.** :    Epidemiologic comparisons between Creutzfeldt-Jakob disease and scrapie in France during the 12-year period 1968-1979,    J. Neurol. Sci., 51 : 329-337, 1981.

**Duffy, P., Wolf, J., Collins, G., DeVoe, A. G., Streeten, B. and Cowen, D.** :    Possible person-to-person transmission of Creutzfeldt-Jakob disease,    N. Engl. J. Med., 290 : 692-693, 1974.

**Farmer, P. M., Kane, W. C. and Hollenberg-Sher, J.** :    Incidence of Creutzfeldt-Jakob disease in Brooklyn and Staten Island,    N. Engl. J. Med., 298 : 283-284, 1978.

**Galves, S., Masters, CM. and Gajdusek, D.C.** :    Descriptive epidemiology of Creutzfeldt-Jakob disease in Chile,    Arch. Neurol., 37 : 11-14, 1980.

**Gibbs, Jr. C. J., Gajdusek, D. C., Asher, D. M., Alpers, M., Beck, E., Daniel, P. M. and Matthews, W. B.** :    Creutzfeldt-Jakob disease (subacute spongiform encephalopathy) : Transmission to the chimpanzee,    Science, 161 : 388-389, 1968.

**Haltia, M., Kovanen, J., Van Crevel, H., Bots, G. Th. A.M. and Stefanko, S.** :    Familial Creutzfeldt-Jakob disease,    J. Neurol. Sci., 42 : 381-389. 1979.

**Kahana, E., Alter, M., Braham, J. and Sofer, D.** :    Creutzfeldt-Jakob disease ; focus among Libyan Jews in Israel,    Science, 183 : 90-91, 1973.

**Kirshbaum, W. R.** :    Jakob-Creutzfeldt Disease,    Elsevier, New York, 1968.

**Kondo, K.** :    Epidemiology of Creutzfeldt-Jakob disease and related disorders,    Brain and Nerve (Japan), 34 : 451-463, 1982.

**Kondo, K. and Kuroiwa, Y.** :    A case-control study of Creutzfeldt-Jakob disease: Association with physical injuries,    Ann. Neurol., 11 : 377-381, 1982.

**Majtényi, G.** :    Creutzfeldt-Jakob disease in Hungary,    J. Neuropathol. Exp. Neurol., 37 : 653, 1978.

**Malmgren, R., Kurland, L. T., Mokri, B. and Kurtzke, J. F.** :    The epidemiology of Creutzfeldt-Jakob disease.    In Slow Transmissible Diseases of the Nervous System, ed by Prusiner SB, Hadlow WJ.    Vol 1, Academic Press, New York, 1979, pp. 93-112.

**Masters, C. L., Harris, J. O., Gajdusek, D. C., Gibbs, Jr. C. J., Bernoulli, C. and Asher, D. M.** :    Creutzfeldt-Jakob disease ; Patterns of world occurrence and the significance of familial and sporadic clustering,    Ann. Neurol., 5 : 177-188, 1979.

**Masters, C. L., Gajdusek, D. C., Gibbs, Jr. C. J., Bernoulli, C. and Asher, D. M.** :    Familial Creutzfeldt-Jakob disease and other familial dementias ; An inquiry into possible modes of transmission of virus-induced familial diseases.    In Slow Transmissible Diseases of the Nervous System, ed by Prusiner SB, Hadlow WJ. Vol 1, Academic Press, New York, 1979 , pp. 143-194.

**Matthews, W. B.** :    Epidemiology of Creutzfeldt-Jakob disease in England and Wales,    J. Neurol. Neurosurg. Psychiatry, 38 : 210-213, 1975.

**Matthews, W. B., Campbell, M., Hughes, J.T. and Tomlinson, A. H.** :    Creutzfeldt-Jakob disease and ferrets,    Lancet, 1 : 828, 1979.

**May, W. W., Itabashi, H. H. and DeJong, R. N.** :    Creutzfeldt-Jakob disease, 2. Clinical pathology and genetic study of family,    Arch. Neurol., 19 : 137-149, 1968.

**Mitrova, E.** :    Focal accumulation of Creutzfeldt-Jakob disease in Slovakia, In Boese A (ed) Search for the Cause of Multiple Sclerosis and Other Chronic Diseases of the Central Nervous System, Verlag Chemie, Weinheim, 1980, pp. 356-366.

**Neugut, R. H., Neugut, A. I., Kahana, E., Stein, Z. and Alter, M.** :    Creutzfeldt-Jakob disease ; familial clustering among Libyan-born Israelis,    Neurology, 29 : 225-231, 1979.

**Nevin, S., McMenemey, W. H., Behrman, S. and Jones, D. P.** :    Subacute spongiform encephalopathy, a subacute form of encephalopathy attributable to vascular dysfunction (spongiform cerebral atrophy), Brain, 83 : 519-564, 1960.

**Packer, R. J., Cornblath, D. R., Gonatas, N. K., Bruno, L. A. and Asbury, A. K.** :  Creutzfeldt-Jakob disease in a 20-year-old woman,  Neurology, 30 : 492-496, 1980.

**Palsson, P. A.** :  Rida (scrapie) in Iceland and its epidemiology.  In Slow Transmissible Diseases of the nervous System, Vol 1, ed by Prusiner SB, Hadlow WJ. Academic Press, New York, 1979, pp. 357-366.

**Prusiner, S. B.** :  Novel proteinaceous infectious particles cause scrapie,  Science, 216 : 136-144, 1982.

**Shinpuku, N., Sugita, T. and Nagayama, K.** :  Presenile dementias in Japan,  Nihon-iji-shinpo, (Japan) No. 2844 : 43-55, 1978.

**Traub, R., Gajdusek, D. C. and Gibbs, Jr. C. J.** :  Transmissible virus dementia : The relation of transmissible spongiform encephalopathy to Creutzfeldt-Jakob disease.  In Aging and Dementia, Spectrum, ed by Kinsbourne M, Smith L. New York, 1977, pp. 91-172.

**Tsuji, S., Kuroiwa, Y. and Ishida, N.** :  The epidemiological and clinical studies of Creutzfeldt-Jakob disease in Japan,  Clin. Neurol. (Japan), 20 : 951-955, 1980.

# CHAPTER III

# Classfication of Clinicopathological Subtypes of Creutzfeldt-Jakob Disease

# Creutzfeldt-Jakob Disease as a Syndrome

Hirotsugu Shiraki, M. D. and Toshio Mizutani, M. D.

Creutzfeldt-Jakob disease is a diffuse degeneration of the central nervous system that almost always occurs in middle-aged and is, as a rule, fatal within several months to several years. The history of the researches on Creutzfeldt-Jakob disease, such as origin of the problem, extended concept, and modern concept and problems of the disease, has already been fully documented in the Chapter I.

As well known, transmission experiments in kuru from New Guinea and in Creutzfeldt-Jakob disease from human beings to animals and from animals to animals have been successful (Gibbs, et al., 1968; Tateishi, et al., 1979). On the basis of these experiments, it has been proposed that the etiologic basis and, possibly, the pathogenesis of the disease is thought to be a slow viral infection.

We should mention at this point, however, that it is our opinion that even though comprehensive descriptions and an acceptable classification of the neuropathologic characteristics of Creutzfeldt-Jakob disease have been given, as determined from well-recognized clinical features, the disease is still not fully clarified, particularly from the morphopathogenetic viewpoint. One reason is that the clinical and neuropathologic characteristic of a new type of the disease, the panencephalopathic type, which is accompanied by severe primary involvement of the cerebral white matter, has only recently been clarified by present authors (Mizutani, et al., 1981a), moreover a similar autopsy case in Japan (Ohta, et al., 1978) has successfully been transmitted to small animals (Tateishi, et al., 1979).

On the basis of previous observations of the disease in the Japanese (Shiraki, 1974; Matsuoka, 1974), mainly on the neuropathologic background, we, at that time, were able to classify the disease in the only following three types; the simple poliodystrophic (inflated neuronal) type, subacute spongiform encephalopathy and thalamic (Stern-Garcin) type.

At that time, the ataxic type (Brownell and Oppenheimer, 1965) of the disease was not

34

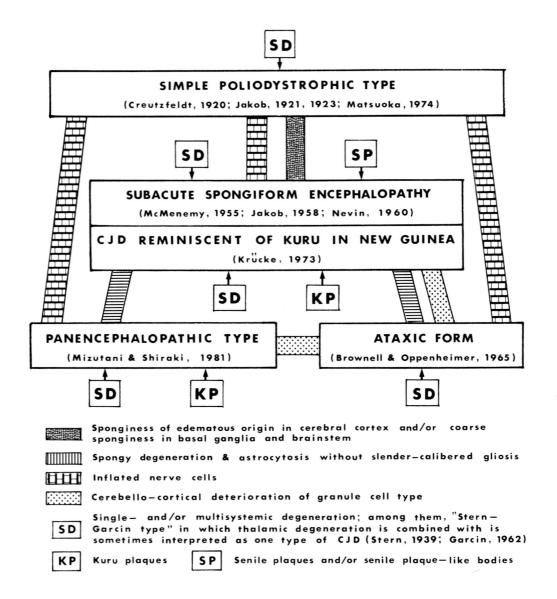

**Fig. 1.** Schematic diagram of the neuropathologic interrelationship of the different types of Creutzfeldt-Jakob disease (CJD) Adapted from Mizutani (1981b). (From: Neuropsychiatric disorders in the elderly: eds., Hirano, A. and Miyoshi, K., Igaku-Shoin, 1983, with permission)

present or at least indefinite in the Japanese.    The panencephalopathic type of the disease
(Mizutani, et al., 1981), on the other hand, has been reported more recently.    Moreover, in
the present text, we also were able to discuss another new type of the disease, the chronic
spongiform encephalopathy with kuru plaques and allied plaques characterized by antecedent and longlasting cerebellar ataxia with or without involvement of cerebral white
matter.    From both the clinical and neuropathologic standpoints, however, not only the
latter two types of Creutzfeldt-Jakob disease but also the other types of the disease have
certain features in common, and thus, it could be understood that various types of
Creutzfeldt-Jakob disease mentioned above were closely interrelated (Fig. 1)

On the other hand, kuru in New Guinea does start during childhood and occurred most
often among preadolescents or young adults, but there are no definite and severe psychic
disturbances in this disease, so it seems distinct clinically from Creutzfeldt-Jakob disease
in presenile people.    However, transmission experiments in kuru from human beings to
animals and from animals to animals have demonstrated that the spongy degeneration and
astrocytosis of the gray matter, that were consistently found in other type of Creutzfeldt
-Jakob disease, except for the simple poliodystrophic type, could be passed from one host
to another.    On this basis, it is conceivable that kuru also is closely related to Creutzfeldt
-Jakob disease in presenile and senile adults.

In any way, it can reasonably be understood that so-called Creutzfeldt-Jakob disease
never comprizes a purely separable disease entity, and so far, this illness can better be
understood in regard to Creutzfeldt-Jakob disease as a syndrome.

The interrelationship of each subtype of Creutzfeldt-Jakob disease mentioned above
will be synthetically discussed in detail later (Chapter III-9).

# REFERENCES

Brownell, B. and Oppenheimer, D. R.: An ataxic form of subacute presenile polioencephalopathy
(Creutzfeldt-Jakob disease), J. Neurol. Neurosurg. Psychiat., 28: 350-361, 1965.
Gibbs, C. J. Jr., Gajdusek, D. C., Asher, D. M., Alpers, M. P., Beck, E., Daniel, P. M. and Matthews,
W. B.: Creutzfeldt-Jakob disease (spongiform encephalopathy): transmission to the chimpanzee, Scien-
ce, 161: 388-389, 1968.
Matsuoka, T.: Creutzfeldt-Jakob disease —— Clinical manifestations and pathological features, Adv.
Neurol. Sci. (Japan), 18: 33-45, 1974.
Mizutani, T., Okumura, A., Oda, M. and Shiraki, H.: Panencephalopathic type of Creutzfeldt-Jakob
disease:   Primary inovolvement of the cerebral white matter, J. Neurol. Neurosurg. Psychiat., 44: 103-115,
1981a.
Mizutani, T.: Neuropathology of Creutzfeldt-Jakob disease in Japan. With special reference to the
panencephalopathic type, Acta Path. Jpn., 31: 903-922, 1981b.
Ohta, M., Koga, M., Tateishi, J., Motomura, S., Yamashita, Y., Kawanami, S., Oda, K. and Kuroiwa,
Y.: An autopsy report of spongiform encephalopathy associated with kuru plaque and leukomalacia,
Adv. Neurol. Sci. (Japan), 22: 487-496, 1978.
Shiraki, H.: The neuropathological background for Creutzfeldt-Jakob disease (Creutzfeldt-Jakob

syndrome), Adv. Neurol. Sci. (Japan), 18: 4-30, 1974.

**Shiraki, H. and Mizutani, T.**: Neuropathologic characteristics of types of Creutzfeldt-Jakob disease with special reference to the panencephalopathic type prevalent among Japanese, In: Neuropsychiatric Disorders in the Elderly, eds. Hirano, A. and Moyoshi, K., Igaku-Shoin, Tokyo, New York, pp. 139-188, 1983.

**Tateishi, J., Ohta, M., Koga, M., Sato, Y. and Kuroiwa, Y.**: Transmission of chronic spongiform encephalopathy with kuru plaques from humans to small rodents, Ann. Neurol., 5: 581-584, 1979.

# Simple Poliodystrophic Type of Creutzfeldt-Jakob Disease

Hirotsugu Shiraki, M. D. and Toshio Mizutani, M. D.

Simple poliodystrophic type of CJD with emphasis on the morphopathogenetic aspects proposed by Shiraki (1974) corresponded well to the previously established subtype of CJD including so-called "classical type" (Creutzfeldt, 1920), Jakob's type with and without muscular atrophy, and amyotrophic type of CJD (Jakob, 1921).

As far as our specimens of this type of CJD were concerned, the most characteristic change is inflation of the nerve cells in combination with alteration of the cytoplasm and eccentricity of the nuclei of these cells; such nuclei and gray matters were widespread in Betz' giant cells (Figs. 1 a, 1 b & 1 c) as well as in other nerve cells, particularly the pyramidal cells, of the cerebral cortex (Fig. 1 d), thalamus, different nuclei and the reticular formation of the brainstem (Figs. 1 e, 2 a & 2 b), the cerebellar dentate nucleus and the anterior horn of the spinal cord (Figs. 2 c & 2 d). The distribution of the inflated nerve cells is illustrated schematically in Figure 4 (Case 3, Table 1).

Disruption of the cerebral cortex due to sponginess, on the other hand, was pronounced in the hippocampal formation, uncus and parahippocampal cortex (Figs. 3 c & 3 d), whereas spongy tissue developed as a result of an edematous process caused by a hemodynamic disturbance and was morphologically distinct from the tissue disruption as seen in the other subtypes of CJD which will be discussed in detail later on. On the other hand, disruption of the globus pallidus and olivary nucleus (Figs. 2 e & 2 f) due to the presence of coarse, spongy tissue could not be attributed solely to an edematous process.

Neuronal disintegration, astrocytosis, neuronophagiae and glial rosettes were generally not evident or questionable, except for in the putamen (Figs. 3 a & 3 b), certain thalamic subnuclei and the end plate of the horn of Ammon (Fig. 3 e).

As far as our specimens were concerned, systemic degeneration, such as the degeneration that occurs predominantly in the distal portions of the corticospinal tract of the spinal cord, which was described in this type of CJD first reported by Creutzfeldt (1920) and Jakob (1921), was not seen.

38

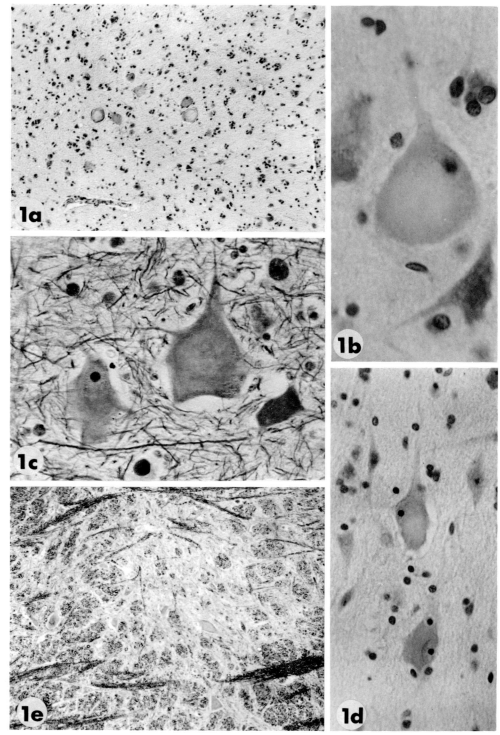

Fig. 1

# Review of References of This Type of CJD in the Japanese

(Each number in italics in the text is corresponded to that in the Table 3 of the Appendix.)

## 1) Clinical features

The number of the cases was 16. There were 12 males and 4 females. The age at death ranged from 29 to 59 years of age, and its average was 46. 8. The total duration of the illness was from 3 to 54 months, and its average was 12. 0.

In the family history there was only one case whose parents had a consanguinous marriage (Matsuoka, et al., 1968, *No. 7*), while no case having relatives or siblings suffered from CJD or similar degenerative disorders was found.

The past history was not remarkable in all cases, except for two; in one case arthritis and some immunological abnormalities were noticed (Matsuoka, et al., 1964, *No. 6*); in another the disease started after the recovery of a car accident with short loss of consciousness (Katayama, et al., 1969, *No. 9*).

The onset of the illness was insidious, as a rule. About a half of the cases had an initial symptom of mental disturbances, such as forgetfulness, personality change, and mental slowness. Some cases started with purely neurological disabilities such as diplopia (Ishino, et al., 1963, *No. 5*), weakness of the lower limbs (Mitsuyama, et al., 1970, *No. 10*) and decreased visual acuity (Sugita, et al., 1977, *No. 14*). In Ishino's case ataxia with positive Romberg's sign, and cerebellar signs and symptoms appeared subsequently, and thus, tumor of the brain or spinal cord was suspected at the early stage. In the other cases mental symptoms and signs, and neurological disabilities developed simultaneously or one after another. Gait disturbance was almost always recognized at the early stage.

Dementia was found in all cases, and showed a progressive worsening. However, various psychic symptoms including emotional incontinence, psychomotor excitement, hallucination, delusion, nocturnal delirium and wandering, and stupor were found from the early stage to the intermediate stage. Cerebral focal signs, such as apraxia, agnosia and aphasia were rather rare in comparison with the other subtypes of CJD.

The clinical conditions appeared to fluctuate, in spite of progressive dementia. This clinical evolution was most characteristic in the simple poliodystrophic type, while other subtypes did not show such a clinical course. Creutzfeldt, on the other hand, already

---

**Fig. 1.** Simple poliodystrophic type of Creutzfeldt-Jakob disease (Table 1). a, b and d: case 1; c and e: case 2.
**(a)** Infragranular layer of precentral cortex; typically and achromatically inflated Betz' giant cells. × 120. **(b)** Highly magnified typically inflated Betz' giant cell. × 950. **(c)** Two conspicuously inflated Betz' giant cells and homogeneously degenerated intracytoplasmic silver fibrils. × 530. **(d)** Deep third layer of the superior frontal cortex; two pyramidal cells of a typical inflation. × 440. **(e)** Reticular formation of the portion of the medulla oblongata; a number of inflated pyramidal cells. × 110. [(a), (b) & (d): Thionine; (c): Bodian; (e): K-B]

40

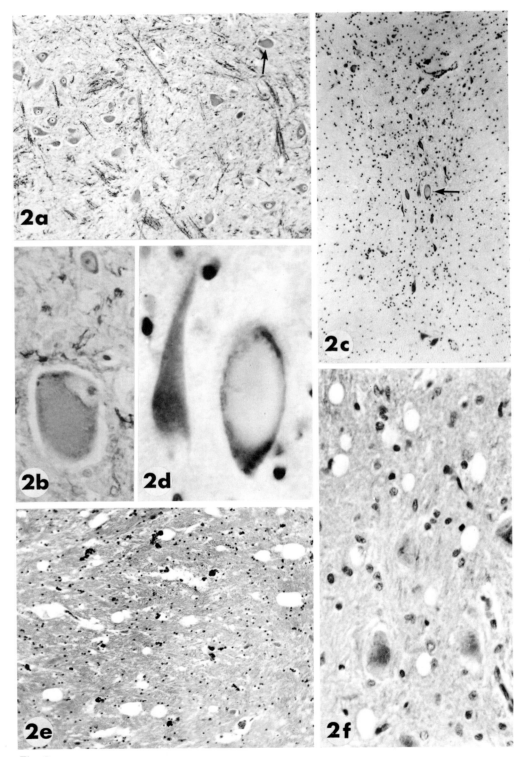

Fig. 2

pointed out the clinical remission and relapse in his case (1921).   This clinical fluctuation was most pronounced in Matsuoka's (*No. 6*) and Yuasa's case (*No. 8*).   In Matsuoka's case (1968, *No. 7*) visual disturbance and unsteady gait as the initial symptom appeared again after the remission for two years. Thereafter, the clinical condition progressively worsened and the patient died four months later after relapse.

Gait disturbance was the most frequent among various neurological signs (94%), particularly outstanding at the early stage.   About a half of the cases with gait disturbance showed an ataxia nature, while some of the other cases demonstrated pyramidal signs, lower motor signs or positive Romberg's sign, and thus, this gait disturbance could be related to the involvement of the spinal cord.   In general the clinical nature of gait disturbance in this type appeared to be more obvious than in the other subtypes.

The lower motor neuron signs including muscular atrophy and fasciculation were also frequently found in this type (31%); this frequency seemed to be rather low, but significantly higher than in the other subtypes.

Distinct cerebellar signs and symptoms were found only in two cases (Ichikawa, et al., 1961, *No. 4*; Ishino, 1963, *No. 5*). Ishino's case also showed Romberg's sign and lower motor neuron signs, while Ichikawa's case had no clinical involvement of the spinal cord. Many of the cases with ataxic gait, on the other hand, showed no obvious signs of cerebellar involvement.

Hand tremor was usually recognized at an early stage, while rigidity of muscles developed at a later stage.   Myoclonus was found only in 6 cases (38%), and this frequency was certainly low in contrast with the other subtypes of CJD.   Periodic synchronous discharge (PSD) was also recorded on EEG only in two cases.

In the later stage the patient fell into a state of akinetic mutism, although in some cases death occurred by intercurrent illnesses, such as gastrointestinal bleeding and paralytic ileus and thus, the completion of akinetic mutism was interrupted.   Para-or tetraplegia in flexion was found only in three cases.

## 2) Neuropathological features

The first autopsy cases of this type of CJD in Japanese were reported by Omaru, et al. (1961, *Nos. 1, 2 & 3*), although case 3 was diagnosed as the presenile dementia of Kraepelin type.   All of them showed a progressive dementia with various psychotic

**Fig. 2.**  Simple poliodystrophic type of Creutzfeldt-Jakob disease (Table 1). a, b, c and d: case 1; e and f: case 2.
**(a)** Trigeminal motor nucleus at the middle portion of the pons; a great majority of the nerve cells of a typical inflation. × 96.  **(b)** Magnified typically and achromatically inflated cytoplasm of the nerve cell with the eccentric nucleus indicated by the arrow in (a). × 513.  **(c)** Anterior horn of the thoracic cord; the arrow indicates the typically inflated nerve cell. × 100.  (d) Highly magnified achromatically inflated nerve cell indicated by the arrow in (c). × 950.  **(e)** Internal segment of the globus pallidus; coarse spongy tissue disruption and a few pseudocalcareous depositions on the capillary walls. × 120.  **(f)** Inferior olivary nucleus; coarse spongy tissue disruption, preserved nerve cells and slightly activated glial nuclei in the parenchyma. × 476.  [(a) & (b): K-B (c) & (d): Thionine; (e) & (f): H-E]

42

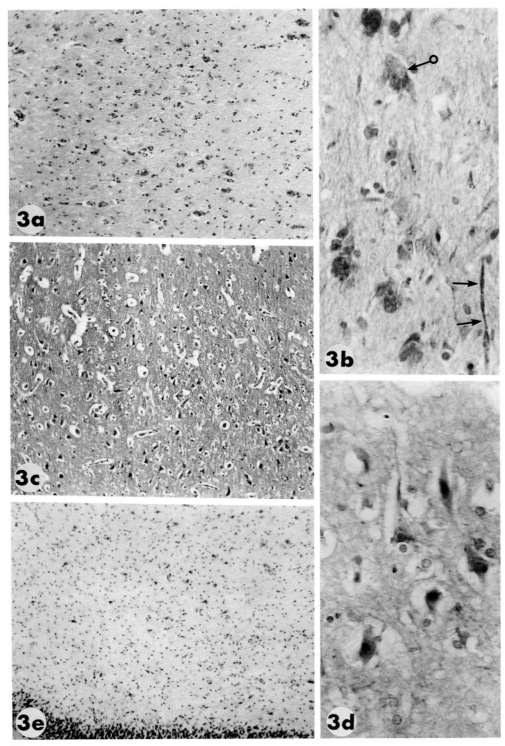

Fig. 3

symptoms including bizarre behaviors, nocturnal delirium, hallucination and delusion, while neurological disturbances comprized unsteady gait with or without positive Romberg's sign, pyramidal sign and lower motor neuron signs, hand tremor, and choreoathetoid movement.    Their neuropathology was a widespread dissemination of inflated neurons in the central nervous system including the precentral cortex, striatum, thalamus, dentate nucleus, pontine nuclei and motor nuclei of the brainstem.    Neuronal depletion and degeneration accompanied by astrocytosis was rather mind in the frontal and temporal cortex.    No definite spongy state was described.    The spinal cord was not examined. In addition case 2 disclosed a calcification of the vascular walls in the striatum, globus pallidus, thalamus, dentate nucleus and cerebral and cerebellar cortex, and thus, this was discussed in a relation to Fahr's disease.    The neuropathology of case 3, however, could be considered to be compatible with that of this of type of CJD, although it has been disputed as to whether Kraepelin's disease is a distinct entity or not.    Ichikawa, et al. (1961, *No. 4*) also reported a case of CJD which, in addition to widespread distribution of inflated neurons, disclosed more severe and diffuse loss of neurons in the frontal, parietal and temporal cortex and striatum, and marked proliferation of astrocytes.

In Ishino's case (1963, *No. 5*), on the other hand, hyperreflexia, fasciculation of the facial and tongue muscles and muscular atrophy of a neurogenic pattern demonstrated by electromyogram were described.    The postmortem examination revealed corticospinal tract degeneration, while the anterior horn cells showed an inflation but no depletion. Similar change were found in Mitsuyama's case (1970, *No. 10*) and Nakazima's case (1976, *No. 15*).    The latter case also showed degeneration of the posterior column as well. Uda's case, on the other hand, disclosed neuronal loss in the anterior horn cells (1972, *No. 12*), while muscular weakness and atrophy were not found clinically.    There were no cases in which change of the skeletal muscles was described.    These cases could be considered in a relation to the amyotrophic form of CJD.    In this type of CJD, however, neuronal depletion of the anterior horn and motor nuclei of the brainstem, such as the hypoglossal nucleus, were slight, while neuronal inflation was greatly predominant.

Recently the autopsy cases of ALS with dementia have been reported.    Several cases showed a subacute clinical course ranging from 4 to 9 months (Mizutani, unpublished cases).    Many cases showed marked increase of the glial nuclei, disproportional to slight loss of neurons there.    Some cases disclosed marked subcortical gliosis comparable with progressive subcortical gliosis (Neuman & Cohn, 1967).    There appeared a clinicopathological dissociation of slight change in the cortical neurons to marked dementia.    The

---

**Fig. 3.**    Simple poliodystrophic type of Creutzfeldt-Jakob disease (Table 1). a, b, c and d: case 2; e: case 1.

**(a)** Putamen; ischemic degenerated nerve cells of both small and large type in which certain of them show neurohophagic process. × 110.    **(b)** Highly magnified area as in (a); neuronophagic nerve cells one example of which is indicated by the arrow with zero; dissemination of the activated rod cell nuclei one example of which is indicated by the arrows. × 440.    **(c)** Subiculum; ischemic shrunken nerve cells, and dilated perineuronal and periadventitial spaces. × 89.    **(d)** Magnified area as in (c); similar to (c) and fine, sieve-like tissue disruption in the parenchyma. × 490.    **(e)** End plate of the Ammon's horn adjacent to the fascia dentata; severely disintegrated nerve cell, remaining darkly shrunken nerve cells and diffusely proliferated glial nuclei in the parenchyma. × 86.    [(a), (c) & (d): H-E; (b): K-B; (e): Thionine]

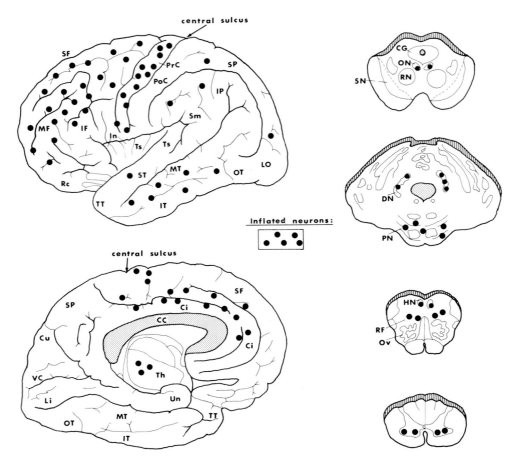

**Fig. 4.** Schematic diagrams of the distribution of the inflated nerve cells in the simple poliodystrophic type of Creutzfeldt-Jakob disease. Adapted from Mizutani(1981), *No. 16* (From: Neuropsychiatric disorders in the elderly: eds., Hirano, A. & Miyoshi, K., Igaku-Shoin, 1983, with permission)

change of the lower motor neurons was more pronounced, while inflated neurons in the cerebral cortex were rare in these cases. It may be assumed that ALS with dementia is located nosologically at the periphery of the simple poliodystrophic type of CJD.

The thalamus was affected in this type of CJD, as in the other subtypes of CJD. The thalamic change in some cases of this type could be regarded as primary thalamic degeneration (Matsuoka, et al., 1968, *No. 7*; Mitsuyama, et al., 1970, *No. 10*; Uda, et al., 1972, *No. 12*). The cerebellar cortex was frequently damaged. Purkinje cell depletion in a slight degree occurred in many cases, while the cortical degeneration of granule cell type was never found. In some cases, the dentate nucleus and inferior olive also showed neuronal loss.

Matsuoka, et al.'s case (1968, *No. 7*) showed spongy state in the cingulate, lateral occipital, middle and inferior temporal cortex, and the hippocampus, as well as neuronal degeneration and inflation, neuronophagiae and glial rosettes, and astrocytosis there.

The authors, on the other hand, commented that spongy state in the cerebral cortex could be considered as a secondary change due to circulatory disturbance.   This problem was also proposed by Ishizaki, et al. (197_, *No. 11*).   They considered their case as an intermediate case between CJD and subacute spongiform encephalopathy.   However, spongy state in the insular cortex of this case showed no clustered and grape-like microcavities but it was of edematous nature.

There was no case in which distinct degeneration of the white matter was described, although Matsuoka's case (1968, *No. 7*) showed diffuse loss of myelin in the centrum semiovale.   Recently the case of the panencephalopathic type of CJD, with widespread distribution of inflated neurons compatible with that of the simple poliodystrophic type of CJD, was reported (Riku, et al., 1983, *No. 117*, see Chapter III-6).

# Discussion

Synthetizing our experiences in this type of CJD together with those clinicopathological findings reported in the references mentioned above, the simple poliodystrophic type showed widespread distribution of the lesions in the central nervous system than that of the other subtypes of CJD, except for the panencephalopathic type which will be discussed in detail later on (Chapter III-6).   In the cerebral cortex the frontal, precentral and temporal cortex, occasionally the parietal cortex were most affected, while the occipital lobe was relatively spared.   The striatum and thalamus were always damaged, as in the other subtypes of CJD.   Purkinje cells, dentate nucleus, motor nuclei of the brainstem, pontine nuclei, inferior olive and anterior horn of the spinal cord were not infrequently damaged in this type, while these structures were usually unaffected in many cases of subacute spongiform encephalopathy.   The main histological change in the simple poliodystrophic type existed in the neurons in which degeneration, such as inflation, sclerosis and pigmentary degeneration, were more predominant than depletion.   Astrocytic reaction and spongy degeneration were less severe than in the other subtypes and if they existed, they were essentially different in nature as compared with those in the other subtypes of CJD.   Actually neuronophagiae and glial rosettes were exclusively  found in the simple poliodystrophic type but usually not in the other subtypes.

In addition to the neuropathology of the simple poliodystrophic type, some clinical characteristics could be pointed out;  Creutzfeldt stated that there was some fluctuation of the clinical pictures (1920), and this was observed particularly in mental symptoms and signs, in spite of progressive worsening of dementia; such fluctuation was seldom recognized in the other subtypes of CJD; moreover, the lower motor neuron signs were found more in this type than in the other subtypes, while myoclonus was less frequent in this type; these clinical features appeared to be somewhat different from those in the other subtypes.

In Japan the autopsy cases of the simple poliodystrophic type of CJD were clustered in the 1960 s, while no cases were reported in the 1980 s.   One reason may be in that the clinicopathological features of this type described above is somewhat different from the main feature of CJD, particularly of subacute spongiform encephalopathy.

The neuropathologic similarities to the simple poliodystrophic type, on the other

**Table 1**

| Case Number, Age (years) and Sex (total duration of illness) Previous History* | Major Clinical Features and Course (——→indicated shift or progression) |
|---|---|
| | Misbehavior——→Pain in right shoulder, fever 1⁺——→Mutism——→Dysphagia ——→Nocturnal delirium, monologue, incontinence, clouded consciousness 1⁺, inertia, mutism, infantile——→*Apallic state, tetraplegia in flexion,* pain in various joints, choreoathetoid movements, foot clonus——→Emaciation, stomatitis——→Miliary bullotic eruptions of skin——→Delirious psycho-motor excitement——→*Myoclonic jerks of whole body, paratonic rigidity* ——→Myoclonic jerks of face, oculogyric movements, nystagmoid and knocking movements——→Convulsive seizures 4⁺——→Semicomatose state, meiosis, stiffness of pupils——→Convulsions——→*Akinetic mutism*——→ Bronchopneumonia, then death |
| | Dementia before and after devotion——→Amnesia 3⁺, dementia, myoclonic jerks ?——→Impairment of gait and vision, inability to work——→Progres-sive dementia, disorientation——→Hyperactive deep-tendon reflexes, de-mentia, *occasional myoclonus-like jerks,* pronounced muscular atrophy of soles and hands——→*Dementia 3⁺*——→Incontinence, inability to sit——→ Fever 1⁺——→Fever 3⁺——→*Muscular rigidity 2⁺*——→High fever, then death |
| | Depression——→Sleeplessness, loss of appetite, inability to concentrate in daily life ——→Inability to stand or walking——→Ability to stand and walk, nocturnal delirum, apathy, misbehavior, foot clonus——→Apathy, impai-red emotion——→Mutism——→Exacerbation of gait impairment, dysarthria ——→*Akinetic mutism,* total incontinence, foot clonus, primitive reflexes ——→*Perianal myoclonic jerks, rigidity of limbs (upper more severe than lower)*——→Conjugate deviation of eyes to right side, *tetraplegia in flexion and extension*——→Bronchopneumonia, then death |

*: Negative family history in all cases.

hand, were occasionally manifested by the development of pellagra neuropsychosis, collagen disease or neurotoxic disorders, such as those due to excessive consumption of alcohol or administration of phenothiazines. In this regard, it should not be overlooked that cases 1 and 2 (Table 1) were accompanied by skin disease during the clinical course of the illness.

Inflated nerve cells were also consistently found and distributed widely in the central nervous system of all other subtypes of CJD, although these cells were usually restricted to the cerebral cortex. Insofar as, the simple poliodystrophic type of CJD may have pathological processes similar to those operating in the other subtypes of the disease, considering that the clinical features of this type more or less closely resembled those of the other subtypes of CJD.

# REFERENCES

Creutzfeldt, H. G.:   Über eine eigenartige herdförmige Erkrunkung des Zentralnervensystems, Z. ges. Neurol. Psychiat., 57: 1-19, 1920.

**Ichikawa, T., Kato, U., Ishikawa, I., Kamei, K. and Sasaki, S.:**   A case of the Creutzfeldt-Jakob disease, Psychiat. Neurol. Jpn., 63: 721-737, 1961.

**Ishino, H.:**   An autopsy case of presenile dementia belonging to the Creutzfeldt-Jakob group, Psychiat. Neurol. Jpn., 65: 589-613, 1963.

**Ishizaki, T., Fukase, K. and Kashimura, H.:**   An intermediate case between Creutzfeldt-Jakob disease and subacute spongiform encephalopathy, Clin. Neurol. (Japan), 11: 601-606, 1971.

**Jakob, A.:**   Über eigenartige Erkrankungen des Zentralnervensystems mit bemerkenswertem anatomische Befunde, Z. ges. Neurol. Psychiat., 64: 147-228, 1921.

**Katayama, Y., Takegoshi, A, Hattori, H., Takeuchi, T., Sakakura, T., Inoue, K. and Tsuda, M.:**   A case of Creutzfeldt-Jakob disease, Adv. Neurol. Sci. (Japan), 13: 198-205, 1969.

**Omaru, I., Hatamoto, N., Yoshida, M. and Tokumitsu, Y.:**   Autopsy findings on the presenile dementia of Jakob-Creutzfeldt and Kraepelin types, Fukuoka Med. J. (Japan), 52: 150-160, 1961.

**Matsuoka, T. and Miyoshi, K.:**   An autopsy case of Creutzfeldt-Jakob disease——A contribution to the understanding of presenile-involutive encephalopathies, Adv. Neurol. Sci. (Japan), 8: 427-438, 1964.

**Matsuoka, T., Mayoshi, K., Saka, K., Kawagoe, T. and Kikuchi, T.:**   A case probably of Creutzfeldt-Jakob's disease——A report of our second case, Psychiat. Neurol. Jpn., 70: 28-39, 1968.

**Mitsuyama, Y., Takamatsu, I and Shinkai, A.:**   Preseniel dementia reminiscent of Creutzfeldt-Jakob disease, Psychiat. Neurol Jpn., 72: 1146-1159, 1970.

**Mizutani, T.:**   Neuropathology of Creutzfeldt-Jakob disease in Japan. With special reference to the panencephalopathic type, Acta Path. Jpn., 31: 903-922, 1981.

**Nakazima, S., Sato, T., Goto, F., Katayama, T. and Matsuyama, H.:**   An autopsy case of Creutzfeldt-Jakob disease group, Clin. Neurol. (Japan), 16: 194, 1976.

**Neuman, M. A. and Cohn, R.:**   Progressive subcortical gliosis, a rare form of presenile dementia, Brain, 90: 405-418, 1967.

**Riku, S., Okamoto, T., Hashizume, Y., Koike, Y. and Sobue, I.:**   Panencephalopathic type of Creutzfeldt-Jakob disease and special reference to its pyramidal tract degeneration, Clin. Neurol. (Japan), 23: 147-151, 1983.

**Shiraki, H.:**   The neuropathological background for Creutzfeldt-Jakob disease (Creutzfeldt-Jakob syndrome), Adv. Neurol. Sci. (Japan), 18: 4-30, 1974.

**Sugita, T., Tadokoro, M., Oikawa, K., Ui, S. and Akikawa, I.:**   An autopsy case of Creutzfeldt-Jakob disease group, Adv. Neurol. Sci. (Japan), 21: 572, 1977.

**Uda, T., Yano, K. and Moro, K.:**   A case of Creutzfeldt-Jakob disease, Adv. Neurol. Sci. (Japan), 16: 543, 1972.

**Yuasa, R. and Kaneko, Z.:**   A case of Creutzfeldt-Jakob disease, Brain and Nerves (Japan), 21: 811-819, 1969.

# Subacute Spongiform Encephalopathy and Creutzfeldt-Jakob Disease in West Germany Reminiscent of Kuru in New Guinea

Hirotsugu Shiraki, M. D. and Toshio Mizutani, M. D.

The history of researches of subacute spongiform encephalopathy (SSE) which could clearly be categorized within CJD has already been well documented in detail in the Chapter I. As will be mentioned in detail later, the autopsy cases of SSE in the Japanese, on the other hand, included a fairly large number and actually comprized 38% of all autopsy cases of CJD.

Besides, in 1978-1979 one of the authors (Shiraki) has had an opportunity to examine the three autopsy cases of CJD in West Germany reminiscent of kuru published by Krücke, et al. (1973), at the Division of Neuropathology, Max-Planck Institute for Brain Research, Frankfurt am Main.

The six autopsy cases of SSE, therefore, consisted of the five representative cases of the Japanese and one case of CJD in West Germany reminiscent of kuru in New Guinea mentioned above, the summary of their clinical features of which is listed in Table 1.

---

**Fig. 1.** Subacute spongiform encephalopathy (Table 1). a: case 1; b: case 2; c, d and e: case 3.
**(a)** Parahippocampal cortex; conspicuous, coalescent spongy tissue disruption in all layers, except for the molecular layer. × 27. **(b)** Supragranular layers of the frontal cortex; conspicuous, coalescent spongy tissue disruption and preservation of interspersed nerve cells and axons. × 86. **(c)** Infragranular layers of the parahippocampal cortex; fine spongy tissue disruption and hypertrophic astroytosis with a coarse gliofiber formation; the arrows indicate senile plaques. × 130. **(d)** Infragranular layers of the visual cortex; phagocytic cells laden with fat granules in all layers but exclusively of fixed type; the cross indicate U fibers. × 89. **(e)** Magnified inflated nerve cell in the infragranular layer of cortex of the temporal tip; several vacuoles in the achromatically swollen cytoplasm (indicated by the arrows) and eccentric nucleus (N). × 1000. [(a): H-E; (b): Bodian; (c): Cajal's gold sublimate; (d): Sudan III; (e): Thionine]

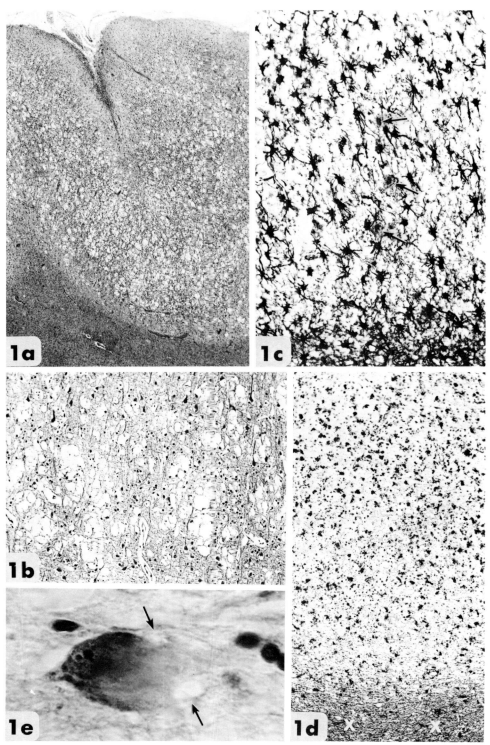

Fig. 1

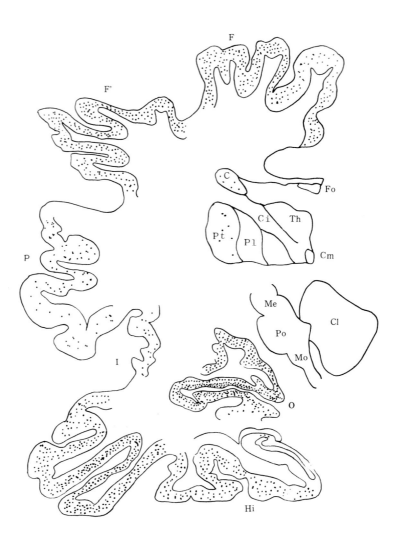

**Fig. 2.** Subacute spongiform encephalopathy (case 1 in Table 1). Adapted from Shiraki & Matsuoka (1963).

Schematic diagram of the distribution pattern of the spongy tissue disruption (dots) in the different cerebral regions.

Most pronounced in the occipital areas (0), followed by the parahipptoampal (Hi), temporal (T), fronto-orbital (F') and fronto-dorsal (F), less pronounced in the parietal (P; area 4) and insula (I), and exceedingly less or even absent in the Ammon's horn; mild in the caudate nucleus (C) and putamen (Pt), and absent in the pallidum (Pl), thalamus (Th) and the brainstem. Fo: fornix; Ci: capsula interna; Cm: corpus mamillare; Me: mesencephalon; Po: pons; Cl: cerebellum; Mo: medulla oblongata.

The basic neuropathologic characteristic of SSE was spongiform degeneration of the cerebral cortex or the subcortical gray matter.   Small or large, grape-like clusters of spongy tissue disruption were distributed in a pseudolaminar or focal pattern in the circumscribed cortical layers, whereas such tissue disruption was occasionally distributed in all cortical layers, even in the crown, between the walls and to the base of the cerebral gyri (Figs. 1a & 1b).   Particularly in the cases with comparatively short duration of the illness, nerve cells, myelin sheaths and axons were fairly well preserved in the septal regions (Fig. 1b).

On the other hand, fine, sieve-like tissue, usually occurring as foci, disrupted the infragranular cortical layers most severely and the supragranular layers least seriously in most cases (Figs. 8a, 8b & 11a).

Although the topographic pattern and severity varied from case to case and from stage to stage, both types of tissue disruption occurred concurrently and were accompanied by disintegration of neurons of variable severity.   The hippocampal formation and uncus were in most cases free of such foci or were involved only slightly; the foci were encountered predominantly in the neocerebral cortex (Fig. 2).

In general, spongy degeneration was also pronounced in the striatum of some cases (Fig. 8c) and less conspicuous in the other (Fig. 2).   The spongy degeneration was less pronounced in the globus pallidus, thalamus, substantia nigra (Fig. 11d) and other structures, and was mild in the tegmentum of the brainstem.

Hypertrophic astrocytes with one or several nuclei and an abundance of cytoplasm were distributed diffusely but were most common in the deteriorated cortex.   Interesting enough, these astrocytes developed a coarse gliofiber formation but never showed fibrillary gliosis with thin gliofibers (Figs. 1c & 11b).   Moreover, phagocytes laden with the by-products of myelin destruction were mobilized but were exclusively of a fixed character, irrespective of the duration of the clinical course (Figs. 1d & 11c).

Both findings clearly indicated certain dysfunction of the astrocytes and microglia throughout the entire clinical course.

In SSE, characteristically inflated neurons, a few of which showed evidence of inclusion body-like structures and vacuole-like structures in their cytoplasm, were found to occur in foci or exist throughout the cerebral cortex of a great majority of the cases studied, although the severity of these changes varied from case to case (Figs. 1e, 4e, 5c, 8c, 10c, 10d & 10e).   The distribution of these neurons closely resembled that seen in both the ataxic and panencephalopathic types, in which inflated neurons were restricted to the cerebrum, as a rule.

In a 35-year-old man who had had the disease for 21 months (case 3, Table 1), atypical and typical plaques with single cores or several cores were extremely abundant, particularly in the cerebellocerebral molecular layers (Figs. 3a, 3b & 3d), followed by other cortical layers (Figs. 1c & 3c) and the striatum.   Some plaques were also visualized in the subcortical white matter, which demonstrated a mild astrocytosis and gliosis there (Fig. 3e).   Considering the age of this patient, the number of plaques was abnormally large, indicating that his brain had become prematurely senile.

The present example (case 4, Table 1) demonstrated symmetric and bilateral, distal-dominant degeneration of the corticospinal tract accompanied by less marked degeneration of the posterior and spinocerebellar tracts of the spinal cord (Figs. 5a & 5b) as well

52

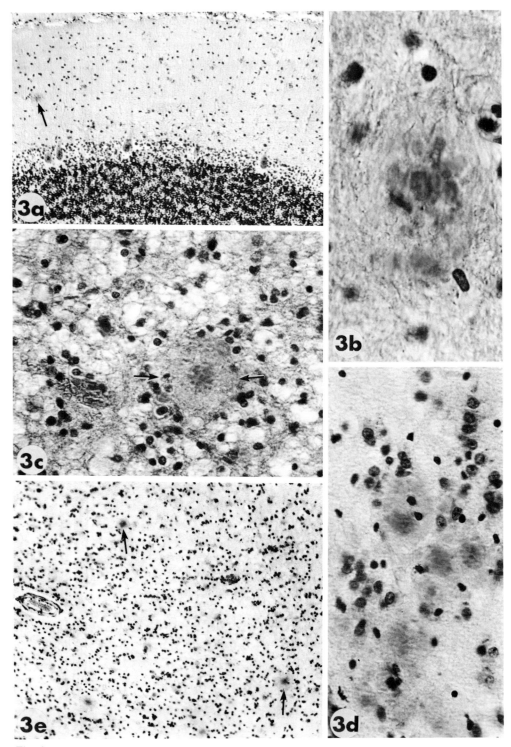

Fig. 3

as degeneration of thalamic subnuclei, such as the dorsalis posterior and anterior, and the formatio medialis and anterior, in which neuronal disintegration, astrocytosis and a few remaining neurons with intracytoplasmic vacuoles were visualized (Figs. 4d & 4e), whereas spongy tissue disruption was extremely insidious.

The distribution of the plaques and other foci of pathologic changes mentioned above in this case is illustrated schematically in Fig. 6.

In this regard, the following case was interesting; in a 49-year-old man who developed abruptly a characteristic clinical course of SSE four years later after the head trauma and subsequent neurosurgical operation (case 5, Table 1); the anterior half of the left hemisphere demonstrated clearly the characteristic neuropathology of the sequelae due to the head trauma and neurosurgical operation (Figs. 7a & 7b); fine, sieve-like tissue disruption, on the other hand, were almost symmetric and bilateral, and widespread in both the cerebral cortex and striatum (Figs. 8a, 8b & 8c); moreover, degeneration was encountered in certain thalamic subnuclei, such as nucleus dorsalis posterior and formatio medials (Fig. 8e), and putamen (Fig. 8d); the degeneration of these gray matters was almost symmetric and bilateral, and consisted of severest disintegration of neurons, conspicuous astrocytosis and very mild spongy tissue disruption, indicating a possibility of occurrence of systemic degeneration of these gray matters.

In this regard, interesting enough was also the cerebellar degeneration in some cases of SSE (Figs. 4a, 4b & 4c); this cerebellar degeneration also occurred symmetrically and bilaterally, and was mostly predominated in the paleocerebellum, such as flocculus and/or vermis.

Typical kuru plaques were found to be numerous, particularly in the cerebellar cortex, in the two cases, whereas only a few were seen in one case; these cases were previously reported by Krücke; et al. (1973) (case 6, Table 1).

The distribution of these kuru plaques in one case is illustrated schematically in Fig. 14.

In this case, the cerebellar degeneration was symmetric and occurred bilaterally, but was restricted to the paleocortex, such as the vermis and flocculus, in which numerous granule cells and some Purkinje cells were moderately to severely disintegrated (Fig. 9a). Moreover, numerous torpedoes (Fig. 9b) and clustered or isolated kuru plaques (Fig. 9c) were distributed throughout almost all the cerebellar foliae in both the paleocerebellum

---

**Fig. 3.** Subacute spongiform encephalopathy (case 3 in Table 1).
**(a)** Neocerebellar cortex; numerous eosinophilic, senile plaque-like bodies of various sizes and with one or several cores, mainly in the molecular layer and to a lesser degree in the Purkinje cell and granular layers. × 120. **(b)** Magnified senile plaque-like body indicated by the arrow in (a); centrally located, multiple eosinophilic cores and faintly stained marginal zone. × 1,000. **(c)** Magnified fourth layer of the second temporal cortex; sieve-like, fine spongy tissue disruption and senile plaque with the central multiple cores and faintly stained marginal zone indicated by the arrows. × 457. **(d)** Magnified molecular layer of the insular cortex; clusters of senile plaques with more or less thioninophilic central cores, and clustered astrocytic nuclei around the senile plaques. × 490. **(e)** Subcortical white matter of the tip of the temporal cortex; more or less thioninophilic senile plaques, two examples of which are indicated by the arrows, and diffusely proliferated glial nuclei in the parenchyma. × 120. [(a), (b) & (c): H-E; (d) & (e):Thionine]

54

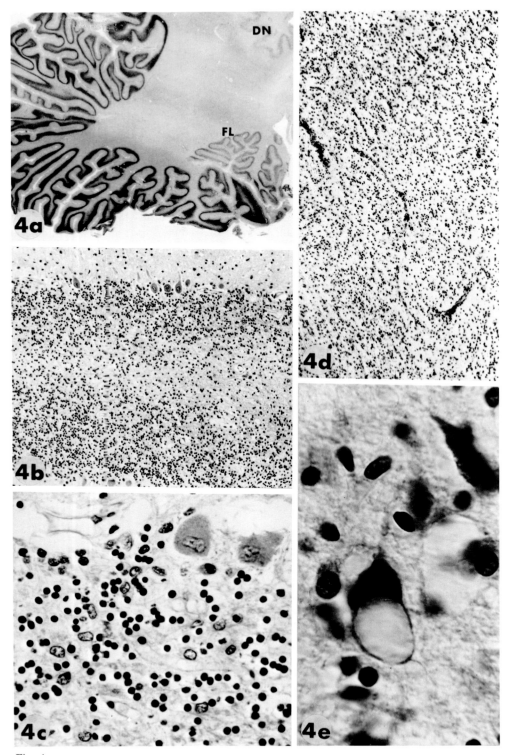

Fig. 4

and the neocerebellum.

In the present example, nerve cells of the cerebellar dentate nucleus were moderately disintegrated, whereas so-called grumorous structures were outstanding not only around the peridendritic areas of the nerve cells, but also around their pericytoplasmic areas (Figs. 9d & 9e). Those structures were also encountered in the many other cases of SSE as well.

In this case, multisystemic degeneration was a well-established coexisting condition. For example, the striopallidal and thalamic systems demonstrated symmetric degeneration that occurred bilaterally accompanied by severe loss of neurons and intense gliosis with thin gliofibers (Figs. 10a & 10b). The latter condition represented a distinct contrast to the hypertrophic astrocytes seen only with coarse gliofibers in the cerebral cortex (Figs. 10b & 11b).

The topographic distribution of the foci of the thalamic subnuclei in this case, on the other hand, was quite similar to that of thalamic degeneration, that is, the Stern-Garcin type of Creutzfeldt-Jakob disease, although the ontogenetically old subnuclei of this case were more or less severely involved as well. The latter disease group, on the other hand, will be discussed in more detail later (Chapter III-4).

The distribution of the foci of the thalamic subnuclei in the present case is illustrated schematically in Figures 14 and 15.

Again in the same case, symmetric, slight to moderate loss of neurons and giant astrocytosis occurred bilaterally in the inferior olivary neurons, in which the remaining neurons contained one or several vacuoles and in which the conspicuously thickened, tortured or tangled dendritic processes originating from these neurons were simultaneously predominant (Figs. 12a, 12b & 12c). Demyelination or hypertrophy of the olivary nucleus was equivocal because this structure showed signs of pseudohypertrophy. In addition, degeneration of the corticospinal tract of the spinal cord, predominantly affecting the distal portions of the tract, was observed (Figs. 13a & 13b).

Different types of foci, including the multisystemic degeneration as seen in the Krücke, et al.'s case are illustrated schematically in Figures 14 and 15.

On the basis of these observations not only of the Krücke, et al.'s case together with those of the other cases of SSE mentioned above, it now could reasonably be concluded that the coexistence of spongy tissue disruption and multisystemic degeneration was not a mere coincidence and that, in fact this finding is very important and a key to an understanding of subacute spongiform encephalopathy.

As far as our specimens examined were concerned, no particular alterations of the

---

**Fig. 4.** Subacute spongiform encephalopathy (Table 1). a: case 4; b and c: case 2; d and e: case 3. **(a)** Cerebellum; slightly disintegrated granular layers in a majority of neocerebellar foliae, and particularly predominant in the flocculus (Fl); DN indicates the dentate nucleus. × 3.1. **(b)** Vermis of the cerebellum; slightly disintegrated granular layers, and well-preserved Purkinje cells. × 125. **(c)** Magnified area in (b); moderately disintegrated granule cells, darkly shrunken remaining granule cells, and activated astrocytic nuclei; preserved Purkinje cells. × 513. **(d)** Nucleus dorsalis posterior of the thalamus; severely disintegrated nerve cells and diffusely proliferated glial nuclei in the parenchyma. × 86. **(e)** Magnified formatio anterior of the thalamus; single large vacuole in the swollen cytoplasm of the nerve cell. × 1,100. [(a), (d) & (e): Thionine; (b) & (c): H-E]

**Table. 1.**

| Case Number, Age (years) and Sex (total duration of illness) Previous and Family History | Major Clinical Features and Course (——→indicates shift or progression) |
|---|---|
| 1<br>59, M<br>(11 months)<br>Heavy drinker, head injury, transient dysphagia & dyspnea, Leischmaniasis during 2nd world war | Difficulty of finding words, paraphasic, iterative speech, impairment of finger-naming, left-right-recognition and calculation, motoric, intentional and clothing apraxias, optic agnosia, closing in figures, deviated optic axis, agraphia, alexia——*Rapid progression of dementia,* incontinence, deteriorated psychic functions 3+, *mutistic,* no remarkable neurological impairments except for suspicious Romberg's sign——Intermittent moderate fever, prupura eruptions of face, hands & legs——Impairment of gait 3+, atactic, stumbles easily——General emaciation——Indifferent, abulic, apathetic——Decubiti——Loss of appetite——Edema of feet, emaciation 3+——*Akinetic-mutistic,* only ocular movements——Weak pulsation, then death<br>*CSF: Wassernann 1 - 2+* |
| 2<br>49, M<br>(14 weeks)<br>Unremarkable | Impairment of vision——Impairment of handwiting——Misbehavior, double vision, impairment of left arm movement——*Dementia 1+*→Delirious excitement——Impairment of conversation——*Bedridden,* incontinence ——Hyperreflexia of arms, hyporeflexia or areflexia of legs——Coma, *occasional fibrillary movements of left shoulder and both arms*——Dyspnea, then death<br>*EEG: Abnormal* |
| 3<br>35, M<br>(21 months)<br>Treated with organic mercury liniment for scabies before the present illness | Shuffling of legs, tendency to stumble, tremor of arms——Atactic gait——Impairment of memory, disorientation, slurring of speech, violent behavior——*Inertia 3+,* bradyphrenia, perseveration 3+, impairment of calculation, alexia and agraphia 1+, dysarthria 3+, weakness of hands (right more severe than left), inability to walk, dysdiadochokinesis 1+, rigidity of arms 3+, "Gehenhalten"——*Coarse tremor, mutism 3+, ataxia 3+,* mask-like face——*Primitive reflexes*—— *Apallic state,* hyperhidrosis, hypersalivation——Positive Babinski's and Gordon's reflexes ——*Paraplegia in flexion*——*Myoclonic jerks of arms,* occasional clonic convulsions ——Decubiti——Generalized weakness, then death<br>*EEG: Periodic synchronous discharge* |
| 4<br>57, M<br>(9 months)<br>Otitis media in childhood | Intoxicated with shellfish, vomitings, diarrhea——Catch cold, bedridden ——Impairment of vision——Double vision, impairment of gait——Concentric constriction of visual field——Unable to walk, confabulatoric, anxiety, distractability, irregular tremor of all limbs——Disorientation to time, space and person, perseveration, decreased spontaneous speech, total incontinence——*Quadriplegia in flexion,* muscular rigidity 3+, *myoclonic jerks of neck, face and trunk to tactile, acoustic and optic stimuli and at voluntary movements,* complained of impairment of vision, dysarthric, dysphagia 3+, total incontinence, hyperaesthsia to all stimuli, moderate fever——High fever, dyspnea, stridor——Bronchopneumonia ——Clouded consciousness——Emaciation——No spontanous speech ——*Apallic syndrome, myoclonic jerks*——Decreased myoclonic jerks, then death<br>*EEG: Periodic synchronous discharge* |

| 5<br>49, M<br>*Head trauma and operation but unknown details; no sequelae left behind, however* | Four years after head trauma, complained of stiff shoulder——→Catch cold, diagnosed as tonsillitis——→No improvement, impairment of speech (suspicious motor aphasia)——→*Involuntary jerks,* apathetic, impairment of sleep, sleeplessness, *demented*——→Poor spontaneous speech, impairment of speech, suspicious motor aphasia, stiff movement, spastic gait, propulsion, hyperreflexias, bilateral positive Chaddock $\pm$, foot clonus of left side $1^+$——→Gradual progression of disorientation, stiff movements, *no spontaneous speech,* total incontinence——→Hyporeflexia, anisocoria (right larger than left), almost no ocular movements, ciliary hyporeflexia, "Gegenhalten"——→*Apallic state,* fibrillary movements, open eye——→Comatose——→ Fever, then death *Wassermann in blood: 3$^+$* |
|---|---|

Creutzfeldt-Jakob disease in West Germany reminiscent of kuru in New guinea*

| 6<br>52, F<br>(54 weeks)<br>Unremarkable | Listlessness, fatigue, fixed facial expression, head tremor, impairment of memory, confusion, disorientation, apathy, wastefulness, weakness of right leg, inability to walk——→*Ataxia, broad-based gait, unsteadiness in heel-knee test 1$^+$, Romberg's sign 1$^+$,* impairment of gait, rigidity of left arm˙$1^+$——→Amimia, coarse tremor of hands——→Monotony, dysarthria and slowness of speech, emaciation, *choreiform and athetoid hyperkinesia to acoustic and tactile stimuli,* dysphagia——→*No spontaneous speech or movements, flexion and adduction of legs,* sideways turning of head, *severe dementia*——→Dysphagia——→Severe wasting, then death |
|---|---|

*: The case from the Division of Neuropathology, Max Planck Institute for Brain Research, Frankfurt.

cerebral white matter were found (Fig. 10a), except for the subcortical gliosis in slight to moderate degree accompanied by no demyelination as well as the intense gliosis of the unilateral Ammon's horn in the Krücke, et al.'s case (Fig. 10b).

58

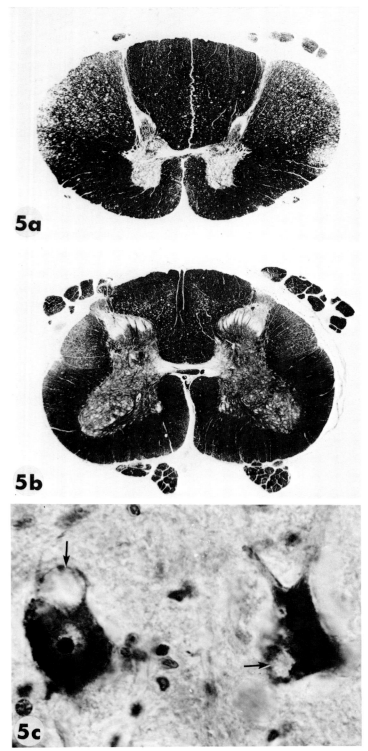

**Fig. 5** (Legend in page 63)

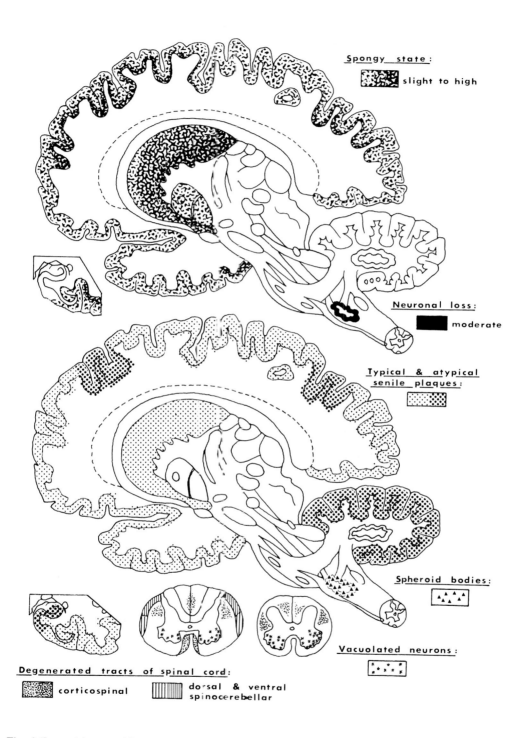

Spongy state:
slight to high

Neuronal loss:
moderate

Typical & atypical
senile plaques:

Spheroid bodies:

Vacuolated neurons:

Degenerated tracts of spinal cord:
corticospinal
dorsal & ventral
spinocerebellar

**Fig. 6** (Legend in page 63)

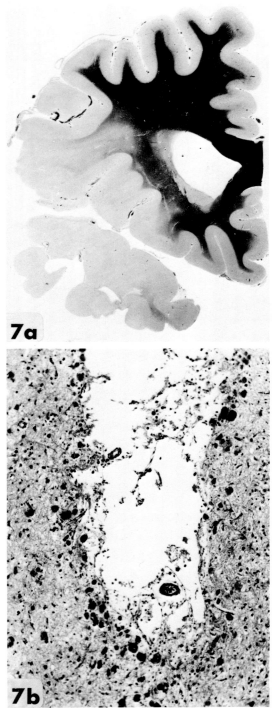

Fig. 7 (Legend in page 63)

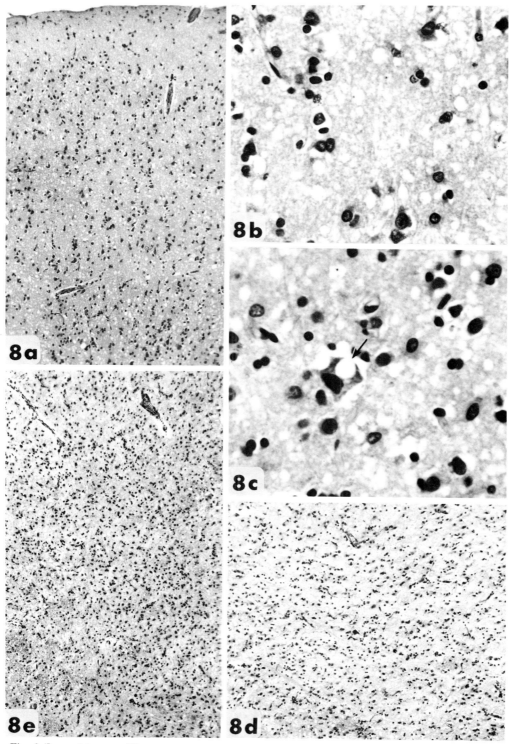

**Fig.** 8 (Legend in page 63)

62

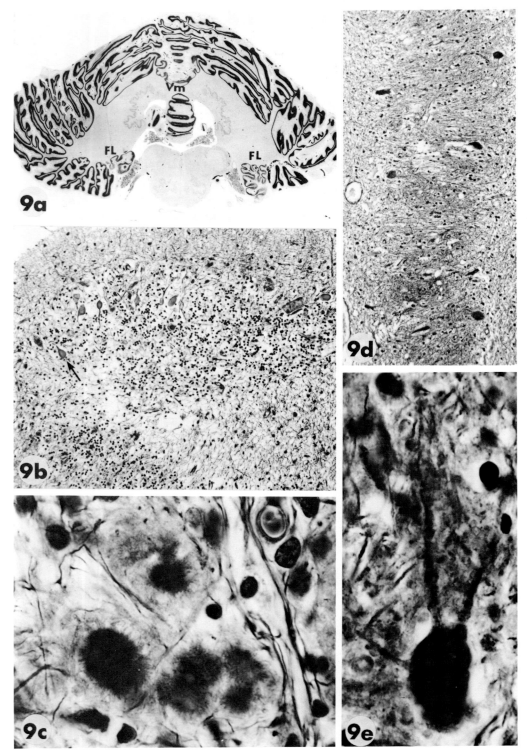

**Fig. 9** (Legend in page 63)

**Fig. 5.** Subacute spongiform encephalepathy (Table 1). a and b: case 3; c: case 4.
**(a)** Thoracic cord; spongy tissue disruption and demyelination symmetrically and bilaterally in the lateral and anterior corticospinal tracts, and both ventral and dorsal spinocerebellar tracts. × 10.0. **(b)** Lumbar cord; symmetrical moderate demyelination in the bilateral lateral corticospinal tracts and minimal spongy tissue disruption in the bilateral posterior tracts. **(c)** Magnified anterior horn of the upper lumbar cord; single or multiple vacuoles (the arrows) in the cytoplasm of the nerve cells. × 950. [(a) & (b): Woelcke myelin; (c): Thionine]

---

**Fig. 6.** Schematic diagrams of the distribution of the different foci in subacute spongiform encephalopathy (same case as case 3 in Table 1 and Figs. 1c - e, 3a - e, 4d, e and 5a, b) (From: Neuropsychiatric disorders in the elderly: eds., Hirano, A. & Miyoshi, K., Igaku-Shoin, 1983, with permission)

---

**Fig. 7.** Subacute spongy form encephalopathy followed by head trauma (case 5 in Table 1)
**(a)** Frontal-cut left-sided hemisphere through the rostral part of the corpus callosum (G); severest ulegyric atrophy of the cortex particularly predominant at the latero-orbital convolutions of the frontal lobe and temporal tip; widespread demyelination of the temporal tip and a part of the centrum semiovale; dilated anterior horn of the lateral ventricle; all of them presumably and partially attributed to the antecedent head trauma and neurosurgical operation. **(b)** Magnified deteriorated cortex and subcortical white matter of the temporal tip in (a); sharply demarcated cystic cavity marginated by the multiple spheroid bodies. × 80. [(a): K-B; (b): H-E]

---

**Fig. 8.** Subacute spongiform encephalopathy followed by head trauma (case 5 in Table 1)
**(a)** Supragranular layers of the left-side first temporal cortex; exceedingly fine, sieve-like spongy tissue disruption of isolated character in all layers; interspersed, well-preserved nerve cells. × 96. **(b)** Magnified area in (a); similar to (a). × 475. **(c)** Magnified left-side putamen; exceedingly fine, sieve-like spongy tissue disruption in the parenchyma interspersed nerve cells; the arrow indicates intracytoplasmic single vacuole in large type of the nerve cell. × 120. **(d)** Magnified left-side caudate nucleus; severely disintegrated nerve cells and diffuse astrocytosis and minimal spongy state in the parenchyma. × 97. **(e)** Formatio medialis of the thalamus; severely disintegrated nerve cells, and conspicuous astrocytosis, and no spongy state in the parenchyma. × 96. [(a), (b), (c), (d) & (e): H-E]

---

**Fig. 9.** Creutzfeldt-Jakob disease in West Germany reminiscent of kuru in New Guinea (MPI. No. 4705; case 6 in Table 1)
**(a)** Cerebellar hemispheres and middle portion of the medulla oblongata; moderate to high disintegration of the cerebellar cortex symmetrically and bilaterally but restricted to the paleocerebellar vermis (Vm) and flocculus (Fl); no remarkable changes in the neocerebellar cortex. **(b)** Magnified flocculus in (a); severely disintegrated granular and Purkinje cell layers, and numerous torpedos, one example indicated by the arrow. **(c)** Magnified neocerebellar granular layer in (a); clusters of kuru plaques of various sizes with the deeply argyrophilic central cores, radially-arranged, fine fibrils and similar but faintly argyrophilic marginal zone. **(d)** Cerebellar dentate nucleus; moderately disintegrated nerve cells and more or less deep argyrophilia in the parenchyma. **(e)** Highly magnified area in (d); faintly argyrophilic, amorphous or fine granular substances closely adjacent to the peridendritic areas of the nerve cell (the cross). [(a): Thionine; (b), (c), (d) & (e): Bodian]

64

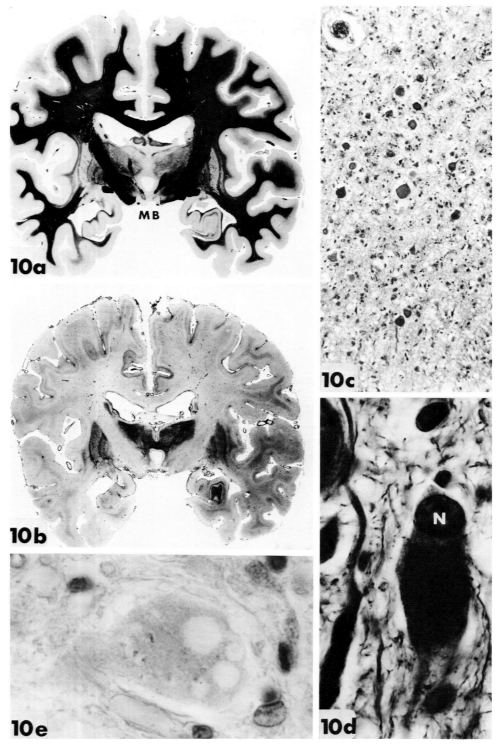

**Fig. 10** (Legend in page 70)

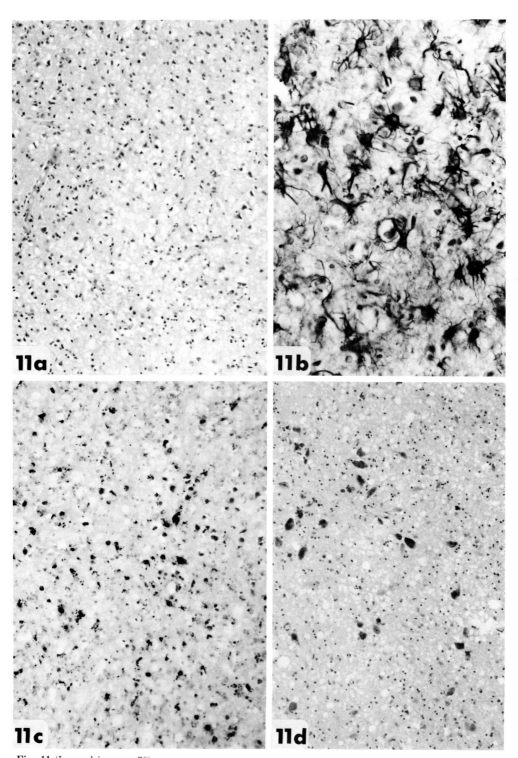

**Fig. 11** (Legend in page 70)

66

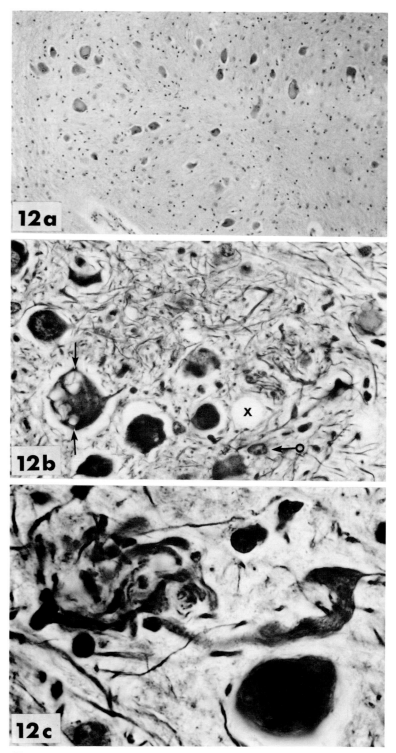

**Fig. 12** (Legend in page 70)

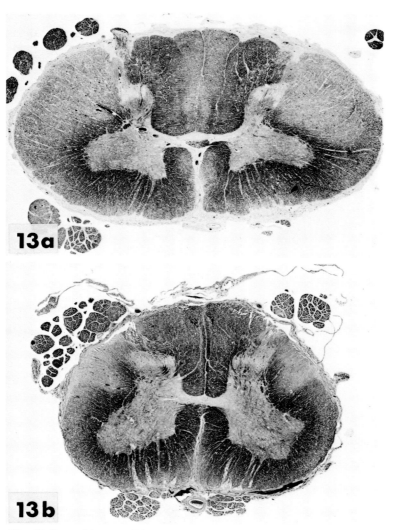

**Fig. 13** (Legend in page 70)

68

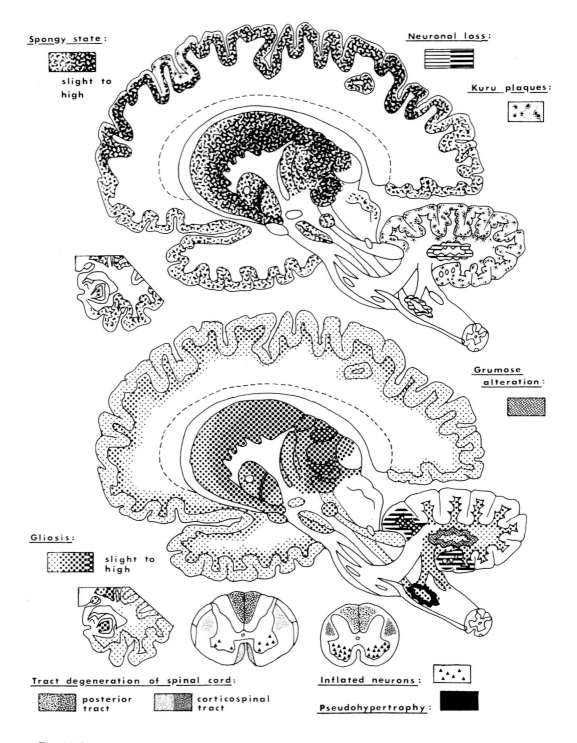

**Spongy state:**

slight to high

**Neuronal loss:**

**Kuru plaques:**

**Grumose alteration:**

**Gliosis:**

slight to high

**Tract degeneration of spinal cord:**

posterior tract

corticospinal tract

**Inflated neurons:**

**Pseudohypertrophy:**

**Fig. 14** (Legend in page 70)

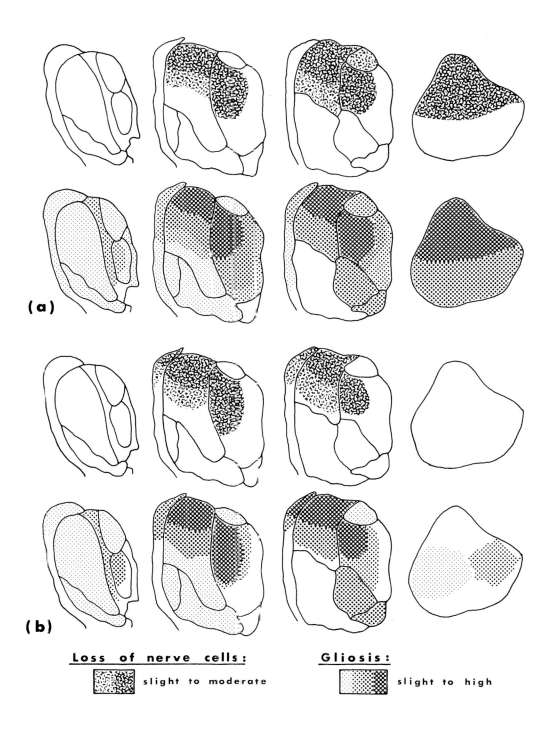

**(a)**

**(b)**

Loss of nerve cells:    slight to moderate    Gliosis:    slight to high

**Fig. 15** (Legend in page 70)

70

**Fig. 10.** Creutzfeldt-Jakob disease in West Germany reminiscent of kuru in New Guinea (MPI. No. 4705; case 6 in Table 1)
**(a)** Frontal-cut cerebral hemispheres through the cranial part of the mammillary body (MB); slight to moderate and widespread cortical atrophy in the both hemispheres but no remarkable change in the white matter and diencephalic nuclei. **(b)** Same section as in (a); moderate gliosis bilaterally in the cingulate cortex and a part of the superior frontal cortex and subcortical white matter; moderate to severe gliosis symmetrically and bilaterally in the caudate nucleus, putamen, globus pallidus, thalamic subnuclei and end plate of the right-side uncus. **(c)** Deep third layer of the cingulate cortex of the prefrontal gyrus; numerous inflated nerve cells. **(d)** Magnified same area as in (c) showing inflated nerve cell and eccentric nucleus (N) with a normal appearance, and deeply argyrophilic, core-like structure in the center of the inflated cytoplasm. **(e)** Almost same area as in (d); different-sized vacuoles in the inflated cytoplasm of the nerve cell and few PAS-positive tiny granules with marginal halo in the cytoplasm. [(a): Woelcke myelin; (b): Holzer; (c) & (d): Bodian; (e): PAS]

**Fig. 11.** Creutzfeldt-Jakob disease in West Germany reminiscent of kuru in New Guinea (MPI. No. 4705; case 6 in Table 1)
**(a)** Supragranular layers of the cingulate cortex; pronounced, fine, sieve-like tissue disruption in all layers showing comparatively good preservation of the nerve cells with the darkly shrunken nuclei. **(b)** Magnified same area as in (a); hypertrophic astrocytes with a coarse gliofiber formation but no gliosis with thin gliofibers. **(c)** Same area as in (a); oil red O-positive granules, mainly in the phagocytic cells, which are exclusively of fixed type. **(d)** Compact zone of the substantia nigra; fine, sieve-like tissue disruption but well-preserved nerve cells laden with melanin pigments. [(a) & (d): H-E; (b): Holzer; (c): Oil red O]

**Fig. 12.** Creutzfeldt-Jakob disease in West Germany reminiscent of kuru in New Guinea (MPI. No. 4705; case 6 in Table 1)
**(a)** Inferior olivary nucleus; more or less achromatically inflated cytoplasm of the remaining nerve cells with the eccentric nuclei and disseminated, enlarged astrocytic nuclei in the parenchyma. **(b)** Magnified area in (a); multiple coalescent vacuoles in the swollen cytoplasm of the nerve cell (the arrows), and single large vacuole presumably derived from a disintegrated nerve cell (the cross); pronounced manifestation of proliferated, hypertrophic and tangled dendritic processes of the nerve cells; the arrow with zero indicates one example of enlarged astrocytic nuclei. **(c)** Highly magnified similar area to (b); exceedingly thick and tangled dendritic processes of nerve cell; the adjacent inflated nerve cell is indicated by the cross. [(a); H-E; (b) & (c): Bodian]

**Fig. 13.** Creutzfeldt-Jakob disease in West Germany reminiscent of kuru in New Guinea (MPI. No. 4705; case 6 in Table 1)
**(a)** Upper cervical cord; moderate demyelination symmetrically and bilaterally in the lateral and anterior corticospinal, and Goll's tracts; slight demyelination in the Burdach's tracts as well. **(b)** Lumbar cord; pronounced demyelination symmetrically and bilaterally in the lateral corticospinal tract but only minimal demyelination throughout almost all of the posterior tracts. [(a) & (b): Woelcke myelin]

**Fig. 14.** Schematic diagrams of the distribution of the different foci in Creutzfeldt-Jakob disease in West Germany reminiscent of kuru in New Guinea (same case as case 6 in Table 1 and Figs. 9-13) (From: Neuropsychiatric disorders in the elderly: eds., Hirano, A. & Miyoshi, K., Igaku-Shoin, 1983, with permission)

**Fig. 15.** Schematic diagrams of the distribution of the thalamic lesions in Creutzfeldt-Jakob disease in West Germany reminiscent of kuru in New Guinea (same case as case 6 in Table 1 and Figs. 9-13) (From: Neuropsychiatric disorders in the elderly: eds., Hirano, A. & Miyoshi, K., Igaku-Shoin, 1983, with permission).

# Review of Reference of SSE in the Japanese

(Each number in italics in the text is corresponded to that in the Table 3 of the Appendix.)

## 1) Clinical features

The number of the autopsy cases of subacute spongiform encephalopathy (SSE) in the Japanese was 47 and comprized about 37% of the all cases of CJD in Japan.   There were 25 males and 22 females.   The total duration of the illness ranged from 2 to 108 months and its average was 14.1 months.   A great majority of the cases of SSE had no remarkable family history, whereas familial CJD was identified in one autopsy case (Oikawa, et al., 1969, *No.25*, see Chapter IV).

The following two cases were remarkable, since there existed some triggering factors before the development of the disease; in Hoshino's case SSE developed about four years later after complete recovery from the head trauma (case 5, Table 1; 1974, *No. 40*); in Hamaguchi's case, on the other hand, the patient was presented with disorientation two days later after the surgical operation for hemorrhoid under lumbar anesthesia (1972, *No. 32*).

The onset of the disease was abrupt or insidious.   The initial symptoms and signs were neurological and/or pyschic and they varied from case to case.   In any case, those cases which started with abrupt onset appeared to show a more rapid downhill course.

Neurological symptoms and signs at the early stage included gait disturbance and visual disturbances, such as loss of visual acuity and diplopia.   One third of the cases with gait disturbance showed ataxic nature, while the others disclosed no obvious pattern of ataxic nature.   Visual disturbance was, as a rule, frequently combined with agnosia and apraxia.   Insofar as the frequency of cerebral focal symptoms and signs were comparatively high as compared with that of the other subtypes of CJD, except fot the panencephalopathic type.

Forgetfulness, decreased daily activity and sleeplessness were found at the early stage.   These symptoms and signs progressively worsened, and subsequently, distinct dementia became obvious.

Rigidity of muscles developed rapidly.   Myoclonus appeared simultaneously or subsequently.   However, the frequency of the latter was lower than that of the panencephalopathic type.   PSD also showed a similar tendency.   Pyramidal signs and/or muscular weakness were noticed in some cases, while hand tremor and choreo-athetoid movement were less frequently found in comparison with those of the simple poliodystrophic type and the panencephalopathic type.

Cerebellar symptoms and signs were also infrequent as those in the ataxic form of CJD.   Taking account of no or less morphological changes in the cerebellum in SSE, on the other hand, the frequency of the cerebellar disturbances appeared to be rather high.

Immediately before the completion of akinetic mutism, one or two psychic disturbances, such as delirium, stupor, hallucination and psychomotor excitement, were almost always found.   In the cases in which obvious dementia was not described, the disturban-ces described above were rather pronounced.   Akinetic mutism particularly at the termi-nal stage was found in many cases, while it was not described in some cases which showed marked disturbance of consciousness, such as coma at the terminal stage.

Para- or tetraplegia in flexion was found in about a half of the cases.   The reasons why this frequency appeared to be rather low may be as follows; one was that there was the cases in which this sign was not described; the other was that the cases without this sign showed usually a rapid downhill course.

## 2) Neuropathological features

The first report of the two autopsy cases of SSE in the Japanese was documented by Shiraki and Matsuoka in 1963 (*Nos. 17 & 18*).   These cases showed typical neuropatholo-gical changes of SSE, although one of them disclosed widespread distribution of senile alterations, such as senile plaques, Alzheimer's neurofibrillary tangles and granulovacuo-lar degenerations.   A dissociation of the pronounced spongy state to the slight loss of neurons was clearly emphasized by the authors, and thus, they could be compatible with the cases described by H. Jakob (1958) rather than the cases by Nevin, et al. (1960).   In the Shiraki and Matsuoka's cases astroytosis was never outstanding.

The paper entitled "Heidenhain's syndrome", on the other hand, was published by Tsujiyama, et al. (1965, *No. 19*).   This case was a 24-year-old man particularly with the protracted clinical course of 43-months' duration.   The autopsy case of Heidenhain's syndrome was reported by Suetsugu, et al. (1973, *No. 33*).   A predominant involvement of the visual cortex was stressed in these cases.   It, however, is certain that the visual cortex was consistently involved in SSE, but spongy degeneration was usually more widespread in the different cerebral cortex.

The frontal and temporal cortex were usually affected but its degree was less severe.   The pre- and postcentral cortex appeared to be far less severely affected or even spared in many cases.   Izaki's case showed predominant change of the cerebral cortex of the left hemisphere (1972, *No. 31*).   There was no obvious evidence to explain such laterality.

In the Heidenhain's paper a predominant loss of the small neurons of the visual cortex was described.   However, there were no Japanese cases in which this finding could clearly be demonstrated.   Although Shiraki and Matsuoka described the finding that there occurred relatively well preservation of the neurons of the cortex, in spite of the conspi-cuous spongy state, this finding was not always pointed out in all other cases of SSE.   In many cases severe neuronal loss was found in the cerebral cortex.   Inflated neurons were also found in many cases of SSE, but they were exclusively restricted to the cerebral cortex.

In the cerebral cortex spongy degeneration occurred mainly in the infragranular layers, but frequently occurred in the supragranular layers as well.   Furthermore, it occurred, irrespective of the gyral crowns and depths of the sulci, and never showed a laminar disruption in true sense of words.   In many cases spongy degeneration of the cortex was never found in the subcortical white matter.   However, astrocytosis usually predominated in the corticomedullary junction.

The spongy degeneration could be differentiated into the two subtypes; one was coarse, grape-likely coalescent microcavities and/or more larger cavitations; the other was very fine, sieve-like spongy state; in the former astrocytosis was less pronounced (Shiraki & Matsuoka, 1963, Nos. 17 & 18), whereas in the latter astrocytes became conspicuously hypertrophied and proliferated; these different morphological aspects of spongy state were frequently found in the different sites of the same cerebrum, and thus, they appeared to reflect the different stages based upon the same process. Astrocytes extended their foot processes but did never form thin-calibered gliofibers.

Masters, et al. stated that gliosis occurred in the cortex of the case with the protracted clinical course (1981), whereas our observations and experiences showed that even in the protracted cases, fibrillary gliosis consisting of a feltwork of thin-calibered gliofibers was never found. Spongy state in the thalamus, however, was occasionally accompained by fibrillary gliosis.

Fat granule cell mobilization was, as a rule, rare in SSE, but in Narita's case (1976, No.43), numerous fat granule cells were disseminated in the cerebral cortex and this finding was also described in case 8 of Nevin's series (1960). Ikuta demonstrated an existence of cholesterol ester in the microcavities of the cerebral cortex of SSE (1974). We, however, failed to demonstrate this substance and also neutral fat in the frozen section of the cerebral cortex (unpublished data).

In Taniguchi's case (1972, No. 30) and Ogasawara's cases (1973, Nos. 36 & 37) spongy degeneration was found in the subcortical white matter. However, its nature and distribution were obscure. In Inoue's case there occurred circumscribed foci of astrocytic proliferation (1981, No. 56). The circumscribed spongy necrotic foci in the panencephalopathic type of CJD, on the other hand, had a marked proliferation of astrocytes.

Oikawa's case showed an important consideration of the development of the white matter change (1969, No. 25). In this case swelling of oligodendrogliae and ameboid change of astrocytes were found in the cerebral white matter, and the cousin of this case showed a typical change of the panencephalopathic type the latter of which will be discussed in the chapter of the familial CJD later (Chapter IV).

The striatum, claustrum and thalamus showed spongy state and astrocytosis almost identical to the cortical change, but its degree was usually less severe. On the other hand, there were no cases in which similar changes were found in the other subcortical nuclei.

The typical primary thalamic degeneration appeared not to be usual in the cases of SSE. There, however, existed several possible cases (Shinfuku, et al., 1965, No. 20; Mizushima, 1978, No. 48; Inoue, et al., 1981, No. 56). The other cases disclosed astrocytosis, spongy state and/or some loss of nerve cells in the medial nucleus of the thalamus.

Pyramidal tract degeneration was found in three cases (Iwase, et al., 1967, No. 22; Hoshino, et al., 1974, No. 40; Ishii, et al., 1977, No. 44). Among them the pyramidal tract degeneration in Hoshino's case has a possibility of secondary degeneration. In the other cases, however, it could be of a primary nature.

The spongy state was also found in the Purkinje cell and molecular layers with or without neuronal loss, but its degree was far less severe than that of the cerebral cortex. Ishida's case revealed activated microglial cells laden with fat droplets in the cerebellar molecular layer (1971, No. 28), which were consistently found in the panencephalopathic type of CJD. In Mukai's case (1978, No. 46) spongy state occurred in the dentate nucleus and substantia nigra as well as the cerebellar cortex, while in Mizushima's case (1978, *No. 48*) it also was disseminated widely in the superior colliculus, central gray of the midbrain and pontine reticular formation.

In Hirai's case idiopathic intracerebral hemorrhage occurred during the course of SSE (1974, *No, 39*). In the discussion of Nevin's paper (1960), a similar case was described.

Senile changes including senile plaques, senile plaque-like bodies, Alzheimer's neurofibrillary tangles and granulovacuolar degeneration were occasionally found in the sponginously degenerated cortex (Shiraki & Matsuoka, 1963, *No. 18*; Matsuoka, et al., 1970, *No. 27*; Ishida, et al., 1971, *No. 28*; Suetsugu, et al., 1973, *No. 34*; Harada, et al., 1979, *No.49*; Nonaka, et al., 1981, *Nos. 53 & 54*; Shirabe, et al., 1982, *Nos. 58 & 59*). Almost all cases showed features compatible with the typical clinical pictures of SSE. Matsuoka's case, however, disclosed a relatively longstanding prodromal period characterized by cerebellar ataxia, which was followed by a rapid deterioration of mental state resulting in akinetic mutism, although the total duration of the illness including the prodromal period was about 21 months. The neuropathology of this case was questionably compatible with SSE, but this case also should be considered in its relation to the chronic spongiform encephalopathy with plaques characterized by antecedent and longstanding cerebellar ataxia which will be discussed in detail later on. Matsuoka's case was categorized into the Gerstmann-Sträussler syndrome by Masters, et al. (1981).

## Discussion

Not only in the Krücke, et al.'s case but also in the other autopsy cases of subacute spongiform encephalopathy mentioned above, the most common neuropathologic features were spongy tissue disruption and astrocytosis of the gray matters, which, as is well known, could be transmitted from human beings to animals and from animals to animals. However, it should be born in mind that transmission experiments have as yet not been fully successcul in reproducing typical and widespread inflated neurons, kuru plaques or senile plaques, although Tateishi, et al. were recently successful in reproducing kuru plaques in small animals (1984).

Single or multiple systemic degenerations which were most beautifully demonstrated in Krücke, et al.'s case (case 6, Table 1) as well as in the other cases of SSE, on the other hand, comprized one of the most essential features of the neuropathology of SSE. As far as we know, this, however, has never been successful in its reproducing in the transmission animal experiments up to date.

It is also noteworthy that the cerebral white matter of the familial CJD reported by Oikawa, et al. (1969, *No. 25*) demonstrated astrocytic metamorphosis, which may certain implications in the development of medullary pallor. This case was also discussed in the Shiraki's paper of CJD in some detail (1974). Actually, the related case (cousin of this patient), which will be discussed by Akai later, demonstrated the characteristic neuropathologic features of the panencephalopathic type of CJD coexisting with severe and widespread medullary degeneration of a primary nature (Chapter IV).

# REFERENCES

Hamaguchi, K., Kato, Y., Nakamura, S. and Matsuyama, H.:  An autopsy case of subacute spongiform encephalopathy, Clin. Neurol. (Japan), 12: 274-281, 1972.

Hirai, T., Masuko, T., Morimatsu, M., Yoshikawa, M. and Nagashima, K.:  An autopsy case of subacute spongiform encephalopathy complicated by idiopathic intracerebral hemorrhage, Clin. Neurol. (Japan), 14: 814, 1974.

Hoshino, K., Kobayashi, H., Kosaka, K., Shibayama, H. and Iwase, M.:  An autopsy case of subacute spongiform encephalopathy developed after head trauma, Adv. Neurol. Sci. (Japan), 18: 222, 1974.

Ikuta, F., Kumanishi, T., Ohashi, T. and Koga, M.:  Studies on Creutzfeldt-Jakob disease - Is this disease a metabolic disorder?, Adv. Neurol. Sci. (Japan), 18: 46-61, 1974.

Inoue, Y. Anraku, S., Okawa, T. Ueda, S., Sato, D. and Kida, H.:  A case of subacute spongiform encephalopathy, Neuropathol. (Japan), 2: 52, 1981.

Ishida, Y., Hashiba, S., Okamoto, K., Hoshi, S. and Takahashi, T.:  An autopsy case of subacute spongiform cerebral atrophy with senile and vascular lesions, Adv. Neurol. Sci. (Japan), 15: 582-591, 1971.

Ishii, T., Kimura, S., Sakai, K., Seyama, S. and Mitsuyama, Y.:  An autopsy case of spongiform encephalopathy with 9-year duration, Adv. Neurol. Sci. (Japan), 21: 571, 1977.

Izaki, K., Fukuda, T., Nakamura, I., Ito, K. and Otsuka, R.:  A case of spongiform encephalopathy with fronto-temporal predominance, Adv. Neurol. Sci. (Japan), 16: 544, 1972.

Iwase, M., Ito, S., Kobayashi, H. and Kosaka, K.:  An autopsy case of subacute spongiform encephalopathy, Adv. Neurol. Sci. (Japan), 11: 845, 1967.

Jacob, H., Eicke, W. and Orthner, H.:  Zur Klinik und Neuropathologie der subakuten praesenilen spongiösen Atrophien mit dyskinetischem Endstadium, Dtsch. Z. Nervenheilk., 178: 330-357, 1958.

Kida, H., Koizumi, H., Anraku, S., Okawa, T., Inoue, Y., Ueda, S. and Kotorii, I.:  An autopsy case of subacute spongiform encephalopathy (Heidenhain type), Adv. Neurol. Sci. (Japan), 24: 375, 1980.

Krücke, W., Beck, E. and Vitzum, H. G.:  Creutzfeldt-Jakob disease; Some unusual features reminiscent of kuru, J. Neurol., 206: 1-24, 1973.

Masters, C. L. and Richardson, E. P. Jr.:  Subacute spongiform encephalopathy (Creutzfeldt-Jakob disease).  The nature and progression of spongiform change, Brain, 101: 333-344, 1978.

Masters, C. L., Gajdusek, D. C. and Gibbs, C. J. Jr.:  Creutzfeldt-Jakob disease virus isolation from the Gerstmann-Sträussler syndrome: With an analysis of the various forms of amyloid plaque deposition in the virus-induced spongiform encephalopathies, Brain, 104: 559-588, 1981.

Matsuoka, T., Hamanaka, T., Taii, S., Tatebayashi, Y., Kijima, S. and Nishikawa, T.:  Subacute spongiform encephalopathy as a subype of Creutzfeldt-Jakob disease-Report of two cases, Psychiat. Neurol. Jpn., 72: 669-680 1970.

Mizushima, S.:  A case of spongiform encephalopathy, Adv. Neurol. Sci. (Japan), 22: 561, 1978.

Mukai, E., Mukoyama, M. and Tamura, J.:  A case of subacute spongiform encephalopathy with special reference to neuropathological comparison with the reported cases in Japan, Adv. Neurol. Sci. (Japan), 22: 561, 1978.

Narita, H., Miyake, H., Masuda, K. and Hara, T.:  An autopsy case of subacute spongiform encephalopathy, Adv. Neurol. Sci. (Japan), 20: 519, 1976.

Nevin, S., McMenemy, W. H., Behrman, S. and Jones, D. P.:  Subacute spongiform encephalo-

76

pathy - A subacute form of encephalopathy attributable to vascular dysfunction (Spongiform cerebral atrophy), Brain, 83: 519-564, 1960.

**Nonaka, H., Kudo, K., Aoyama, A., Fukunaga, N., Ito, K., Wada, F. and Kinoshita, M.:** Two autopsyc cases of Creutzfeldt-Jakob disease with plaques, Neuropathol. (Japan), 2: 54, 1981.

**Ogasawara, S., Ito, T. and Tanaka, K.:** Two cases of Cruetzfeldt-Jakob disease group, Adv. Neurol. Sci. (Japan), 17: 402, 1973.

**Oikawa, K., Fukazawa, K., Hasegawa, K., Sasaki, M. and Shinfuku, N.:** An autopsy case of subacute spongiform cerebral atrophy, Adv. Neurol. Sci. (Japan), 13: 392, 1969.

**Shinfuku, N., Ishino, H., Kadowaki, T. and Gomyoda, M.:** An autopsy case of subacute spongiform encephalopathy, Psychiat. Neurol. Jpn., 67: 816-829, 1965.

**Shirabe, T., Nasu, Y., Yasuda, Y., Morimoto, K. and Terao, A.:** Two autopsy cases of Creutzfeldt-Jakob disease, Neuropathol. (Japan), 3: 126, 1982.

**Shiraki, H. and Matsuoka, T.:** Two autopsy cases of the subacute spongiform encephalopathy. A contribution to the understanding of presenile or senile psychosis, Psychiat. Neurol. Jpn., 65: 989-1013, 1963.

**Suetsugu, M. and Mitsuyama, Y.:** An autopsy case of subacute spongiform encephalopathy (Heidenhain's syndrom) - On the correlation with Creutzfeldt-Jakob's disease, Clin. Neurol. (Japan), 13: 499-505, 1973.

**Suetsugu, M., Sato, Y. and Tateishi, J.:** A case of subacute spongiform encephalopathy with kuru plaques, Adv. Neurol. Sci. (Japan), 24: 376, 1980.

**Taniguchi, K.:** A case belonging to Creutzfeldt-Jakob disease, Clin. Neurol. (Japan), 12: 237, 1972.

**Tateishi, J., Sato, Y., Nagara, H. and Boellaald, J. W.:** Experimental transmission of human subacute spongiform encephalopathy to small rodents. IV. Positive transmission from a typical case of Gerstmann-Straüssler-Scheinker's disease, Acta neuropathol., 64: 85-88, 1984.

**Tsujiyama, Y., Otsuka, T., Sato, T., Matsuno, M. and Ariizumi, M.:** A case of Heidenhain's syndrome, Adv. Neurol. Sci. (Japan), 9: 137-140, 1965.

# Stern-Gracin Type (Thalamic Type) of Creutzfeldt-Jakob Disease

Hirotsugu Shiraki, M. D. and Toshio Mizutani, M. D.

The history of the researches of this type of CJD has already been fully documented in the Chapter I. Although the autopsy cases of this type of CJD were extremely rare, throughout all countries of the world, the five autopsy cases of the disease in the Japanese have been reported by us and others (Oda, et al., 1973; Shiraki, 1974; Iwata, et al., 1979), and they could be divided into the two subtypes; two cases of thalamic degeneration of presumable secondary nature combined with other systemic degeneration; three cases of thalamic degeneration of presumable primary nature combined with other systemic degeneration.

## 1. Thalamic Degeneration of Presumable Secondary Nature Combined with Other Systemic Degeneration

The cases consist of the two (cases 1 and 2) and the summary of their clinical features is listed in Table 1.

One of the most outstanding neuropathology in this subtype of the disease was the thalamic degeneration in which different thalamic subnuclei were symmetrically and bilaterally affected; nerve cells in these nuclei were, as a rule, slightly to moderately disintegrated, whereas astrocytosis and gliosis, as a rule, were more severe and distributed more widely than disintegration of the nerve cells (Figs. 1a, 1b, 4a, 4b, 4c & 4d). The disintegration of nerve cells of the thalamic subnuclei was mostly pronounced in the formatio medialis and followed by nucleus dorsalis posterior, anterior, and pulvinar of the thalamus. This finding indicated that the affected thalamic subnuclei were of an ontogenetically recent origin.

The distribution of the foci in the thalamic subnuclei mentioned above is illustrated schematically in Figs. 8, 9, and 10. In the latter, it was remarked that the gliosis was more widespread in different thalamic subnuclei, including those of ontogenetically old origin, than that of the neuronal disintegration (Fig. 10).

Another characteristic of this group, on the other hand, was that disintegration of the cortical neurons were predominant in the prefrontal, frontal and parietooccipital cortex (Figs. 3a, 3c, 3d, 4a, 5a, 5b, 6a & 6b). Although a diffuse pallor of the cerebral white matter was widespread in the almost entire areas of both hemispheres, this was particularly predominant in the cortical areas, corresponding to the cortical devastation mentioned above. The subcortical gliosis simulating that of progressive subcortical gliosis (Neuman & Cohn, 1967) was also pronounced in these areas (Figs. 3b & 4d). Considering the fact that the topography of cortical disintegration and thalamic degeneration and a dissociation of the severe and widespread astrocytosis and gliosis to slight and/or moderate disintegration of nerve cells of thalamic subnuclei in the two cases here as well as a well established normal neuroanatomy of the presence of corticothalamic projection fibers were visualized, the degeneration of the thalamic subnuclei of this subtype may be mainly of a secondary nature.

In case 1, disintegration of the Betz' giant cells occurred in certain convolution of the precentral cortex, whereas the internal capsule and corticospinal tract of the brainstem were distal-dominantly affected (Figs. 1a, 1c, 1d, 2a & 2b), although the spinal cord was not dissected. Moreover, these changes were symmetric and occurred bilaterally. Interesting enough was a coexistence of Lafora body and/or Lafora body-like structures and they were sporadically but restricted mainly to the precentral cortex (Figs. 2c, 2d & 8).

In case 2, on the other hand, the compact zone of the substantia nigra was moderately to severely involved bilaterally, and astrocytosis and gliosis were pronounced there (Figs. 4d & 7c). In this case, typical inflated nerve cells were sporadically disseminated in the claustrum and cerebral cortex (Figs. 7a & 7b).

The corticomedullary and some systemic degenerations in the two cases are also illustrated schematically in Figures 8 and 9.

---

**Fig. 1.** Thalamic degeneration of presumable secondary nature combined with other systemic degeneration (Table 1). a, b, c and d: case 1.
**(a)** Frontal-cut cerebral hemisphere through the subthalamus; conspicuous atrophy of the cortex, white matter and corpus callosum, and resultant dilatation of the lateral ventricles; diffusely pallored white matter, particularly predominant in its deep portion; moderately to slightly disintegrated myelinoarchitecture of the formatio medialis and nucleus dorsalis posterior of the thalamus; pallored cerebral peduncle and ventral part of the internal capsule (the arrows). × 1.0. **(b)** Magnified formatio medialis of the thalamus; moderately to severely disintegrated nerve cells, and conspicuously and diffusely proliferated glial nuclei in the parenchyma. × 89. **(c)** Infragranular layers of the precentral cortex; darkly shrunken but still preserved Betz' giant cells. × 89. **(d)** Same area as in (c) but at different convolution; completely disintegrated Betz' giant cell replaced by a coarse spongy state and widespread proliferation of glial nuclei in all layers. × 89. [(a), (b), (c), & (d): K-B]

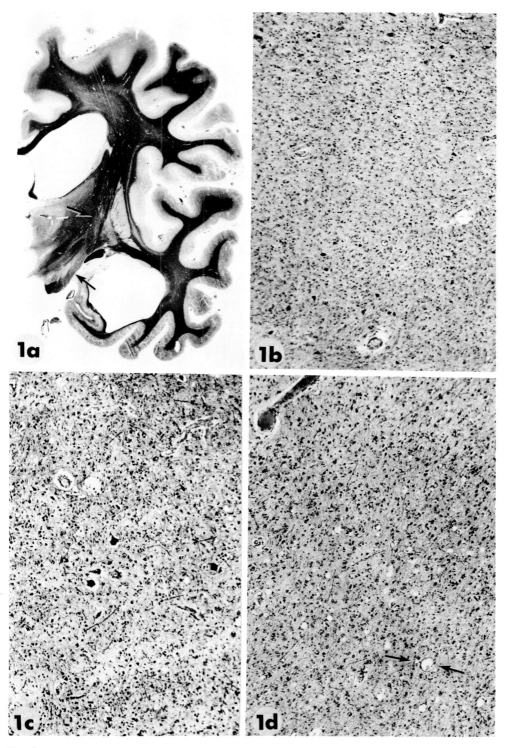

Fig. 1

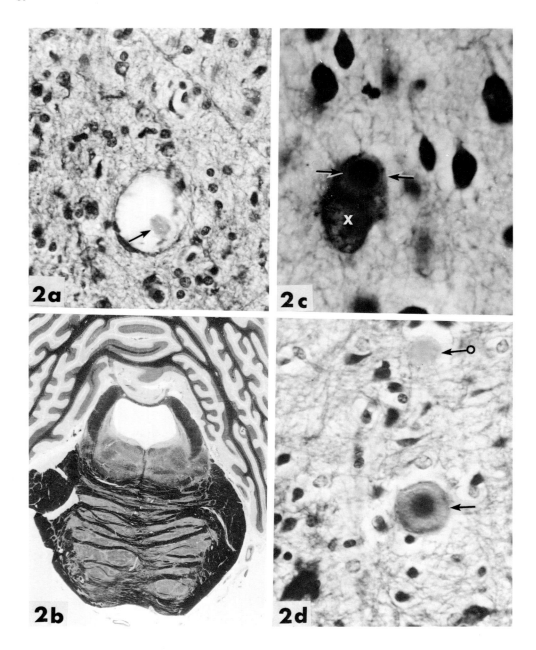

**Fig. 2.** Thalamic degeneration of presumable secondary nature combined with other systemic degeneration (Table 1).  a, b, c and d: case 1.

**(a)** Magnified area indicated by the arrows in Fig. 1d; the arrow indicates the residue of the cell body of the disintegrated Betz' giant cell.  × 525.  **(b)** Cranial portion of the pons; slightly to moderately pallored corticospinal tracts symmetrically and bilaterally.  **(c)** Magnified fronto-parietal cortex; the arrows indicate a Lafora body closely adjacent to the enlarged astrocytic nucleus (cross).  × 1150.  **(d)** Almost same area as in (c); the arrow indicates a Lafora body; the arrow with zero indicates the cytoplasm of the inflated nerve cell.  × 600.    [(a), (b), (c) & (d): K–B]

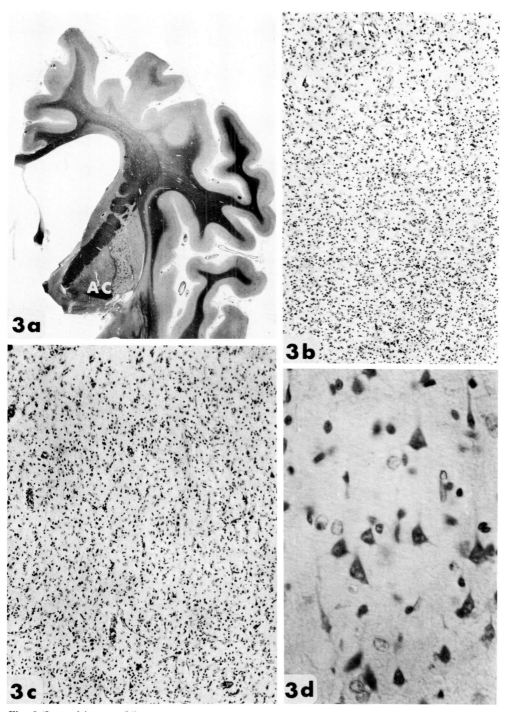

**Fig. 3** (Legend in page 84)

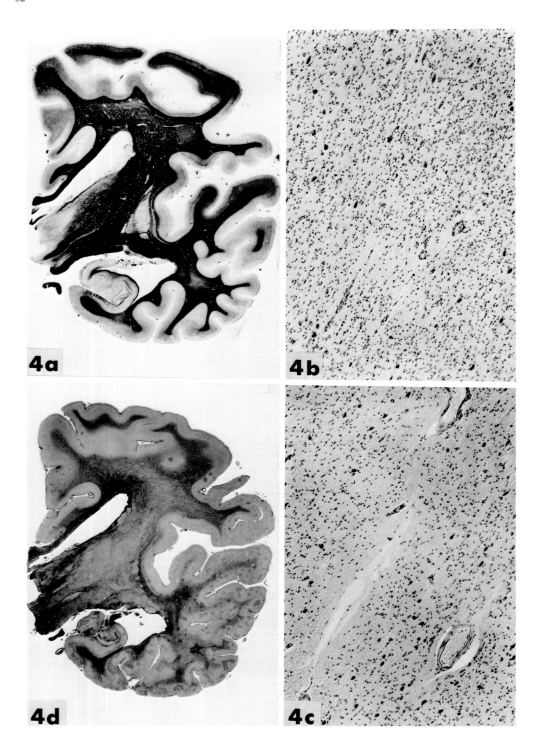

**Fig. 4** (Legend in page 84)

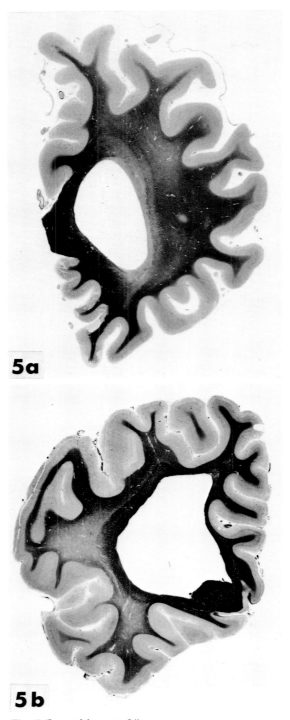

**5a**

**5b**

**Fig. 5** (Legend in page 84)

**Fig. 3.** Thalamic degeneration of presumable secondary nature combined with other systemic degeneration (Table 1). a, b, c and d: case 1.

**(a)** Frontal-cut cerebral hemisphere through the anterior commissure (AC); similar to Fig. 1a; conspicuous cortical atrophy and pallored subcortical white matter, particularly predominant in the superior (SF), medial (MF) and inferior frontal gyrus (IF), and precentral gyrus (Pr). × 1.2. **(b)** Magnified border area of the subcortical white matter to the deepest layer of the medial frontal cortex; conspicuously and diffusely proliferated glial nuclei in the subcortical white matter continuous into the cortical layer. × 89. **(c)** Magnified supragranular layers of the medial frontal cortex in (a); moderately to severely disintegrated nerve cells; conspicuous and diffuse proliferation of both the activated astrocytic and rod cell nuclei. × 89. **(d)** Magnified third layer in (c); similar to (c), while still-preserved nerve cells but darkly shrunken. × 525. [(a), (b), (c) & (d): K-B]

**Fig. 4.** Thalamic degeneration of presumable secondary nature combined with other systemic degeneration (Table 1). a, b, c and d: case 2.

**(a)** Frontal-cut cerebral hemisphere through the uncus; conspicuous atrophy of the cortex, white matter and corpus callosum, and resultant dilatation of the lateral ventricles; diffusely pallored white matter, particularly predominant in its deep portion; moderately to severely disintegrated myelinoarchitecture of the formatio medialis and most dorsal part of the nucleus dorsalis anterior of the thalamus. × 1.4. **(b)** Magnified formatio medialis of the thalamus in (a); moderately disintegrated nerve cells; conspicuosly and diffusely proliferated glial nuclei in the parenchyma. × 89. **(c)** Magnified nucleus dorsalis anterior of the thalamus in (a); similar to (b), while less pronounced proliferation of glial nuclei in the parenchyma. × 89. **(d)** Frontal-cut cerebral hemisphere through the subthalamus; moderate to intense gliosis widespread in the white matter, particularly predominant in the subcortical white matter and corpus callosum; moderate to intense gliosis also in the formatio medialis and nucleus dorsalis anterior of the thalamus, and substantia nigra. × 1.4. [(a), (b) & (c): K-B; (d): Holzer]

**Fig. 5.** Thalamic degeneration of presumable secondary nature combined with other systemic degeneration (Table 1). a and b: case 2.

**(a)** Frontal-cut hemisphere through the most rostral part of the corpus callosum; conspicuous atrophy of the cortex and white matter, and resultant dilatation of the cerebral sulci and anterior horn of the lateral ventricle; diffuse pallor of the white matter, particularly predominant in its deep portion. × 1.4. **(b)** Occipital gyri; diffuse pallor of the white matter, particularly predominant in its lateroventral portion; conspicuously dilated posterior horn of the lateral ventricle. × 1.4. [(a) & (b): K-B]

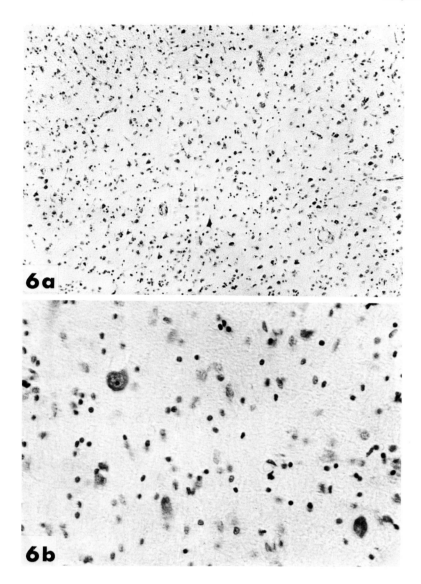

**Fig. 6.** Thalamic degeneration of presumable secondary nature combined with other systemic degeneration (Table 1).   a and b: case 2.
**(a)** Magnified third layer of the frontal cortex; slightly disintegrated nerve cells, and slightly activated astrocytic and rod cell nuclei.   × 120.   **(b)** More magnified area in (a); similar to (a).   × 490.   [(a) & (b): Thionine]

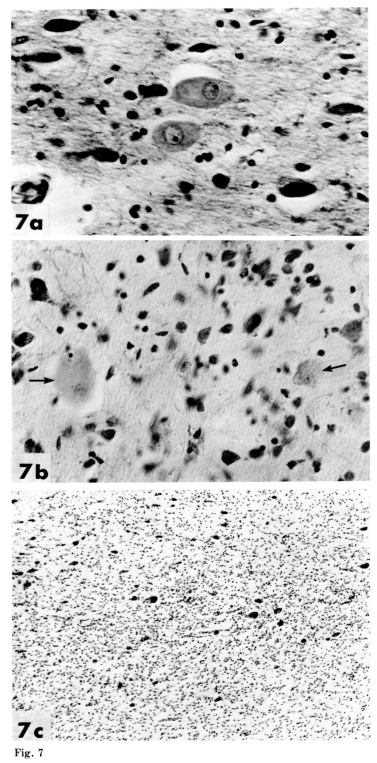

**Fig. 7**

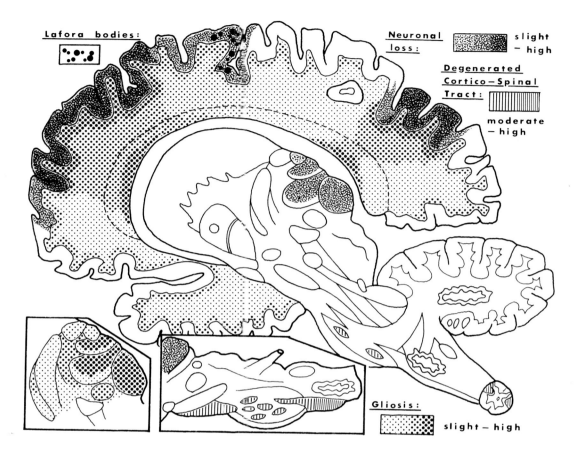

Lafora bodies:

Neuronal loss:    slight – high

Degenerated Cortico–Spinal Tract:    moderate – high

Gliosis:    slight – high

**Fig. 8.** Schematic diagrams of the distribution of the foci in thalamic degeneration of presumable secondary nature combined with other systemic degeneration (same case as case 1 in Table 1 and Figs. 1-3)

**Fig. 7.** Thalamic degeneration of presumable secondary nature combined with other systemic degeneration (Table 1). a, b and c: case 2.
**(a)** Magnified claustrum; two nerve cells with the achromatically inflated cytoplasm and vesicularly enlarged nucleus; darkly shrunken other nerve cells. × 950. **(b)** Magnified cortex at the temporal tip; the arrow indicate two inflated nerve cells. × 590. **(c)** Lateral one third of the compact zone of the substantia nigra; severely disintegrated pigmented cells, and conspicuously and diffusely proliferated glial nuclei in the parenchyma. × 89.    [(a) & (b): K–B; (c): Thionine]

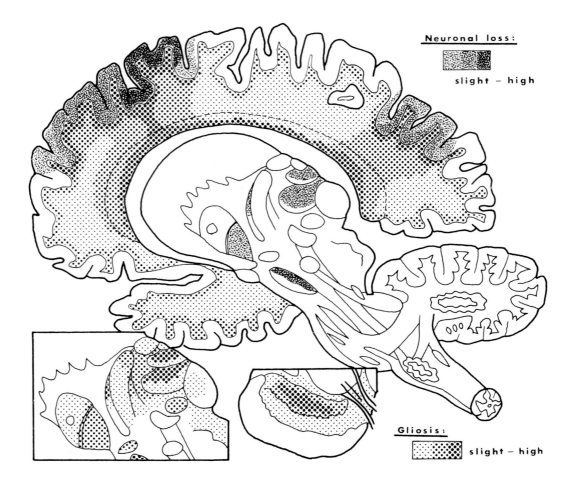

**Fig. 9.** Schematic diagrams of the distribution of the foci in thalamic degeneration of presumable secondary nature combined with other systemic degeneration (same case as case 2 in Table 1 and Figs. 4-7)

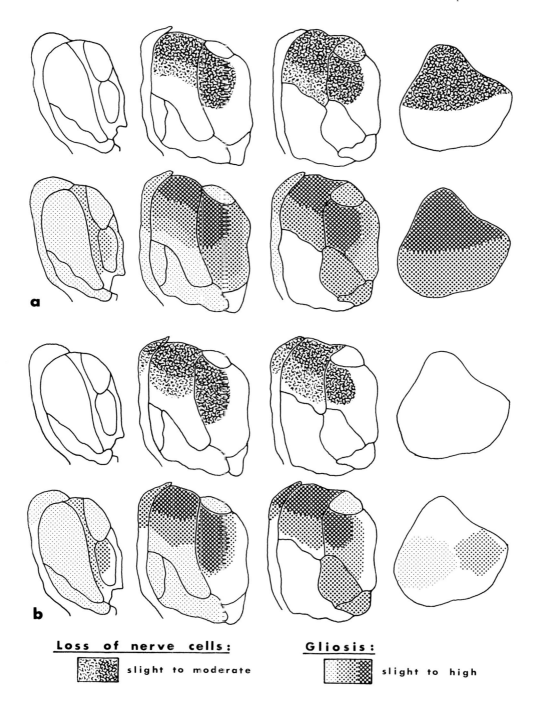

Loss of nerve cells:
slight to moderate

Gliosis:
slight to high

Fig. 10. Schematic diagrams of the distribution of the frontal-cut thalamic foci in thalamic degeneration of presumable secondary nature combined with other systemic degeneration.
(a) Same case as case 1 in Table 1 and Fig. 8.   (b) Same case as case 2 in Table 1 and Fig. 9.

**Table. 1.** Thalamic Degeneration of Presumable Secondary Nature Combined with Other Systemic Degeneration

| Case Number, Age (years) and Sex (total duration of illness) Previous and Family History* | Major Clinical Features and Course (——→indicates shift or progression) |
|---|---|
| 1<br>41, M<br>(3 years)<br>Unremarkable | Amnestic, inertia, disorientation, disturbed daily life——→Difficulty in walking, mutistic, disorientation——→*Mutism, indifferent*, perseveration, forced laughing and grasping, hypobulic, "leeres Lachen", incontinence, *spastic gait, elevated knee jerks (right more pronounced than left), bilateral foot clonus 1⁺ (right more pronounced than left), atrophy of limbs,* dysphagia, *mask-like face,* dilated ventricles with PEG——→Suspected Pick's disease ——→Emaciation, pneumonia, then death. *Wassermann in blood: 0; EEG: Abnormal; Brain weight: 1040 grams* |
| 2<br>62, M<br>(4 years)<br>Unremarkable | Slow motion, apathetic, indifferent, amnestic, inertia——→Restlessness, wandering, occasional bizzare behaviors, loss of self control, verbigeration, repetition of same words, perseveration, amnestic syndrome, finger agnosia, right-left agnosia ——→Transient dirty and irritable behaviors ——→*Mutism, reaction loss to surroundings,* dysphagia, *parkinsonian syndrome such as tremor, muscular rigidity, seborrehoeic face*——→*Akinetic mutism, primitive reflexes, contractured posture,* beddriden——→General wasting, pneumonia, then death |

*: Negative family history in all cases

## 2. Thalamic Degeneration of Presumable Primary Nature Combined with Other Systemic Degeneration

The cases consist of the three (cases 1, 2 and 3) and the summary of their clinical features is listed in Table 2.

One of the most outstanding neuropathology in this subtype of the disease was also the thalamic degeneration in which different thalamic subnuclei were symmetrically and bilaterally affected; nerve cells in these nuclei were, as a rule, moderately to severely disintegrated and there occurred a pallor of the myelinoarchitecture, whereas gliosis, as a rule, was less severe than disintegration of the nerve cells or equal to the latter (Figs. 11a, 11b, 11c & 11d). This disintegration of nerve cells of the thalamic subnuclei was mostly pronounced in the formatio medialis and followed by nucleus dorsalis posterior, anterior, and pulvinar of the thalamus. This finding indicated that the affected thalamic subnuclei mentioned above were also of an ontogenetically recent origin.

The distribution of the foci in the thalamic subnuclei mentioned above is illustrated schematically in Figures 19a, 19b, 19c, 20, 21 and 22.

In the two cases (Figs. 19a, 19b, 20 & 21), the formatio anterior of the thalamus were more or less affected (Fig. 12c), whereas in the one case (Figs. 19c & 22), it was free of lesions. As seen in Table 1, Korsakoff's syndrome, on the other hand, became more or less pronounced, particularly from the initial to the intermediate stage in the former two cases, whereas Korsakoff's syndrome was never observed throughout the entire clinical course of the latter case. Therefore, it could reasonably be assumed that the developmental mechanism of Korsakoff's syndrome was more or less closely associated with the involvement of formatio anterior of the thalamus.

In the two cases in which the total duration of the illness ranged from 14 months to 19 months (cases 1 and 2), a large number of fat granule cells and fatty metamorphosis of the myelin sheaths were mobilized in the deteriorated thalamic subnuclei (Figs. 12a & 12b), whereas in the other cases in which the total duration of the illness ranged 7 years they were not.

Another characteristic of this subtype, on the other hand, was that there were no disintegration of the cortical neurons or pallor of the cerebral white matter, except for circumscribed deteriorated foci restricted to the superior frontal cortex in case 3. This characteristic of this subtype, thus, demonstrated a clear contrast to the former subtype of the disease mentioned above. Insofar as, it could reasonably be concluded that the thalamic degeneration of the present subtype was clearly of a primary nature.

The degeneration of the olivopontocerebellar system was encountered in all three cases, and was symmetric and occurred bilaterally, although the pontine nuclei and related system were spared in the two cases (cases 1 and 2).

The inferior olivary nucleus was consistently involved; nerve cells were moderately to severely disintegrated and astrocytosis and activation of the microglial nuclei were pronounced (Figs. 13b & 13d); in some cases, a clear-cut neuronophagia occurred (Fig. 13c), whereas fat granule cells and fatty metamorphosis of the myelin sheaths were mobilized particularly in the adjacent white matter of this nucleus (Fig. 13e); thus, it was no doubt that severe gliosis was particularly predominant in and outside of this nucleus (Figs. 13a & 18b). In these cases, a moderate to intense gliosis also occurred bilaterally at the fourth ventricular base including the vestibular nucleus as well as in the restiform body (Fig. 13a).

In two cases (cases 2 and 3), degeneration of the olivospinal tract occurred symmetrically and bilaterally, and the fat granule cells were mobilized there in case 2 (Figs. 14a, 14b, 19b & 19c).

In all cases, particularly case 3, atrophy of the cerebellar white matter was conspicuous and widespread in both the paleocerebellum and neocerebellum, and thus, demyelination and gliosis were most outstanding there (Figs. 15a & 15b). Fat granule cells were abundant in the cerebellar white matter in the two cases with a compatively short duration of the illness (Fig. 15c). Disintegration of the cerebellar cortex were more or less found in all cases, but the severity was less marked and torpedoes were occasionally disseminated in the granular layer.

Moreover, in case 3, the severe disintegration of neurons of the pontine nuclei occurred bilaterally (Fig. 16b), whereas the transverse fibers and brachium pontis were also severely involved (Fig. 16a).

Although the above-mentioned degeneration of the spinoolivopontocerebellar system varied from case to case in the severity of the foci and the topography of the involved nuclei and tracts, the degeneration of this system demonstrated clearly a systemic nature, and this is illustrated schematically in Figures 19a, 19b and 19c.

The pallidonigral system was also involved in a systemic way in all cases examined,

**Table. 2.** Thalamic Degeneration of Presumable Primary Nature Combined with Other Systemic Degeneration

| Case Number, Age (years) and Sex (total duration of illness) Previous and Family History | Major Clinical Features and Course (——→indicates shift or progression) |
|---|---|
| 1<br>18, F<br>(14 months)<br>The paternal grandmother exhibited excitement, nocturnal wandering, abnormal behaviors and personality change at 63 years of age; the father had epileptic convulsions at 20 years of age: Inborn retarded mental development of the patient; worker in vinyl factory | *Amenorrhoea*——→Severe diarrhoea, emaciation, loss of appetite——→Tremor of limbs, stiff gait, disturbed memory, inertia, *nervousness,* anxiety, sleeplessness——→Disturbed vision, *progressive nervousness,* high fever, decubiti——→Pronounced disorientation, hypersalivation——→*Highly emaciated (body weight, 50kg——→31kg)*——→Stiff mimic, ptosis 1⁺, tremor of whole body, monotonous and slurred speech, stiff movements and posture, voluntary hyperkinesis, hyperactive deep tendon reflexes, positive bilateral Rossolimo's, Babinski's and Chaddock's signs, rigospasticity of legs, absolute stiffness of pupils, negative convergence, constipation, urinary disturbance, hyperhidrosis, hypersalivation; *disturbed memory particularly of recent origin 3⁺, disorientation 3⁺, verbigeration, confabulation, oversensitiveness,* distractability, poor concentration, restlessness, poor mimic, infantile, unstable, easy crying, *hypnagogic hallucination, episodes of dreamy experiences,* no cerebral focal signs except for the presence of *optic agnosia*——→Spastic paraplegia (right severer than left), *broad-based atactic gait,* unable to walk, *adiadochokinesis, disturbed finger to finger and finger to nose tests*——→High fever, somnolence, illusions, hallucinations——→*Primitive oversensitiveness*——→*Primitive reflexes*——→Positive pyramidal signs, *locomotive ataxia,* anisocoria (right larger than left), nystagmoid oscillating ocular movements, tremor, hyperkinesis——→ Emaciation 3⁺, decubiti 3⁺, hidrosis 3⁺——→High fever, coma, then death<br>*Brain weight: 1080 g* |
| 2<br>33, M<br>(19 months)<br>Worker in cellophanefactory for over 10 years; several episodes of acute keratitis, headache, fatigue feeling, gastrointestinal discomforts and frequent coughings | Minor tremor of whole body——→Emaciation, fatigue, anxiety, loss of appetite——→Disturbed concentration and memory——→Laziness, abulic, *mutistic*——→Slowness, progressed tremor, bizzare gait and behaviors ——→Double vision——→Suspicious delirious state, disturbed memory and writing, misbehaviors——→Apathetic, semistupor, *disturbed memory and orientation 3⁺,* seborrhoeic face, rigidity 1⁺, tremor 1⁺, sluggish pupillary reflex, miosis, hyperactive deep tendon reflexes, foot clonus, positive Babinski's sign on left and slightly on right, *adiadochokinesis (left more pronounced than right), disturbed coordination,* more or less slow waves of EEG——→*Parkinsonian syndrome,* automatic hyperkinesis, *cerebellar ataxia,* hyperreflexia, positive foot clonus and Babinski's sign 1⁺, urinary incontinence——→Chronic paralytic ileus, constipation, disturbed memory and orientation, *tendency to Korsakoff's syndrome,* nocturnal delirium, psychomotor excitement, somnolence, sopor, personality change——→ *Akinetic mutism or apallic state*——→Decubiti, fever, amnesia——→Laparatomy to ileus——→Transient collapse——→Irregular respiration, Chyne-Stokes——→Fever, then death<br>*EEG: Abnormal and paradoxical pattern during sleep* |

| 3<br>57, M<br>(7 years)<br>Unremarkable Worker in iron factory; transient neuroasthenic state at 20 years of age | *Personality change* such as circumstantiality and timid, discharged from professional life ——→Elevated appetite, rough, misbehaviors, amnestic ——→Shuffled legs, disturbed writing, tremor of fingers——→Disturbed memory, *dementia (WAIS; IQ 59)*, euphoria, indifferent, delusion, *parkinsonian syndrome*, hyperactive deep tendon reflexes, muscular weakness (right more pronounced than left), sluggish pupillary reflexes, disturbed left auditory acuity——→Suspicious right hemiparesis——→Total incontinence——→*Gerstmann's or Balint's syndrome*, perseveration, *finger agnosia, right-left disturbances, suspicious acalculia and agraphia*, fixed ocular movements ——→Trismus, fasciculations——→Decubiti, *Akinetic mutism*, beddridden, contracture of all limbs, occasional fits of coma——→Coma, convulsions, subsequent clouded consciousness——→High fever, then death<br>*Note: Negative or minimal cerebellar signs and symptoms and Korsakoff's syndrome through entire clinical course* |
|---|---|

although its severity varied from case to case; for example, nerve cells of the globus pallidus were moderately to severely involved and pallor of the myelinoarchitecture and gliosis occurred there (Figs. 11b, 16c & 16d); the compact zone of the substantia nigra was also slightly to severely disintegrated (Fig. 16e). In case 3, dorsal half of the external segment of the pallidum as well as the subthalamus were also involved, and slight to moderate neuronal loss and gliosis occurred bilaterally, although the severity of the latter was less pronounced (Figs. 11b & 19c).

In this subtype of the disease, not only the pallidonigral system but also the striopallidonigroluysian system was also degenerated in a systemic way. The degeneration of this system is illustrated schematically in Figures 9a, 9b and 9c as well.

Another systemic degeneration occurred in case 3, but this was rather exceptional; the tegmentum of the brainstem including the reticular formation and the rubroolivary tract became conspicuously atrophic and this change was symmetric and bilateral, whereas this degeneration was particularly predominant in the pons and medulla oblongata; nerve cells were moderately to severely disintegrated; astrocytosis with moderate to intense gliosis, activation of the microglial nuclei and less pronounced mobilization of the fat granule cells were identified (Figs. 17a, 17b, 18a & 18b).

In the present subtype of the thalamic degeneration, it is extraordinarily remarked that multisystemic degeneration was closely combined with the presumable primary thalamic degeneration.

This characteristic pattern of the multisystemic degeneration combined with the thalamic degeneration is again illustrated schematically in Figures 19a, 19b and 19c.

# 3. Discussion

As has been mentioned in detail, the thalamic degeneration, irrespective of its presumable secondary and primary natures, was closely combined with the other systemic degeneration; in the former, the corticospinal tract and/or nigral degeneration were closely combined with; in the latter, multisystemic degeneration, such as spinoolivopontocerebellar and striopallidonigroluysian atrophy as well as tegmental atrophy of the brainstem also occurred simulataneously. It, therefore, seems not to be curious that thalamic degeneration itself was actually of a systemic nature, whereas the corticomedullary degeneration in the former subtype of the disease was also interpreted in the same way.

In our previous paper (Shiraki, & Mizutani, 1983), on the other hand, the chapter has not included these subtypes of the Stern-Garcin syndrome of Creutzfeldt-Jakob disease, and the reasons were summarized as follows:

The severe psychiatric disturbances attributed to the thalamic involvement were manifested in these subtype, but were encountered in combination with the pyramidal, extrapyramidal and/or cerebellar signs and symptoms due to degeneration of the cortico-spinal, striopallidonigral or spinoolivopontocerebellar systems. However, from a clinical standpoint, the myoclonic jerks, clear-cut existence of paraplegia or tetraplegia in flexion and extension, and periodic synchronous discharges seen on electroencephalograms, which are the major clinical features of the different types of Creutzfeldt-Jakob disease mentioned above, were in most cases not seen or were questionable in the Stern-Garcin type. Also, there was no spongy tissue disruption, astrocytosis or kuru plaques in the cerebral cortex or white matter.

However, the neuropathologic characteristics of the thalamic and other forms of systemic degeneration in this type were very clearly or more or less identical to those in the other types of the disease, particularly beautifully demonstrated in the Krücke, et al.'s case of the subacute spongiform encephalopathy as well as in a great majority of the cases of the panencephalopathic type of CJD.

Therefore, it should be emphasized that the so-called thalamic type of Creutzfeldt-Jakob disease nevertheless has one of the most important roles in an understanding of the different types of CJD. This, however, will be discussed again in more detail later.

# REFERENCES

Iwata, T., Kaiya, T., Yoshimura, T., Moriuchi, I., Nanba, M., Kato, M., Ojima, A. and Tamai, Y.: Creutzfeldt-Jakob disease with severe change in thalamus, Adv. Neurol. Sci. (Japan), 23: 551, 1979.

Oda, M., Yoshimura, T. and Okumura, A.: Degeneration of the central nervous system enhanced in the thalamus, Adv. Neurol. Sci. (Japan), 17: 238-255, 1973.

Neuman, M. A. and Cohn, R.: Progressive subcortical gliosis, a rare form of presenile dementia, Brain, 90: 405-418, 1967.

Shiraki, H.: The neuropathological background for Creutzfeldt-Jakob disease (Creutzfeldt-Jakob syndrome), Adv. Neurol. Sci. (Japan), 18: 4-30, 1974.

Shiraki, H. and Mizutani, T.: Neuropathologic characteristics of types of Creutzfeldt-Jakob disease with special reference to the panencephalopathic type prevalent among Japanese, In: Neuropsychiatric disorders in the elderly, eds. Hirano, A. & Miyoshi, K., Igaku-Shoin, Tokyo, New York, pp. 139-188, 1983.

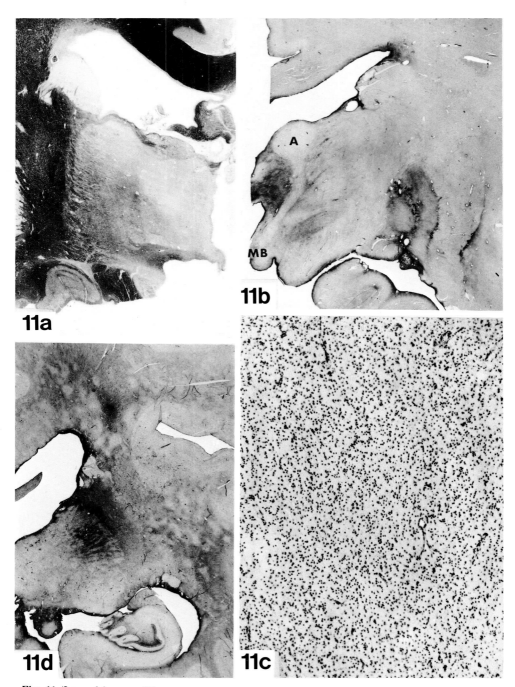

Fig. 11 (Legend in page 98)

96

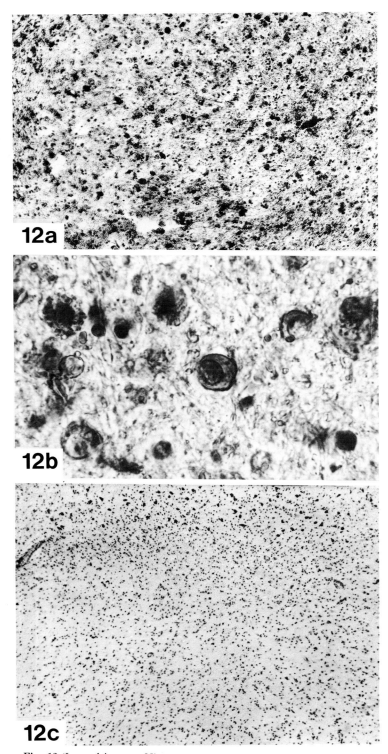

**Fig. 12** (Legend in page 98)

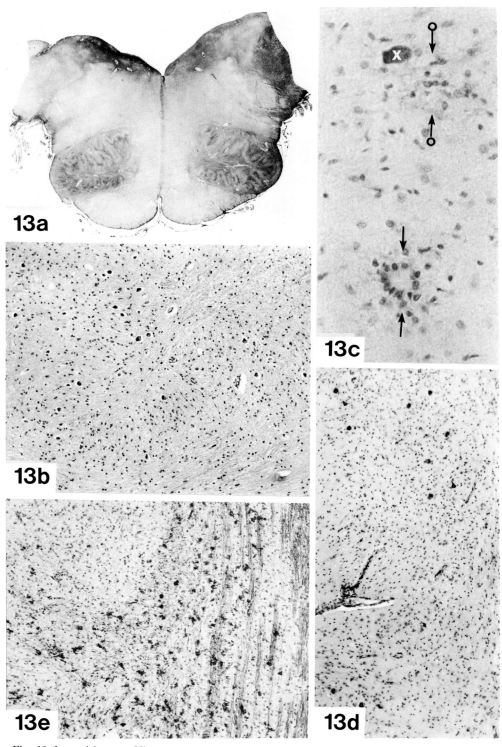

**Fig. 13** (Legend in page 98)

**Fig. 11.** Thalamic degeneration of presumable primary nature combined with other systemic degeneration (Table 2). a and b: case 3; c: case 2; d: case 1.
**(a)** Frontal-cut diencephalon through the lateral geniculate body; severely disintegrated myelinoarchitecture of the formatio medialis and nucleus dorsalis posterior of the thalamus, and slightly in other thalamic subnuclei. × 2.0. **(b)** Frontal-cut contralateral diencephalon through the subthalamus; severe gliosis particularly predominant in the formatio medialis of the thalamus, while less pronounced in the nucleus dorsalis anterior of the thalamus; no gliosis in the formatio anterior of the thalamus (A), mamillothalamic tract and mammillary body (MB); slight to moderate gliosis in the subthalamus and globus pallidus as well. × 2.0. **(c)** Magnified formatio medialis of the thalamus; severely disintegrated nerve cells, particularly predominant in its central part; conspicuously and diffusely proliferated glial nuclei in the parenchyma. × 89. **(d)** Frontal-cut diencephalon through the Ammon's horn; pronounced gliosis restricted to the lateral part of the pulvinar thalami and slight gliosis in other pulvinar areas; slight to moderate gliosis in the cerebral white matter, end plate of the Ammon's horn and elsewhere. × 2.0.
  [(a): Woelcke myelin; (b) & (d); Holzer; (c): Thionine]

---

**Fig. 12.** Thalamic degeneration of presumable primary nature combined with other systemic degeneration (Table 2). a, b and c: case 2.
**(a)** Magnified formatio medialis of the thalamus in (Fig. 11a); an exceedingly large number of the fat granules and phagocytic cells laden with the fat granules. × 89. **(b)** More magnified area in (a); the arrow indicates one example of phagocytes laden with the fat granules; the arrow with zero indicates one example of a swollen fatty metamorphosis of the nerve fibers. × 900. **(c)** Formatio anterior of the thalamus; severely disintegrated nerve cells, particularly predominant in its deep portion, and conspicuously and diffusely proliferated glial nuclei in the parenchyma. × 89. [(a) & (b): Sudan III; (c): Thionine]

---

**Fig. 13.** Thalamic degeneration of presumable primary nature combined with other systemic degeneration (Table 2). a and b: case 3; c: case 1; d and e: case 2.
**(a)** Middle portion of the medulla oblongata; moderate to intense gliosis symmetrically and bilaterally and particularly predominant in the marginal white matter of the inferior olivary nucleus; intense gliosis in the fourth ventricular base and vestibular nucleus, and particularly in the unilateral restiform body. × 3.6. **(b)** Magnified inferior olivary nucleus in (a); moderately to highly disintegrated nerve cells and diffusely proliferated glial nuclei in the parenchyma. × 90. **(c)** Highly magnified inferior olivary nucleus; the arrow indicates the degenerated nereve cell with a neuronophagia; the arrow with zero indicates the loosely proliferated activated astrocytic and rod cell nuclei adjacent to the degenerated nerve cell (cross). × 460. **(d)** Magnified lateral part of the inferior olivary nucleus; severely disintegrated nerve cells, and conspicuously and diffusely proliferated glial nuclei not only in the gray matter but also in the adjacent white matter. × 100. **(e)** Almost same areas as in (d); a large number of the phagocytic cells laden with the fat granules in the adjacent white matter, while a less number of the fat granule cells in the gray matter. × 97. [(a): Holzer; (b): H-E; (c) & (d): Thionine; (e): Sudan III]

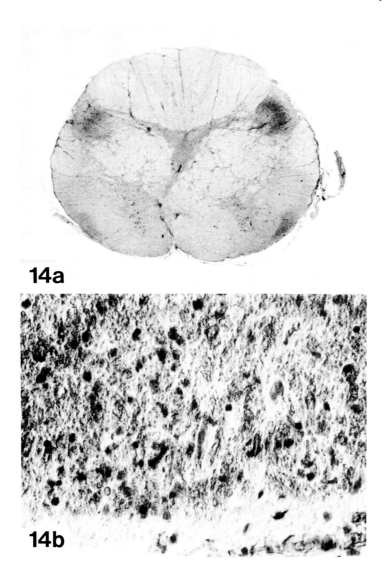

**Fig. 14.** Thalamic degeneration of presumable primary nature combined with other systemic degeneration (Table 2). a and b: case 4.

**(a)** Most caudal part of the medulla oblongata; a rich cellularity symmetrically and bilaterally in the olivospinal tract. × 7.0. **(b)** Magnified olivospinal tract in (a); a large number of the phagocytes laden with the fat granules. × 510. [(a): Thionine; (b): Sudan III]

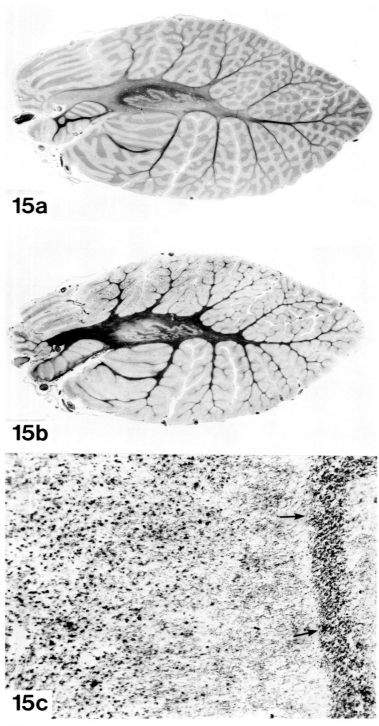

**15a**

**15b**

**15c**

Fig. 15 (Legend in page 105)

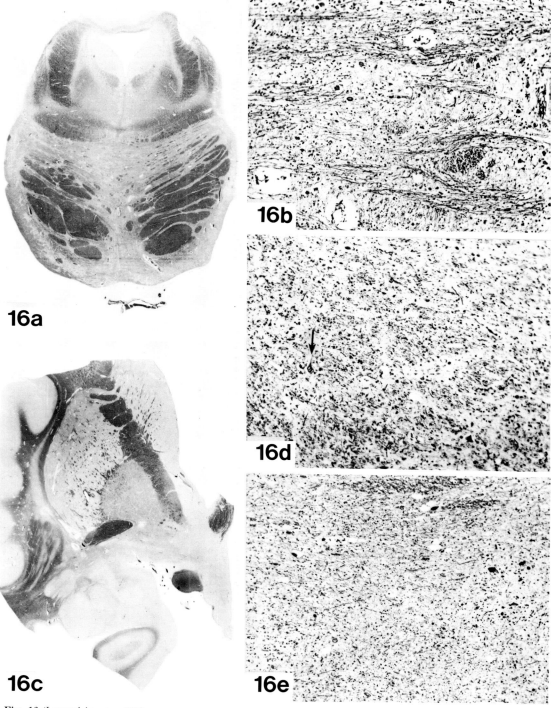

**16a**

**16b**

**16c**

**16d**

**16e**

**Fig. 16** (Legend in page 105)

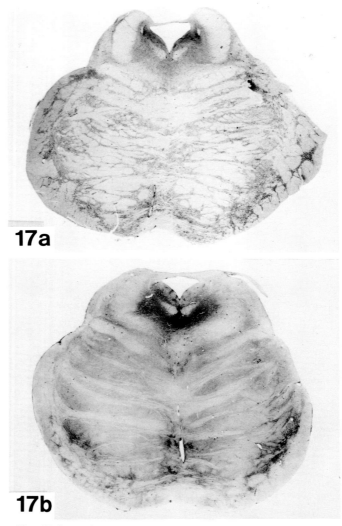

**17a**

**17b**

**Fig. 17** (Legend in page 105)

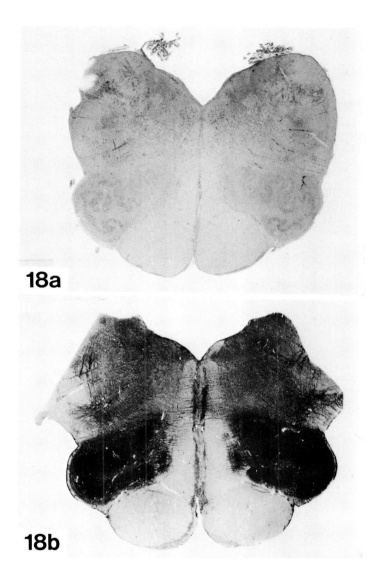

**18a**

**18b**

**Fig. 18** (Legend in page 105)

104

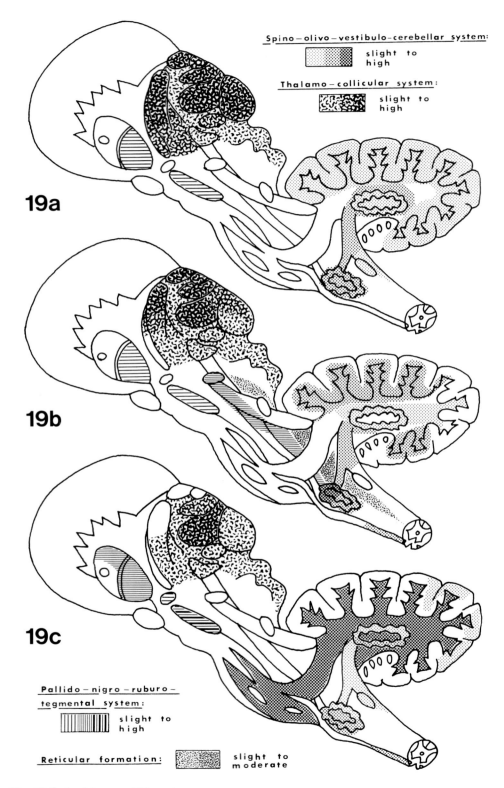

Spino—olivo—vestibulo—cerebellar system:

slight to high

Thalamo—collicular system:

slight to high

19a

19b

19c

Pallido—nigro—ruburo—
tegmental system:

slight to high

Reticular formation:

slight to moderate

**Fig. 19** (Ledend in page 105)

**Fig. 15.**   Thalamic degeneration of presumable primary nature combined with other systemic degeneration (Table 2).   a and b: case 3;   c: case 1
**(a)** Horizontal-cut cerebellar hemisphere; severe atrophy and demyelination in almost the entire white matters, except for the narrow zone around the dentate nucleus.   × 1.7.   **(b)** Same section as in (a); severe gliosis restricted to the white matter.   × 1.7.   **(c)** Cerebellar subcortical white matter; a large number of the phagocytes laden with the fat granules; the arrows indicate the granular layer.   × 70.
[(a): Woelcke myelin;   (b): Holzer;   (c): Sudan III]

---

**Fig. 16.**   Thalamic degeneration of presumable primary nature combined with other systemic degeneration (Table 2).   a, b, c, d and e: case 3.
**(a)** Cranial part of the pons; symmetrical and bilateral atrophy restricted to the basis in which all transverse fibers are severely demyelinated.   × 3.0.   **(b)** Magnified pontine nuclei in (a); severely disintegrated nerve cells.   × 97.   **(c)** Frontal-cut diencephalon through the anterior commissure (AC); moderate pallor of the globus pallidus.   × 2.2.   **(d)** Magnified internal segment of the globus pallidus in (c); disintegrated nerve cells; one remaining pyramidal cell indicated by the arrow; diffusely proliferated glial nuclei in the parenchyma.   × 115.   **(e)** Magnified middle one third of the compact zone of the substantia nigra; severely disintegrated pigmented cells and diffusely proliferated glial nuclei.   × 86.
[(a), (b), (c), (d) & (e): K–B]

---

**Fig. 17.**   Thalamic degeneration of presumable primary nature combined with other systemic degeneration (Table 2).   a and b: case 2.
**(a)** Cranial part of the pons; conspicuous atrophy and cell-richness symmetrically and bilaterally in the tegmentum, except for the brachium conjunctivum and fasciculus longitudinalis medialis.   × 3.2.   **(b)** Almost same section as in (a); conspicuous gliosis symmetrically and bilaterally in the tegmentum.   × 3.0.   [(a): Thionine;   (b): Holzer]

---

**Fig. 18.**   Thalamic degeneration of presumable primary nature combined with other systemic degeneration (Table 2).   a and b: case 2.
**(a)** Middle portion of the medulla oblongata; an exceedingly cell-richness symmetrically and bilaterally in the fourth ventricular base, tegmentum and inferior olivary nucleus.   × 5.0.   **(b)** Almost same section as in (a); intense gliosis particularly predominant in the bilateral inferior olivary nuclei and followed by the fourth ventricular base and tegmentum, except for the medial lemniscus.   × 5.0.   [(a): Thionine; (b): Holzer]

---

**Fig. 19.**   Schematic diagrams of the distribution of the systemic degeneration of the diencephalon, brainstem and cerebellum in three cases of thalamic degeneration of presumable primary nature combined with other systemic degeneration (Table 2).
**(a)** Case 2.   **(b)** Case 2.   **(c)** Case 3.

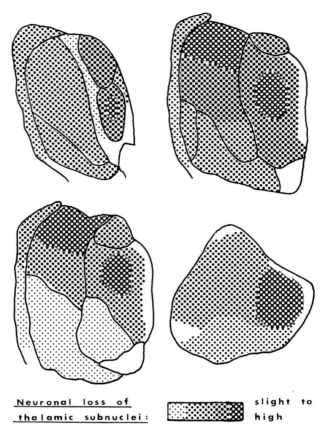

Neuronal loss of
thalamic subnuclei:      slight to
high

**Fig. 20.** Schematic diagrams of the distribution of the foci in the frontal-cut thalamic subnuclei in case 1 (Table 2).

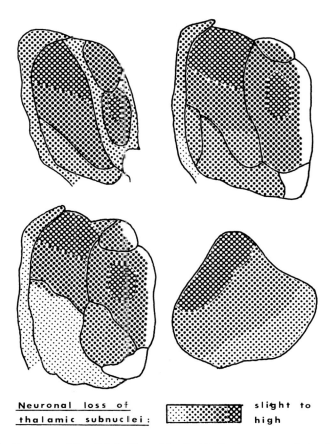

Fig. 21. Schematic diagrams of the distribution of the foci in the frontal-cut thalamic subnuclei in case 2 (Table 2).

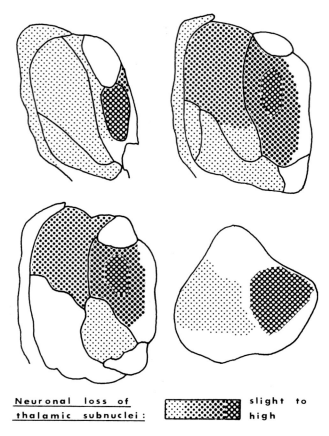

Neuronal loss of
thalamic subnuclei :  slight to high

**Fig. 22.** Schematic diagrams of the distribution of the foci in the frontal-cut thalamic subnuclei in case 3 (Table 2).

# Chapter III-5

# Ataxic Form of Creutzfeldt-Jakob Disease

Hirotsugu Shiraki, M. D. and Toshio Mizutani, M. D.

As has been mentioned before (Chapter I), the ataxic form of CJD was firstly proposed by Brownell and Oppenheimer (1965).

In 1979 one of the authors (Shiraki) has had an opportunity to examine the four published and one unpublished cases of this type of CJD examined by Brownell and Oppenheimer at the Radcliff Infirmary, Oxford. The authors are particularly grateful to Prof. Oppenheimer for permission to examine his materials of this type of CJD.

The six autopsy cases of this type actually consisted of the Brownell and Oppenheimer's five cases and one case of the Japanese, the summary of their clinical features of which is listed in Table 1.

As far as the cases of this type mentioned above were concerned, the most common neuropathologic features were related to cerebellar involvements and consisted of the following:

One characteristic was that the cerebellar cortex, irrespective of both the paleo- and neocerebellum, was moderately to severely involved in all cases (Fig. 1a). In the crown as well as between the walls and deep in the cerebellar foliae, conspicuous atrophy of the cortex was symmetric and occurred bilaterally. The granular layers, in which granule cells were severely disintegrated but in which Golgi type II cells were fairly well preserved, were most prominently involved. Granule cells just beneath the Purkinje cell layer, which appeared more or less spared and which developed, as a rule, a number of torpedoes (Fig. 1d), were spared in most cases (Fig. 1b). Moreover, the disintegrated granular layers manifested diffuse tissue loosening or even cystic cavitation, particularly in the deep layer, which was occasionally continuous into the subcortical white matter as well (Figs.1b and 1e). Fine, sieve-like tissue disruption, on the other hand, was restricted to the molecular layer (Fig. 1c).

Surprizing enough, a single typical kuru plaque was found in a single section from one

**Table. 1**

| Case Number, Age (years) and Sex (total duration of illness) Previous and Family History | Major Clinical Features and Course (———▸indicates shift or progression) |
|---|---|
| 1*<br>60, F<br>(8 months)<br>Unremarkable | *Difficulty in walking,* weak voice——▸Vague and forgetful but oriented, dysarthria 1+, *vertical nystagmus, gross intention tremor of arms, gross ataxia in standing, unsteady gait 3+*——▸*Dementia 2+, inability to stand or walking without support*——▸*Much worsened mental confusion and ataxia,* dysphagia——▸Helplessness, incomprehensibility, total incontinence——▸ *Athetoid movements of left arm, positive extensor plantar reflexes*——▸ Chest infection, then death |
| 2*<br>55, F<br>(7 months)<br>Head injury 1+,<br>8 months ago | Unsteady gait, numbness in left hand, staggering gait, nystagmus, limb and trunk ataxia, euphoria 1+, slight dysarthria, some tutibation of head——▸ *Rapid development of dementia,* dysphagia, dysarthria 3+, *continuous nystagmus, grossly ataxic gait, choreiform movements of face and limbs* ——▸*Mutism,* uncooperativeness, incontinence——▸*Myoclonic jerks with synchronous discharges of EEG*——▸Decreased rhythmic jerks, *stiffness of limbs at first in flexion, later extension*——▸Bronchopneumonia, then death |
| 3*<br>47, F<br>(2.5 months)<br>Unremarkable | Unsteadiness in walking, feeling shaky——▸Weakness of left arm, *unsteadiness of legs, slurring of speech*——▸Disoriented, dysphagia, dysarthria, *coarse tremor of arms,* abnormal mental state——▸Less responsive, not eating and drinking——▸*Given electroconvulsive therapy (E.C.T.)*——▸Kind of stupor, *mute,* incontinent, uncooperative, alternately restless and rigidity, opistotonic——▸*Daily E.C.T. for 8 days, rigid in all limbs, generalized coarse tremor on stimulation*——▸*Comatose, inconstant clonic movements of left arm and leg*——▸*Abnormal EEG,* twitching movements mainly on left ——▸Sudden death |
| 4*<br>60, M<br>(4 months)<br>Unremarkable | *Ataxic impairments*——▸Progression of ataxia——▸*Gross ataxia, mental confusion,* memory disturbance but still able to make conversation——▸ Progression of physical and mental deterioration——▸Became more aggravated ——▸Death |
| 5*<br>49, M<br>(8 months)<br>Unremarkable | Numbness and tingling in left hand, *gradually increased unsteadiness of legs,* occasional spasm of all limbs, *bilateral nystagmus, ataxia with increasing tone in all limbs, unsteadiness of gait, positive Romberg's sign,* general impairment of sensation to pinprick, dilataion of lateral ventricles with PEG 1+, *slow activity of EEG* ——▸Steadily deteriorated——▸ *Mute, akinetic,* doubly incontinent, *spastic limbs, bilateral extensor plantar responses*——▸Death |
| 6*<br>29, M<br>(22 weeks)<br>Unremarkable | Double vision, slurring of speech, tremor of limbs (right severer than left), impairment of handwriting, *ataxic gait*——▸*Mutism,* euphoria, perseveration, impairment of memory, calculation and comprehension, mask-like face, *slurring and explosiveness of speech, horizontal nystagmus, twitchings of left periorbicular region, hypermetria, intention tremor, dysdiadochokinesis (right worse than left), positive Romberg's sign,* hyperreflexia, ankle clonus 1+, *spasticity and ataxia of gait*——▸Total incontinence, semicoma, *myoclonic jerks of right arms,* positive Babinski's reflex, Rossolimo's reflex and foot clonus——▸ Hypersecretion, bronchopneumonia *Tetraplegia in extension*——▸General weakness, then death |

*: The cases from the Department of Neuropathology, Radcliffe Infirmary, Oxford.

case (case 1, Table 1).

In the case 3 (Table 1), the ischemically degenerated Purkinje cells with or without a neuronophasic process were predominant in the circumscribed foliae at the depth of the sulci (Fig. 2a).   In the same case Purkinje cells were completely disintegrated and left a coarse cavitic formation, whereas triangle-shaped necrotic focus occurred in the molecular layer (Fig. 2b).   Those pathological changes were quite different from the cerebellocortical degeneration in the other cases mentioned above.   This, however, could be attributed to the fact in which, in the present example (Table 1), the several electroshock treatments were performed and thus, those cerebellar changes were essentially of an ischemic origin.

In almost all cases the cerebellar dentate nucleus was involved; although the number of the nerve cells remained normal or was slightly decreased, the so-called grumorous structures were pronounced not only around the peridendritic areas of the nerve cells but also around their pericytoplasmic areas (Figs. 2c, 2d & 2e).

Another characteristic was that spongy tissue disruption of the cerebral cortex was generally no severe, showing a fine, sieve-like pattern and occurring only sporadically (Fig. 3a), whereas hypertrophic astrocytes with a coarse gliofiber formation were more prominent in the infragranular layers than in the supragranular layers (Figs. 4a & 4c).   This characteristic change of the cerebral cortex was seen in the striatum as well (Fig. 3b).   In some cases typical grape-like, clustered sponginess occurred in the supragranular layers of the occipital cortex (Fig. 3c), but this was rather exceptional.   In one case a laminarily distributed tissue loosening or even cystic cavitation of the cerebral cortex developed in the circumscribed gyrus, such as parahippocampus (Fig. 3d).

In this type of CJD, characteristically inflated neurons, a few of which showed evidence of inclusion body-like structures in their cytoplasm, were focally or diffusely disseminated throughout the cerebral cortex in every cases studied, and their distribution coincided well with that of the structures in both the subacute spongiform encephalopathy and the panencephalopathic type of CJD (Figs. 4b, 4c & 4d).   Single or coalescent vacuoles were frequently found in the inflated cytopalsm of the nerve cells, particularly predominant in the nerve cells of large type of the striatum (Fig. 4e).

In the case of one Japanese man (case 6, Table 1), the systemic degeneration was symmetric and occurred bilaterally in the corticospinal tract of the spinal cord, whereas degeneration of both the posterior and spinocerebellar tracts of the spinal cord showed a perfect distal-dominant pattern (Figs. 5a & 5b).

In one case of the Brownell and Oppenheimer's cases (case 4, Table 1), multiple, different-sized, more or less deeply argentophilic spheroid bodies were disseminated or clustered, particularly in the medioventral portion of the anterior horn of the lumbar cord, and they were clearly abnormal as compared with those of the age-matched control (Figs. 6a & 6b).   A higher magnification of them may indicate that some of those spheroid bodies developed at the axon terminal and/or preterminal areas (Figs. 6c & 6d).

112

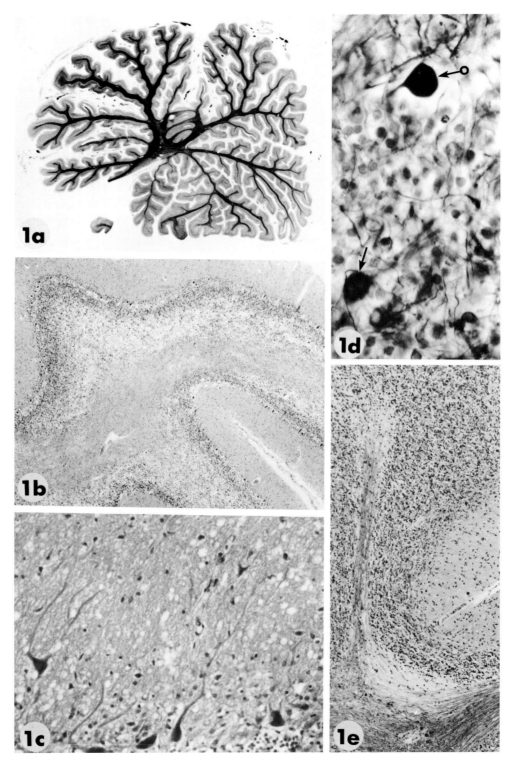

**Fig. 1** (Legend in page 116)

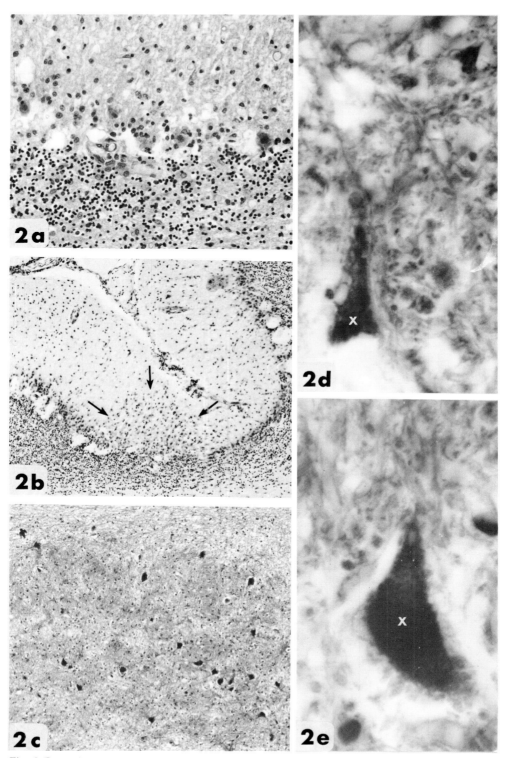

**Fig. 2** (Legend in page 116)

114

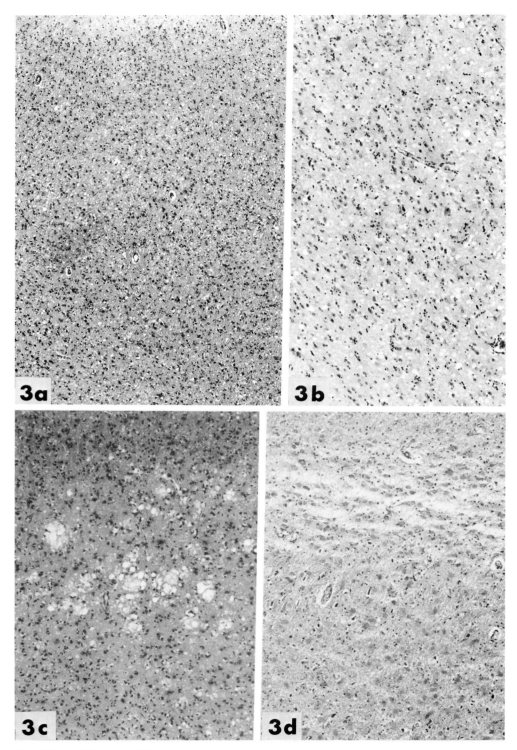

**Fig. 3** (Legend in page 116)

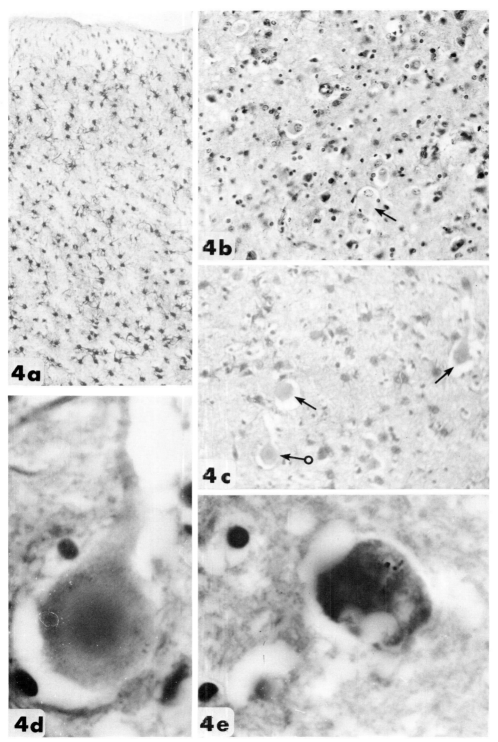

**Fig. 4** (Legend in page 116)

**Fig. 1.** Ataxic type of Creutzfeldt-Jakob disease (Table 1). a,c and e: case 1; b and d: case 2.
**(a)** Cerebellar hemisphere: conspicuous cortical atrophy widespread in both the paleocerebellar and neocerebellar foliae. **(b)** Magnified neocerebellum at the crown; coalescent and/or cystic tissue disruption or loosening, particularly pronounced in the deep portion of the granular layers but comparatively good preservation of Purkinje cells. **(c)** Magnified molecular layer of the neocerebellum; fine, sievelike tissue disruption. **(d)** Magnified granular layer of the cerebellum; the arrow with zero indicates a torpedo; the arrow indicates a Golgi type II cell. **(e)** Magnified neocerebellum; two sharply-defined cystic cavitations from the deepest portion of the granular layer to the subcortical white matter. [(a), (c) & (e): K-B; (b): H-E; (d): Palmgren silver]

---

**Fig. 2.** Ataxic type of Creutzfeldt-Jakob disease (Table 1). a and b: case 3; c: case 1; d and e: case 4.
**(a)** Magnified neocerebellum; vacuolarly disrupted Purkinje cells, ischemically degenerated remaining Purkinje cells and moderately disintegrated granule cells. **(b)** Magnified neocerebellum; vacuolarly and completely disrupted Purkinje cells, proliferated glial nuclei in both the Purkinje cell and granular layers; the arrows indicate triangle-shaped softening focus in the molecular layer. **(c)** Cerebellar dentate nucleus; slightly disintegrated nerve cells and pronounced grumorous structures in the peridendritic and pericytoplasmic areas. **(d)** Magnified dentate nucleus; conspicuous grumorous structures mainly in the peridendritic areas of the darkly shrunken nerve cell (cross). **(e)** Similar area to (d); similar to (d), but with pericytoplasmic grumorous structures as well; the cross indicates the darkly shrunken nerve cell. [(a) & (b): H-E; (c), (d) & (e): PTAH]

---

**Fig. 3.** Ataxic type of Creutzfeldt-Jakob disease (Table 1). a and b: case 6; c: case 3; d: case 5.
**(a)** Both supra- and infragranular layers of the frontal cortex; less pronounced, fine, sieve-like tissue disruption, astrocytosis and less pronounced disintegration of nerve cells. **(b)** Caudate nucleus; pronounced, fine, sieve-like tissue disruption, less pronounced astrocytosis and comparatively good preservation of nerve cells. × 80. **(c)** Supragranular layers of the occipital cortex at lateral convexity; grape-like clusters, coarse sponginess, particularly pronounced in the third layer. **(d)** Parahippocampal cortex; severely disintegrated nerve cells in all layers; laminarily distributed, cystic tissue disruption accompanied by conspicuous hypertrophic astrocytosis in the superficial layers; a large number of the hypertrophic astrocytes in the deep layers. [(a) & (b): H-E; (c) & (d): PTAH]

---

**Fig. 4.** Ataxic type of Creutzfeldt-Jakob disease (Table 1). a, c and d: case 2; b: case 6; e: case 1.
**(a)** Supragranular layers of the middle temporal cortex; astrocytosis with a less pronounced gliofiber formation in all layers. **(b)** Deep third layers of the cingulate cortex; clusters of typical inflated nerve cells, an example indicated by the arrow. × 200. **(c)** Third layer of the cingulate cortex; widespread hypertrophic astrocytosis; the arrows indicate three inflated nerve cells. **(d)** Magnified inflated nerve cell indicated by arrow with zero (c); ill-defined inclusion body-like structure in the inflated cytoplasm of the nerve cell. **(e)** Magnified nerve cell of large type of the putamen; multiple vacuoles in the inflated cytoplasm of the nerve cell; fine, sieve-like tissue disruption as well in the adjacent parenchyma. [(a): Cajal's gold sublimate; (b) & (e): H-E; (c) & (d): PTAH]

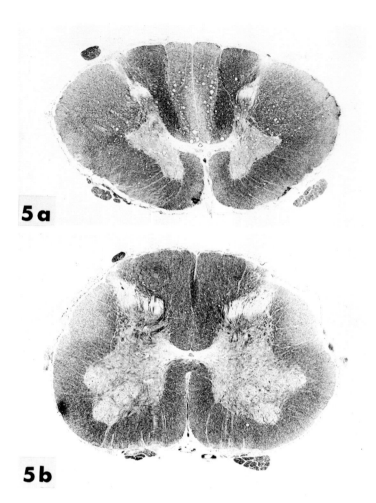

**Fig. 5.**   Ataxic type of Creutzfeldt-Jakob disease (Table 1).   a and b: case 6.
**(a)** Lower cervical cord; symmetric and bilateral demyelination, predominantly in the Goll's tract and to a lesser degree in the lateral and anterior corticospinal tracts as well as in both the dorsal and ventral spinocerebellar tracts.   **(b)** Upper lumbar cord; symmetric and bilateral demyelination, predominantly in the lateral corticospinal tract and minimal demyelination in the entire areas of the posterior tract.
  [(a) & (b): Woelcke myelin]

---

**Fig. 6.**   Ataxic type of Creutzfeldt-Jakob disease (Table 1).   a, b, c and d: case 4.
**(a)** Medioventral portion of the anterior horn of the lumber cord; multiple, clustered spheroid bodies.   **(b)** Magnified area in (a); multiple, deeply argentophilic, different-sized, and clustered spheroid bodies.   **(c)** Highly magnified ventral portion in (b); two different-sized, foamy spheroid bodies near to the nerve cell (cross); the arrows indicate the axonal structure connected to one of the spheroid bodies.   **(d)** Some area but at the different focus as in (c); triangle-shaped, foamy spheroid body closely attached to the nerve cell (cross) and connected with the very slender-calibered axonal structure to another spheroid body (arrows with double zeros).   [(a),(b), (c) & (d): Palmgren silver]

118

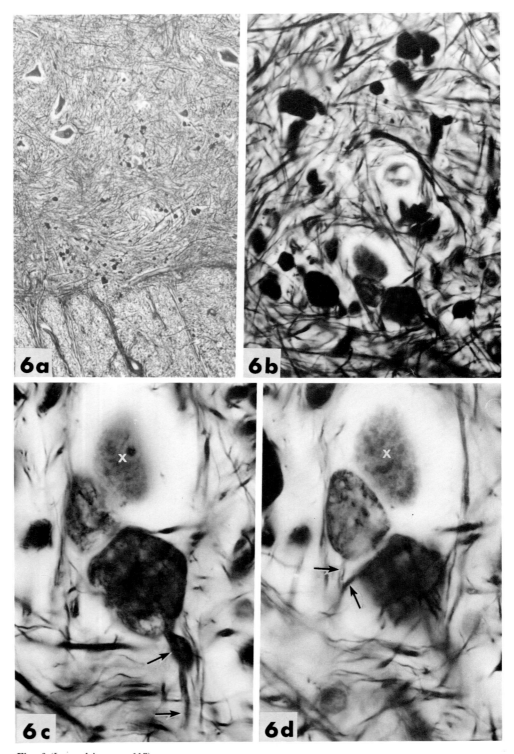

**Fig. 6** (Legend in page 117)

# Review of References of This Type of CJD in the Japanese

(Each number in italics in the text is corresponded to that in the Table 3 of the Appendix.)

## 1) Clinical features

There were 9 autopsy cases of the ataxic form of CJD in the Japanese. There were 8 males and 1 female. The age at death ranged from 29 to 72, and its average was 58. The total duration of the illness was from 3 to 14 months and its average was 7.5 months.

Only one case had the family history in which the two nephews expired of a similar degenerative disorder but the pathological confirmation was not performed (Araki, et al., 1980, *No. 70*), while the other cases had no remarkable history. There was no remarkable past history in all cases, except for one who had suffered from chronic rheumatoid arthritis (*No. 70*). Trauma as a possible triggering factor was recognized in the two cases; in one case the disease started after head trauma (Otsuka, et al., 1967, *No. 64*); in the other (Kuroiwa, 1975, *No. 66*), unsteady gait developed after falling off a chair.

The onset of the illness was rather abrupt and in many cases the disease started frequently with the neurological symptoms and signs. The initial neurological disturbances were unsteady gait, numbness of the limb, and visual disturbance including diplopia and decreased visual acuity. In two cases, on the other hand, mental symptoms and signs were predominate during the total clinical course (Nakazato, et al., 1977, *No. 67* ; Akai, et al., 1980, *No. 68*).

The clinical features of this type in the Japanese was characterized by scanty or even negative cerebellar and/or ataxic symptoms and signs during the total clinical course, although the pathological involvement of the cerebellar cortex was quite definite, as mentioned below. This characteristic was quite different from that of the Brownell and Oppenheimer's cases (1965). In the latter cerebellar and/or ataxic pictures were more or less pronounced from the intermediate even to the later stage. The two cases in the Japanese (Arai, et al., 1969, *No. 65;* Kuroiwa, 1975, *No. 66*), however, were relatively compatible with the clinical features described originally by Brownell and Oppenheimer. In the Arai's case diplopia appeared abruptly. Subsequently dysarthria, hand tremor and difficulty to write, and unsteady gait were noticed. The neurological examinations revealed definite cerebellar disturbances, positive Romberg's sign, and spastic and ataxic gait. Rigidity developed at the later stage and then, cerebellar disturbances became difficult to recognize. Disturbance of consciousness and myoclonus were also found, and the patient fell into a state of akinetic mutism. The Kuroiwa's case also showed a similar clinical course. The one case (Ogawa, et al., 1982, *No. 72*) showed gait disturbance, while cerebellar and/or ataxic symptoms and signs were not found.

The clinical course was steadily progressive, irrespective of the presence or the absence of cerebellar and/or ataxic disturbances. In all cases progressive deterioration of mental disturbance resulted in akinetic mutism or apallic state without exception. Rigidity of muscles, myoclonic jerks and periodic synchronous discharge (PSD) were

120

found in a great majority of the cases.

As described above, it was remarked that the frequencies of cerebellar and/or ataxic disturbances were rather low. The clinical involvement of the cerebellum, on the other hand, was recognized not only in the ataxic form but also in the other subtypes of CJD, although the frequency of cerebellar involvement was variable from one subtype to the other, and this was, as a rule, low in all subtypes of CJD (Mizutani, et al., 1984). As far as the cases of CJD in the Japanese were concerned, this finding, therefore, could support the view that cerebellar disturbances never comprized a differential diagnosis of the ataxic form from the other subtypes of CJD. In this regard, Tsuji and Kuroiwa reported that the cerebellar signs and symptoms were found in about a half of the clinical cases of CJD (1983). Thus, it is not surprizing that much difference existed in the data of the clinical cases from that of the autopsy cases.

As a consequence, typical cases of the ataxic form in the Japanese compatible with the Brownell and Oppenheimer's cases were only three among which only one case could be almost completely compatible with the Brownell and Oppenheimer's cases.


## 2) Neuropathological features

The cerebello-cortical degeneration of granule cell type, characteristic of the ataxic form of CJD, was also found in the panencephalopathic type of CJD. The former disclosed no pathological changes in the cerebral white matter, while the latter had a primary involvement of the white matter.

The first autopsy case with the cerebello-cortical degeneration of granule cell type in the Japanese was published by Otsuka, et al. (1967, No. 64), although the authors did not refer to this subtype of CJD. The clinical features were completely compatible with CJD, whereas no obvious signs and symptoms of the cerebellar involvement were detected. The brain weight ranged only 875 g and conspicuous atrophy of the cerebrum and cerebellum occurred. The cerebellar cortex disclosed marked loss of the granule cells and moderate loss of the Purkinje cells with a proliferation of Bergmann's glial nuclei. Marked thinning of the molecular layer also occurred. The cerebellar white matter showed slight loss of myelin. There occurred slight loss of the neurons of the dentate nucleus, while the pontine nuclei and the inferior olive revealed severe neuronal loss, astrocytosis and fat granule cell mobilization. The cerebellar peduncles showed no particular change. The spinal cord also disclosed no remarkable changes. In the cerebral cortex, on the other hand, coarse spongy state, astrocytosis and fat granule cell mobilization occurred, particularly pronounced in the occipital cortex, whereas severe neuronal depletion was predominate in the temporal cortex and less severe in the frontal cortex. The striatum and thalamus showed only slight degeneration of the neurons. No changes were found in the cerebral white matter.

The other cases, except for one (Arai, et al., 1969, No. 65), showed conspicuous degeneration in the cerebral cortex and striatum. Thus, the cerebral changes seemed to be almost equal to or more conspicuous than the cerebellar change in almost all cases of the ataxic form of CJD. The Brownell and Oppenheimer's cases, on the other hand, showed that the cerebellar involvement far exceeded the cerebral changes (1965). The

Arai's case, on the other hand, could be comparable with the Brownell and Oppenheimer's cases (Table 1, case 6).

The systemic degeneration in the brainstem and spinal cord was found in some cases one of which Otsuka's case was mentioned above.  In the Koya's case (1980, *No. 69*) the similar degeneration of the pontine nuclei and inferior olive was also described.   In this case there occurred marked gliosis in the pontine tegmentum as well.   The degeneration of the corticospinal tract was found in one case (Nakazato, et al., 1977, *No. 67*), whereas the degeneration of the posterior column was described in the Arai's case.   Inflated neurons in motor nuclei of the brainstem and the anterior horn of the spinal cord were found in two cases (Otsuka, et al., 1967, *No. 64;* Miyake, et al., 1980, *No. 71*), whereas inflated neurons in the cerebral cortex were found in many cases.   There was no case with typical thalamic degeneration, however.

## Discussion

As far as the Brownell and Oppenheimer's cases (cases 1-5, Table 1) and one Japanese case (case 6, Table 1) of this type of CJD described above were concerned, their clinicopathologic features coincided well in each; the cerebellar foci were far more severe than those in the cerebral cortex and striatum; thus, the involvement of the cerebellum was clinically the most outstanding feature, and sign of this involvement were evident until death, even when moderate to severe psychiatric disturbances developed at a subsequent stage.

In a great majority of the autopsy cases of this type in the Japanese, on the other hand, the cerebellar involvements were almost equal to those of the former group, but the involvements, particularly of the cerebral cortex, were far more predominant than those of the cerebellum and thus, it could reasonably be assumed that the cerebellar signs and symptoms became insidious or even masked.

The clinical characteristics of the ataxic form of CJD were similar to those of subacute spongiform encephalopathy and panencephalopathic type of CJD in the following; presence of apallic state or akinetic mutism particularly at the terminal stage, myoclonic jerks, PSD on EEG and tetraplegia in flexion etc., although their frequencies varied from case to case.

The neuropathological characteristics of this type, on the other hand, also disclosed a great similarities to those of the other subtypes of CJD including the simple poliodystrophic type.   The existence of the inflated neurons which comprized the most outstanding characteristics of the simple poliodystrophic type was again identified in all cases of the ataxic type examined.

# REFERENCES

**Akai, J. and Nezu, M.**: An autopsy case of Creutzfeldt-Jakob disease, Clin. Neurol. (Japan), 20: 308, 1980.

**Arai, et al.**: An autopsy case of extensive degeneration of the gray matter of the brain with subacute course, Adv. Neurol. Sci. (Japan), 13: 391, 1969.

**Araki, J., Kishikawa, M., Nomura, K. and Akashi, M.**: Creutzfeldt-Jakob disease developed during the clinical course of chronic rheumatoid arthritis, Adv. Neurol. Sci. (Japan), 24:.377. 1980.

**Brownell, B. and Oppenheimer, D. R.**: An ataxic form of presenile polioencephalopathy (Creutzfeldt-Jakob disease), J. Neurol. Neurosurg. Psychiat., 28: 350-361, 1965.

**Koya, G.**: An autopsy case of Creutzfeldt-Jakob disease, Clin. Neurol. (Japan), 20: 854, 1980.

**Kuroiwa, Y.**: An autopsy case of the ataxic form of subacute spongiform encephalopathy, The 1975 Annual Report of the Study Team of the Department of Welfare Concerning Creutzfeldt-Jakob Disease and Slow Virus Infections, 1975.

**Miyake, K., Kuroda, S., Hosaka, K., Taguchi, K. and Morioka, E.**: An autopsy case of Creutzfeldt-Jakob disease, The 8th Annual Meeting of Clinical Neuropathology, 1980.

**Mizutani, T., Morimatsu, Y. and Shiraki, H.**: Clinical pictures of Creutzfeldt-Jakob disease based on 97 autopsy cases in Japan——With special reference to clinicopathological correlation of cerebellar symptoms, Clin. Neurol. (Japan), 24: 23-32, 1984.

**Nakazato, Y., Ishida, Y., Okamoto, K., Hori, S. and Hirano, M.**: An autopsy case of subacute spongiform encephalopathy, Adv. Neurol. Sci. (Japan), 21: 571, 1977.

**Otsuka, R., Isaki, K. and Yagi, H.**: An autopsy case of subacute spongiform encephalopathy, Psychiat. Neurol. Jpn., 69: 637-648, 1967.

**Tsuji, S. and Kuroiwa, Y.**: Clinical pictures of Creutzfeldt-Jakob disease in Japan——Analysis of national survery, Clin. Neurol. (Japan), 23: 70-74, 1983.

# Panencephalopathic Type of Creutzfeldt-Jakob Disease

Toshio Mizutani, M. D.

The reason why the term of "panencephalopathic type" of CJD was proposed is in that this type shows the changes of both the gray and white matter, while the other subtypes were considered as "polioencephalopathy" which affects exclusively the gray matter, but not the white matter (Mizutani, 1977; Mizutani, et al., 1981a; Mizutani, 1981b; Shiraki & Mizutani, 1983). However, the view of primary involvement of the white matter raised arguments in relation to morphopathogenesis and nosological situation, since CJD has been defined as a degenerative disorder of the gray matter of the central nervous system. Secondary degeneration of the myelin of the cerebral hemispheres and brainstem based upon atrophy of the cerebral and cerebellar cortex has been reported (Meyer, et al., 1954; Foley & Denny-Brown, 1955). Thus, the panencephalopathic type is explained in such a way in which this may be a very atypical CJD, particularly of subacute spongiform encephalopathy (SSE), and this may be outside the spectrum of CJD.

Nevertheless, in our opinion, it is distinct enough to categorize this type into one of the subtypes of CJD, from careful consideration of several clinical and neuropathological aspects, together with the successful experimental transmission to the rat (see Chapter V). It also is not surprising that primary involvement of the white matter can occur in CJD, because Jacob predicted it in 1958. He described the white matter change in his case 1 in which foci were found in the centrum semiovlae, cerebellar peduncles, medial lemiscus, inferior longitudinal fasciculus, external arcuate fibers, pyramidal tracts and posterior column of the spinal cord, and he suggested the possibility that a more widespread involvement of the white matter may be found in the future. He also speculated that such change may be found in the longer-surviving cases. In our opinion, he might consider the white matter change as coexistence of both primary and secondary degeneration. To our knowledge, it may be suggested that the changes described by Jacob included system degeneration in the cerebellum, brainstem and spinal cord.

It seems that the panencephalopathic type occurred preferentially in the Japanese at least up to date.  Among 127 neuropathologically verified autopsy cases of CJD in Japan from 1961 to 1983, 48 cases were classified into this type (38%) (see Appendix, Mizutani, et al., 1984).  Recently, however, five cases of CJD accompanied by extensive degeneration of the white matter were reported from the United States (Park, et al., 1980; Monreal, et al., 1981; Schoene, et al., 1981), France (Buge, et al., 1978; Vallat, et al., 1983) and Italy (Macchi, et al., 1984).  Particularly the two cases in France were the members of the same family.  Although a question as to whether this type is prevailing in Japanese or not is still open at this moment, it is certain that CJD in Japan can be characterized by a high incidence of this type.

# 1. Clinical Features

There were 24 males and 24 females.  The age at death ranged from 41 to 73 years and the average was 56.0 years.  The total duration of illness ranged from 4.5 to 108 months and the average was 18.6 months.  There were no cases having family history except three which will be discussed in Chapter IV.

The clinical symptomatology was most typical among the subtypes of CJD, although some variety was present from case to case.  Thus, organic mental symptoms resulting in akinetic mutism or apallic state from the intermediate to the terminal stage, rigidity of muscles, myoclonic jerks, gait disturbance and para- or tetraplegia in flexion were cosistently found.  Periodic synchronous discharge (PSD) on EEG was recorded in almost all cases (75%).  In addition it was remarked that in spite of distinct evidence of cerebello-cortical degeneration of granule cell type (see Chapter III-5), cerebellar and/or ataxic symptoms and signs were exceedingly scanty or obscure (22%) and, even if present, they never comprized the main feature not only at the early stage but also at the later stage (Mizutani, et al., 1984).  These observations are quite different from that in the ataxic form in which cerebellar and/or ataxic symptoms were the most predominant feature throughout all stages (Brownell & Oppenheimer, 1965).  This will be discussed clinicopathologically later on (also see Chapter III-5).

The total duration of illness was variable from case to case, but its clinical course was characteristic (Fig. 1).  The early stage showed rapidly progressive neuropsychic deterioration leading to akinetic mutism, while after the completion of akinetic mutism, the clinical condition of the patient remained rather stationary and not always downhill.  The duration of the illness from the onset to the completion of akinetic mutsim was approximately 2 to 3 months in a great majority of the cases, while the duration from the completion of akinetic mutism to death was considerably variable from case to case.  This may probably reflect the patient's general condition including various complications of infections, malnutritional state mainly due to neurological disabilities, and medical care.  It, therefore, is emphasized that the rapidly progressive downhill course at the early stage followed by the non-progressive and stationary condition shows the most characteristic clinical feature of this type, since the other subtypes of CJD disclosed, as a rule, a progressive downhill course.

Recently serial computerized tomograms (CT) revealed some interesting aspects of dynamic changes of cerebral atrophy in relation to clinical features (Rao, et al., 1977; Kashiwamura, et al., 1981; Kawai, et al., 1981; Kishida, et al., 1981; Nagura, et al., 1983). Many authors stated that after full development of mental deterioration, cerebral atrophy from CT still went on for several months. It was also pointed out that there existed a discrepancy between slight cerebral atrophy on CT and marked mental deterioration. A reason for this discrepancy could be attributed to the fact that a rapid shrinkage of the brain occurred at the more or less later stage and myoclonus became infrequent and PSD was less marked. Another reason is that functional disturbance precedes morphological change on CT. In the case of this type as shown in Fig. 2 (*No. 119*) serial CTs demonstrated that a rapid progress of brain atrophy occurred from the third to the fifth month of the illness, while akinetic mutism was already completed from the second to the third month (Fig. 1c). It should be remarked that the degree of brain atrophy during three months at the early stage was more pronounced than that during seventeen months at the later stage. It seems more likely that during short duration of the acute stage a rapid shrinkage of the brain occurs. A similar finding on CT was reported by Ueno, et al. (1983). In their case cerebral atrophy was noticed three months later after the onset.

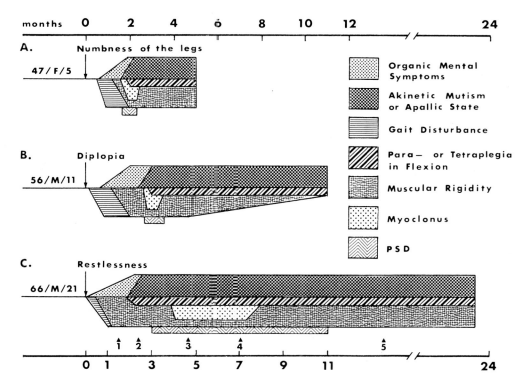

**Fig. 1.** Characteristic clinical course of the panencephalopathic type. Age at death/Sex/Total duration of illnes. Arrow indicates the onset of the disease and the initial symptom. Each triangle in C indicates the time when CT survey was performed (see Fig. 2). (A: *No. 82*; B: *No. 76*; C: *No. 119*)

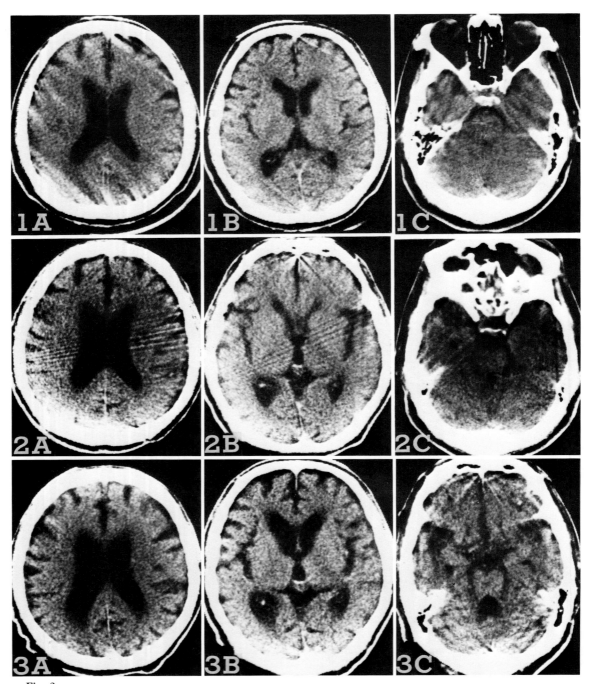

Fig. 2

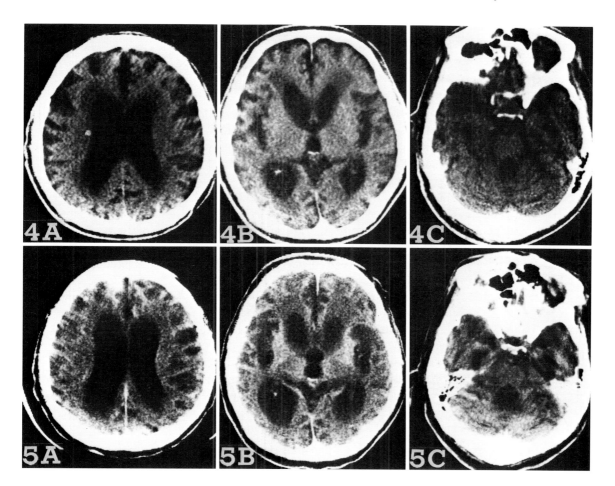

**Fig. 2.** Serial CT findings in the panencephalopathic type (*No. 119*).   Each triangle in Fig. 1C indicates the time when CT survey was performed: 1. 1.5 months after the onset; 2. 2.5 months; 3. 4.5 months; 4. 7. 5 months; 5. 15 months. See text !

## 2. Neuropathological Features

### 1) Macroscopic findings

Both cerebrum and cerebellum showed moderate to severe atrophy. Brain weight ranged from 1320 to 623 g and the average was 912 g, which was the lowest among all subtypes of CJD. It is noted that the degree of the brain weight of this type was proportional to the length of the total duration of illness, but not true in the other subtypes of CJD (see Appendix). The cerebral cortex, except for the hippocampus and amygdala, became extremely thin (Figs. 3, 9A, 9B, 11A & 14A), and showed laminar or pseudolaminar tissue disruption. Although the cerebral atrophy was more or less diffuse, its consistent distribution pattern was found in all cases. The atrophy was more marked in the frontal and parieto-temporal lobes, and in the lateral convexity than in the medial surface. The frontal lobe became atrophic and more pronounced in the pole, where the orbital area was also involved severely (Fig. 3A). In the temporal lobe except for the hippocampal formation, atrophy of the superior temporal gyrus was less marked than of the other gyri (Figs. 9 & 11A). The central region including the precentral and postcentral gyri disclosed minimal atrophy in all lobes of the cerebrum. The lateral ventricle was dilated symmetrically and bilaterally. The caudate nucleus and putamen showed conspicuous atrophy, but the globus pallidus disclosed far less severe atrophy. The thalamus became markedly atrophic, particularly predominant in the medial nucleus, accompanied by dilatation of the third ventricle (Figs. 3B & 14A). The cerebral white matter became soft, but no obvious softening foci nor cystic formation were found anywhere (Figs. 3A, B & C). The cerebllum became small and its foliae were atrophied conspicuously (Figs. 3D & 17A).

### 2) Microscopical findings

Cerebral Cortex: The cortical changes were conspicuously extensive and destructive. They were particularly predominant in the depths and walls of the sulci (Figs. 3A & 5). In these areas all layers except for the molecular layer were affected (Fig. 4A). The change consisted of marked loss of nerve cells, activated microglia with fat droplets, and sieve-like tissue loosening and more severely, cleft-like tissue disruption which tended to coalesce in laminar distribution or cystic cavitation (Figs. 4A, 4C, 4D & 9A). Similar but less severe changes developed at the gyral crowns in a laminar fashion, particularly in the third layer (Fig. 10A). In the mildly affected cortex, the nerve cells were comparatively well preserved in contrast with pronounced proliferation of astrocytes (Fig. 4B). Nerve cells, particularly in the deeper layers, showed a swollen and pale cytoplasm with eccentric nucleus (Figs. 6A, B & C). Some of them had an ill-defined, eosinophilic inclusion-like structure in their cytoplasm, which showed very weak argentophilia and thus, was different obviously from Pick's body (Figs. 6B & C). They occasionally showed vacuolar degeneration. The inflated neurons were widespread in the cortex, particularly of the cingulate, inferior frontal and insular cortex (Fig. 7). However, this was never found below the level of the diencephalon. It seems that this distribution pattern was different

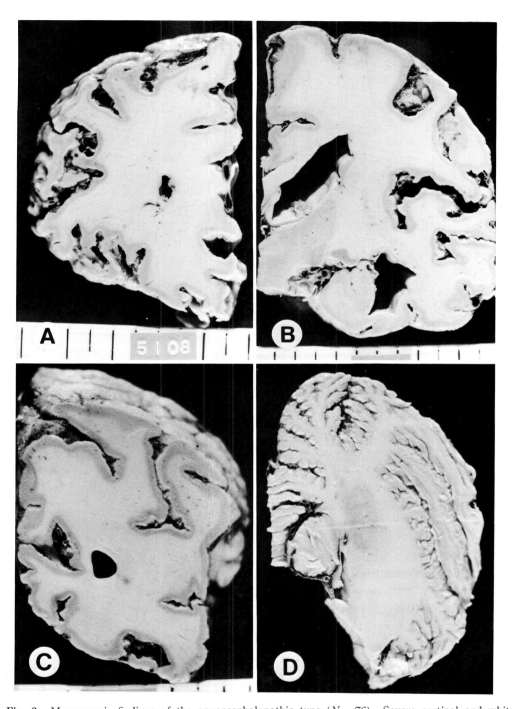

**Fig. 3.** Macroscopic findings of the panencephalopathic type (*No. 76*). Severe cortical and white matter atrophy with dilation of the ventricular system. Conspicuous narrowing of the cortical ribbons particularly accentuated in the wall and depth of the sulcus. Relatively well preserved hippocampal formation. Atrophy of the caudate nucleus, putamen, thalamus and lateral geniculate body. Marked atrophy of the cerebellum, particularly of the cerebellar foliae.

from that of the simple poliodystrophic type of CJD (see Chapter III-2). In the case recently reported by Riku, et al., however, (1983) inflated neurons were scattered not only in the cerebrum but also in the spinal cord (*No. 117*, Figs. 6D, E & F). Therefore, the present case had the panencephalopathic type conjoined with the aspect of the simple poliodystrophic type.

Although the hippocampal formation showed no obvious neuronal loss, there occurred fine, sieve-like spongy state and slight astrocytosis in all cases without exception. This was also found in the other subtypes of CJD. In this regard, although it seems macroscopically that the hippocampus is completely spared in CJD, the microscopic observations reveal that the hippocampus is extremely less severe but always affected.

It was remarked that in the cerebral cortex astocytes markedly proliferated and extended their foot processes but did never form thin-caliberd gliofibers (Figs. 8A & B). Moreover, there was no evidence of the tendency for the accumulation of fat granule cells around the vessels, irrespective of the length of the total duration of the illness (Fig. 4D).

Cerebral White Matter: Its change consisted of two morphologically different types: circumscribed foci and diffuse lesions (Figs. 9, 10, 11 & 12). The circumscribed focus, the most characteristic of the white matter change in this type, was a sharpy-demarcated, coarse spongy necrotic one. It occurred preferentially at the subcortical white matter of the gyral crowns (Figs. 5, 9B & 10A), although it frequently extended into the subcortex at the walls and depths of the sucli. This focus showed a conspicuously necrotic tendency in which both myelin sheaths and axons disappeared almost completely (Figs. 10C, D, E & F). While numerous empty microcavities were found in H-E stained preparation, fat droplets phagocytosed by activated microglial and gitter cells were observed in Sudan III stained frozen section. Marked proliferation of astrocytes, many of which were gemistocytic, was found. No changes of the blood vessels in the focus were found. The U-fiber was comparatively well preserved and the cortical change never spread into the circumscribed focus (Figs. 10B & F). Some foci showed conspicuous proliferation and hypertrophy of astrocytes and less marked spongy state (Fig. 10D). In other foci marked spongy state accompained by phagocytic cells laden with fat droplets was marked, while astrocytosis was far less severe and some astrocytes showed a regressive change (Fig. 10E). The foci of this variety occurred independently of the severity of the diffuse lesion, as a rule. For example, there were the cases in which numerous subcortical foci coexisted with diffuse lesion in slight degree, and those cases had a relatvely short duration of illness. In the case with long duration of illness, on the other hand, marked and extensive, diffuse lesions were superimposed on circumscribed foci, and thus, the latter were difficult to recognize (Fig. 10F).

---

**Fig. 4.** Cortical lesion of the cerebrum. **A:** Severe devastation of all layers except the upper two layers at the depth of the sulcus. Marked neuronal loss, tissue destruction, proliferation of astrocytes and mobilization of fat granule cells. Numerals indicate the number of the cortical layer. × 80. *No. 76.* **B:** Relatively well preserved cortex at the crown of the gyrus. Marked proliferation of astrocytes with minor loss of neurons. Arrow indicates inflated neuron. × 80. *No. 76.* **C:** Marked microcavitation in the frontal cortex except for the molecular layer. × 100. *No. 98.* **D:** Numerous fat granule cells scattered in the entire cerebral cortex. × 45. *No. 82.* (A, B & C: H-E; D: Sudan III)

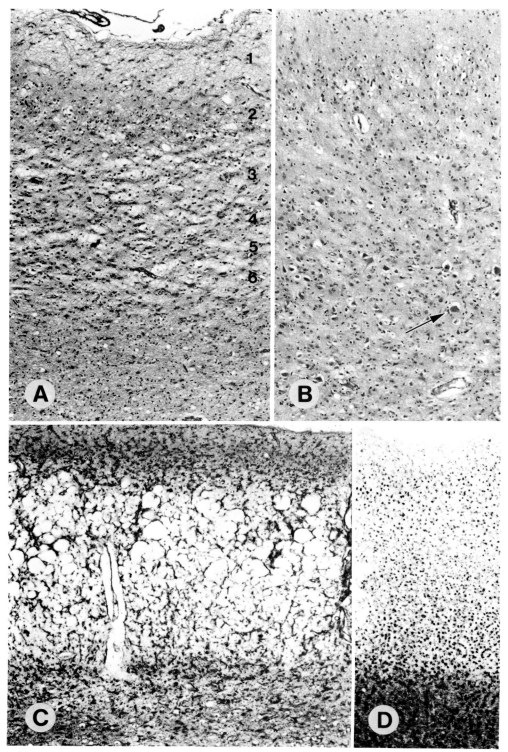

Fig. 4

Circumscribed foci were also found in the internal capsule, cerebral peduncle and lateral column of the spinal cord (Figs. 11A, 11E & 19B). In the internal capsule spongy microcavitions in various sizes were found (Fig. 11B). The focus showed an edematous swelling in general (Fig. 11E). As seen in those of the subcortical white matter, both myelin sheath and axon were depleted severely. Axonal swellings were found (Figs. 11C & D). Astrocytic proliferation was rather mild and a few fat granule cells were disseminated. The corticospinal tract below the focus showed secondary degeneration (Fig. 11F). However, this degeneration appeared to be more marked than that of secondary degeneration due to physical transection of the tract, for example, by cerebral hemorrhage or infarct and thus, the corticospinal tract degeneration in this type of CJD may have resulted from a coexistence of Wallerian degeneration and primary circumscribed foci.

The diffuse lesion was an extensive pallor of myelin, decreased number of axons, scattered fat granule cells, and proliferation of astrocytes (Figs. 12A & B). Even in the case without obvious loss of myelin, there occurred proliferation of astrocytes and a few fat granule cells. The white matter of the advanced case showed almost complete loss of nerve fibers, but no cystic formation occurred (Fig. 9A). Only a few remaining axons showed swelling (Fig. 12C). It also is remarkable that the fat granule cells had no tendency to accumulate around the vessels, as seen in the cortex. There occasionally occurred an infiltration of lymphocytes probably secondary to tissue damage in the severely affected white matter. Many of astrocytes revealed a regressive change. No fibrillary gliosis consisting of a feltwork of thin-calibered gliofibers was found. In the protracted cases, however, fibrillary gliosis occurred particularly pronounced in the subcortical white matter. The deep white matter showed slight or even absent fibrillary gliosis. The change was particularly predominant in the centrum semiovale and temporal white matter, although its severity was roughly parallel to that of the cortical change (Fig. 5). The corpus callosum was also damaged and markedly reduced in thickness. However, the internal capsule was never involved in a great majority of the cases, although circumscribed focus mentioned above occasionally occurred there (Figs. 9 & 11A). Secondary degeneration to the change of the white matter seldom developed in the corticospinal tract.

Subcortical Gray Matters: The caudate nucleus, putamen and claustrum were damaged in decreasing order. They disclosed identical alterations with the cortical deterioration, although neuronal loss was less severe in these nuclei (Fig. 13A). The globus pallidus, on the other hand, showed no outstanding alterations except for a diffuse pallor of myelin and increased number of glial nuclei (Fig. 13B); in some cases, however, severe neuronal loss and marked fibrillary gliosis occurred there, combined with degeneration of the subthalamus and substantia nigra (Fig. 11A).

The thalamus was consistently affected. Although the severity of the lesions in each thalamic subnuclei varied from case to case, both the dorsomedial (DM) and lateral dorsal (LD) nuclei and dorsal portion of the ventral lateral nucleus (VL) were constantly affected (Fig. 15). The changes in them were identical with the cortical degeneration, although neuronal loss was less severe (Figs. 14A & C). The pulvinar thalami showed similar but less severe degeneration. The lateral geniculate body was not infrequently involved (Figs. 3B & 9A). Almost complete loss of neurons with astrocytic proliferation and fat granule cell mobilization was found (Fig. 14D), accompanied frequently by degeneration of

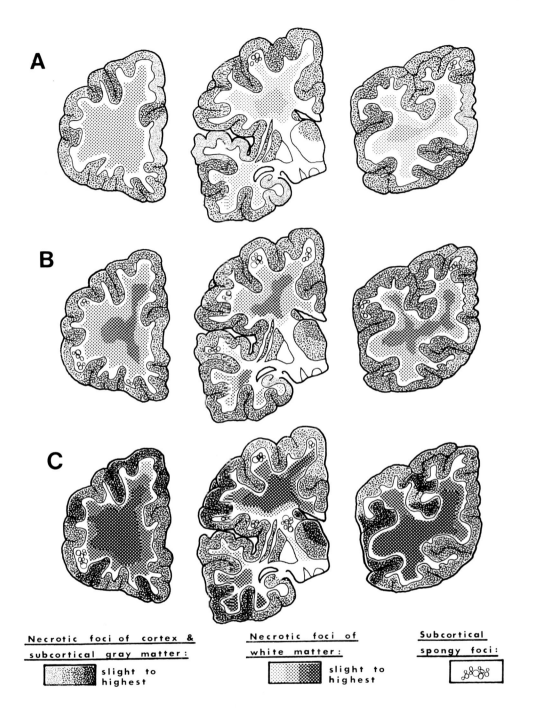

**Fig. 5.**   Schematic distribution of the lesions   (A: *No. 82*;   B: *No. 76*;   C: *No. 110*)   (From: Neuropsychiatric Disorders of the Elderly, eds., Hirano, A. & Miyoshi, K., Igaku-Shoin, 1983, with permission)

both the optic tract and optic radiation (Fig. 9B).   In addition to these features of the thalamus, different pathological changes were found in some cases; severe neuronal loss and conspicuous fibrillary gliosis occurred particularly predominant in the dorsomedial nucleus symmetrically and bilaterally (Figs. 8C, 14A & 15).   In one case of this type (*No. 79*) only one but typical kuru plaque was found in the dorsomedial nucleus of the thalamus.

The subthalamus was spared, as a rule.   In some cases, however, conspicuous degeneration with fibrillary gliosis occurred (Fig. 16D), frequently combined with degeneration of the globus pallidus and substantia nigra.

Cerebellum: Cortical degeneration was found in all cases without exception (Fig. 3D). It consisted of pronounced loss of the granule cells and relatively well preservation of Purkinje cells (Figs. 17A & 18A).   Marked subpial rarefaction resulting into the reduction of the molecular layer was frequent and phagocytic cells with fat droplets were interspersed (Fig. 17B).   An increased number of glial nuclei was also found.   Proliferation of Bergmann's glia occurred in the Purkinje cell layer.   Torpedo formation was frequently observed (Fig. 17C), but cactus was rarely found.   The granule cell layer showed a diffuse loss particularly pronounced in the area adjacent to the subcortical white matter, and thus, only a few granule cells were found just below the Purkinje cell layer in the advanced cases.   Phagocytic cells laden with fat droplets were also scattered in the granule cell layer (Fig. 17B).   No kuru plaques were found anywhere.   There occurred conspicuous proliferation of astrocytes in the cortex, which extended into the subcortical white matter. Fibrillary gliosis in slight degree was found only in the protracted cases.   The cortical degeneration was more predominant in the superficial foliae than in the deeper ones.   It occurred symmetrically and bilaterally, irrespective of paleo- and neocerebellum (Fig. 18A).   The deep white matter showed no obvious loss of myelin with slight to moderate astrocytosis, as a rule.   In the severe cases, on the other hand, marked degeneration with fat granule cell mobilization occurred and extended into the middle cerebellar peduncle. The dentate nucleus showed no remarkable changes, except for occasional "grumose alteration".   However, there were the cases in which marked degeneration of the dentate nucleus and its hilus extended into the brachium conjunctivum and occasionally into the red nucleus (Fig. 17D).

Brainstem and Spinal Cord: Although there certainly existed the cases in which these structures were never involved, they were not infrequently affected.   The posterior commissure, superior and inferior colliculi showed marked atrophy, loss of myelinoarchitecture, neuronal loss and astrocytic proliferation.   The substantia nigra was severely damaged.   Marked neuronal vacuolation was common (Figs. 16A, B & C).   Neuronal loss was severe and gitter cells with neuromelanin pigments were disseminated.   No Lewy bodies nor neurofibrillary tangles were found.   The red nucleus occasionally dislcosed marked astrocytosis with some loss of neurons (Fig. 16E).   The changes in the cerebellar peduncles and pontine base were combined frequently with the cerebellar lesions.   There occurred severe neuronal loss of the pontine nuclei with degeneration of the transverse fibers and middle cerebellar peduncle (Fig. 17E).   The inferior olive not infrequently showed neuronal loss and fibrillary gliosis.   In some cases olivary hypertrophy was found, in spite of intact central tegmental tracts (Fig. 18A).   In these cases neuronal loss was severe, and the remaining nerve cells showed marked inflation of their cytoplasm.   Some

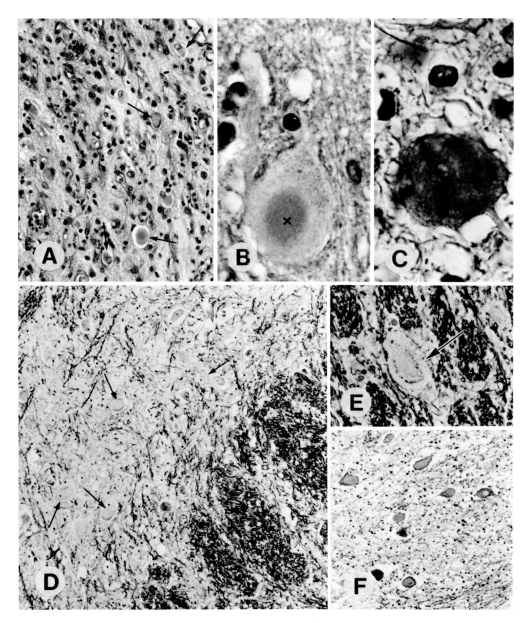

**Fig. 6.** Inflated neurons. **A:** Many inflated neurons scattered in the deeper layers of the superior frontal cortex (arrows). × 200. *No. 88.* **B:** Large inflated neuron in the insular cortex. Eosinophilic inclusion-like structure in the cytoplasm (cross). × 1000. *No. 73.* **C:** Inflated neuron with argentophilia in the parahippocampal cortex. No distinct Pick's body. × 1000. *No. 117.* **D:** Inflated neurons in the oculomotor nucleus (arrows). × 1000, *No. 117.* **E:** Inflated neuron of the pontine reticular formation (arrow). × 250. *No. 117.* **F:** Inflated neurons in the anterior horn of the cervical cord. × 100. *No. 117.* (A & B: H-E; C: Bodian; D, E & F: K-B)

neurons developed intracytoplasmic single or multiple vacuoles. Thickened dendritic processes of the remaining neurons and tangles of argyrophilic fibers (so-called glomerular structures) around the nerve cells were observed (Fig. 18D). Besides, there were many bizarre and giant astrocytes with single or multiple eosinophilic inclusions in their cytopalsm (Fig. 18C). In addition to olivary hypertrophy *No. 79* showed comparatively well-defined degeneration developed in the white matter symmetrically and bilaterally along the lateral border of the severely affected dentate and emboliform nuclei (Fig. 18A). This degeneration became more pronounced in the ventral portion of the dentate nucleus and was continuous into the restiform body. The motor nuclei of the brainstem including the ocular motor, trigeminal motor, facial nuclei and dorsal motor nucleus of the vagal nerve disclosed no remarkable change, as a rule, except one (*No. 117*).

Corticospinal tract degeneration seldom occurred, in spite of the extensive degeneration of the cerebral white matter. In most cases with the degeneration, clearly distal-dominant nature was demonstrated, being more predominant at the lumbar cord than at the cevical level (Fig. 19). The anterior horn cells, Clarke's column and posterior root ganglion cells showed no remarkable changes.


## 3. Discussion

### 1) Panencephalopathic type as a distinct subtype differentiated from other subtypes of CJD

Panencephalopathic type prevailed in the presenile and senile period, the onset of the disease developed subacutely, and the total duration of illness ranged within one and a half years in most cases, although several cases disclosed an exceptionally protracted clinical course. The clinical pictures included various neurological and mental symptoms and signs, while the following symptoms were consistently found in all cases without exception: severe mental deterioration resulting into akinetic mutism, para-, or tetraplegia in flexion, myoclonus, gait disturbance and PSD on EEG; actually they are most essential in CJD in general. On the contray, the clinical course of the panencephalopathic type was atypical: acute deterioration for 2 to 3 months at the initial stage followed by stationary condition for variable durations.

Pathologically there were not only severe cerebro-cerebellar degeneration with conspicuous astrocytosis without fibrillary gliosis but also severe degeneration of the white matter as well. Cerebello-cortical degeneration of granule cell type also occurred without exception and almost identical with that in the ataxic form of CJD, while cerebral

---

**Fig. 7.** Schematic distribution of the inflated neuron. Inflated neurons were scattered exclusively in the cerebral cortex, particularly in the cingulate, inferior frontal and insular cortex, as a rule. (From: Neuropsychiatric Disorders of the Elderly, eds., Hirano, A. & Miyoshi, K., Igaku-Schoin, 1983, with permission)

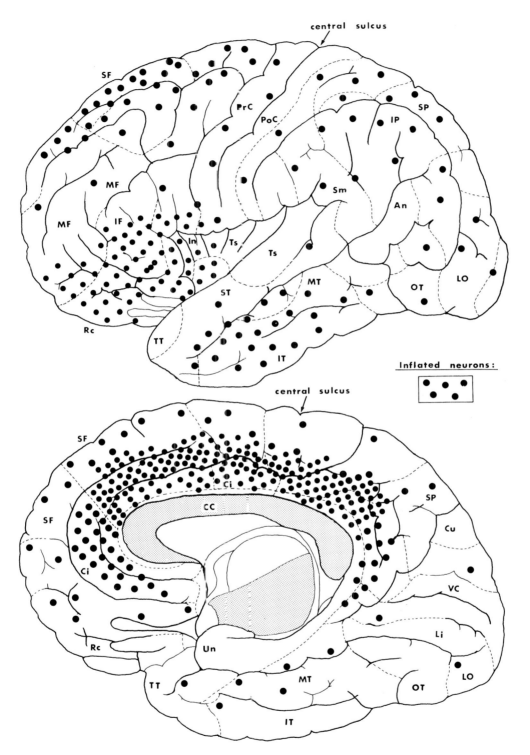

Fig. 7

138

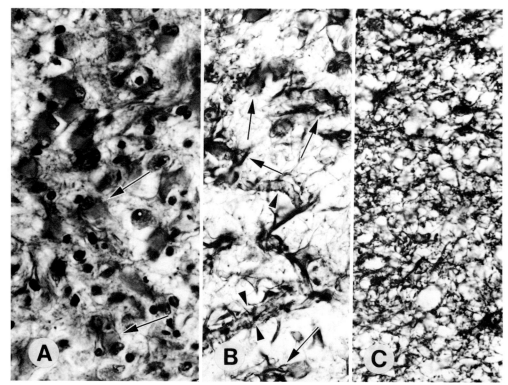

**Fig. 8** (Legend in page 142)

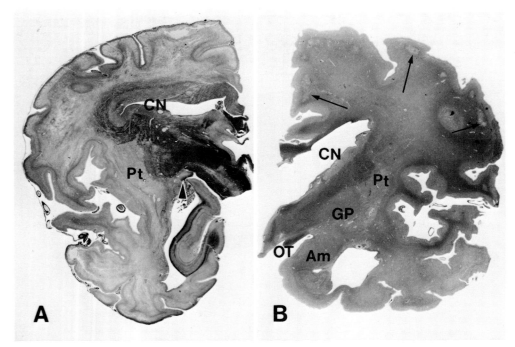

**Fig. 9** (Legend in page 142)

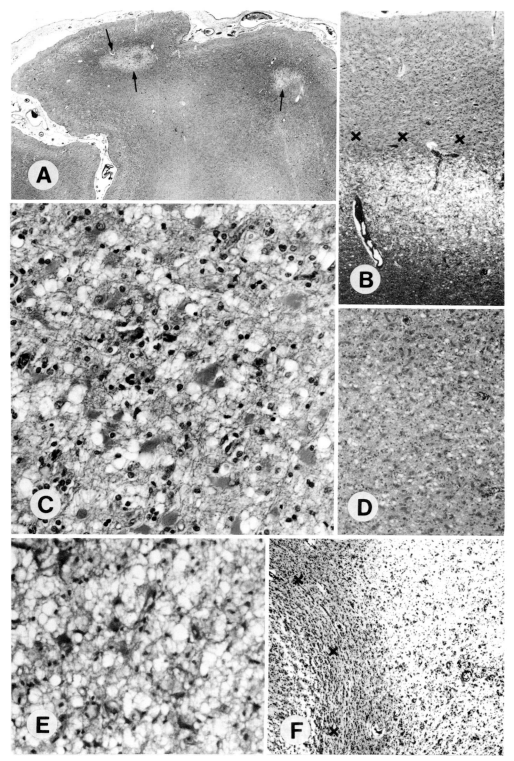

**Fig. 10** (Legend in page 142)

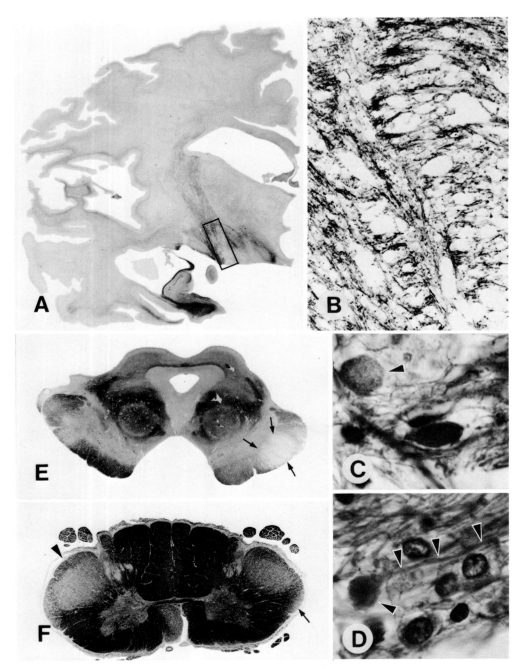

**Fig. 11** (Legend in page 142)

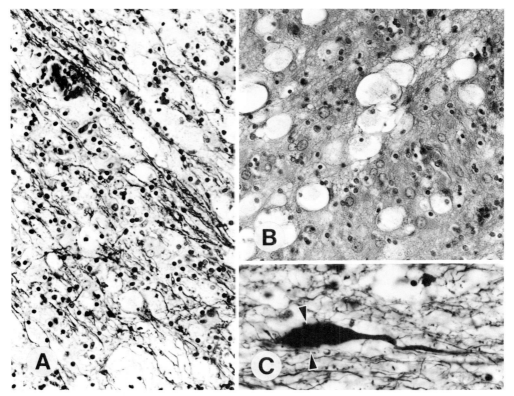

**Fig. 12** (Legend in page 142)

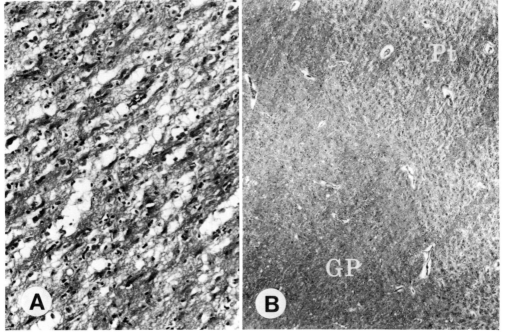

**Fig. 13** (Legend in page 142)

**Fig. 8.** Different aspects of astrocytes. Infraparietal cortex (A & B) and thalamus (*No. 117*). **A:** Marked hypertrophy of astrocytes (arrows). × 50. **B:** Astrocytes formed their foot processes but did not form thin-calibered gliofibers (arrows). Arrow-heads indicate capillaries. × 50. **C:** Isomorphic gliosis consisting of thin-calibered gliofibers in the dorsomedial nucleus of the thalamus. × 50. (A:H-E; B & C: Holzer)

---

**Fig. 9.** White matter change. **A:** Diffuse loss of myelin in the centrum smiovale and temporal white matter with well preserved internal capsule. Microcavitation in the cerebral cortex and well presevation of the hippocampus. *No. 98.* **B:** Circumscribed foci preferentially situated at the subcortex of the gyral crown (arrows). Marked atrophy of the optic tract (OT). *No. 76.* Abbreviations: Am: Amygdaloid nucleus; CN: Caudate nucleus; GP: Globus pallidus; OT: Optic tract; Pt: Putamen. (A: K-B; B: H-E)

---

**Fig. 10.** Circumscribed foci in the cerebral white matter. **A:** Sharply-demarcated spongy foci at the subcortex of the gyral crown (arrows) of the frontal lobe. × 3. *No. 76.* **B:** Relatively intact U-fibers (crosses). Note the absence of spongy state in the frontal cortex. × 34. *No. 76.* **C:** Numerous spongy microcavities with or without fat granule cells, and hypertrophy of astrocytes in the focus of the frontal white matter. × 250. *No. 77.* **D:** Pronounced astrocytic proliferation and hypertrophy with less marked spongy state in the focus of the occipital white matter. × 87. *No. 77.* **E:** Marked spongy state with far less severe astrocytosis in the focus of the frontal white matter. × 360. *No. 76.* **F:** Marked degeneration with hypertrophic astrocytes and fat granule cells with relatively well preserved U-fibers (croses). × 40. (*unpublished case*) (A: Masson's trichrome; B, C, D, E & F: H-E)

---

**Fig. 11.** Circumscribed foci in the pyramidal tract (*No. 117*). **A:** Almost complete loss of myelin in the centrum semiovale, corpus callosum and temporal white matter except for the hippocampus. Circumscribed spongy focus in the less severe degeneration in the internal capsule (square). B: Square in A. Coarse spongy cavities in various sizes and relatively intact myelinated fibers among them. × 100. **C & D:** Axonal swellings in the focus (arrows). × 1000. **E:** Circumscirbed spongy focus with edematous swelling in the cerebral peduncle at the midbrain (arrows). **F:** Wallerian degeneration of the corticospinal tract at the cervical cord. Degeneration of the ventral (arrow) and dorsal (arrow-head) spinocerebellar tracts. (A & B: K-B; C & D: H-E; E & F: K-B)

---

**Fig. 12.** Diffuse lesion of the cerebral white matter. **A:** Severe degeneration of the centrum semiovale with relatively intact myelinated fibers. × 250. *No. 100.* **B:** Marked mobilization of fat granule cells, and proliferation of astrocytes, many of which had large and pale nucleus and large eosinophilic cytoplasm. So-called "Wetterwinkel". × 250. *No. 100.* **C:** Axonal swelling of the remaining nerve fiber in the centrum semiovale. × 550. *No. 79.* (A: K-B; B: H-E; C: Bodian)

---

**Fig. 13.** Striatum (*No. 76*). **A:** Marked degeneration almost identical to the cortical lesion in the caudate nucleus. × 220, **B:** Similar but less severe change in the putamen (Pt). Increased number of glia without spongy degeneration in the globus pallidus (GP). × 35. (A & B: H-E).

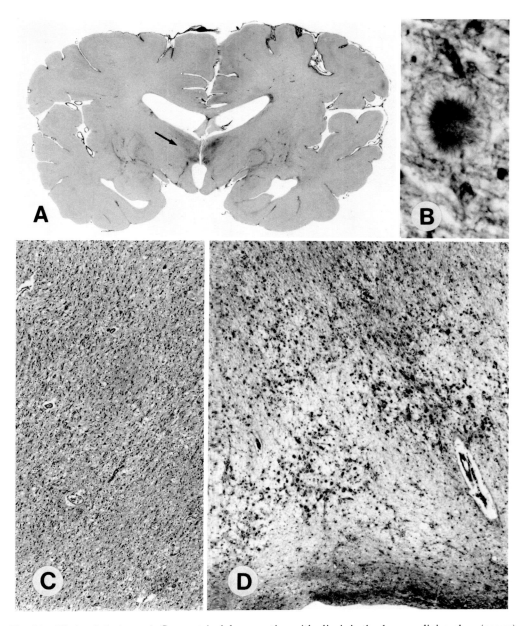

**Fig. 14.** Thalamic lesion.  **A:** Symmetrical degeneration with gliosis in the dorsomedial nucleus (arrow). *No. 119.*  **B:** Only one typical kuru plaque found in the dorsomedial nucleus of the thalamus of *No. 79.*  × 800.  **C:** Severe neuronal depletion and conspicuous fibrillary gliosis in the dorsomedial nucleus of the thalamus. × 50.  *No. 79.*  **D:** Almost complete loss of neurons and destruction of the cytoarchitecture of the lateral geniculate body.  × 4.  *No. 117.*  (A: Holzer;   B, C & D: H-E)

144

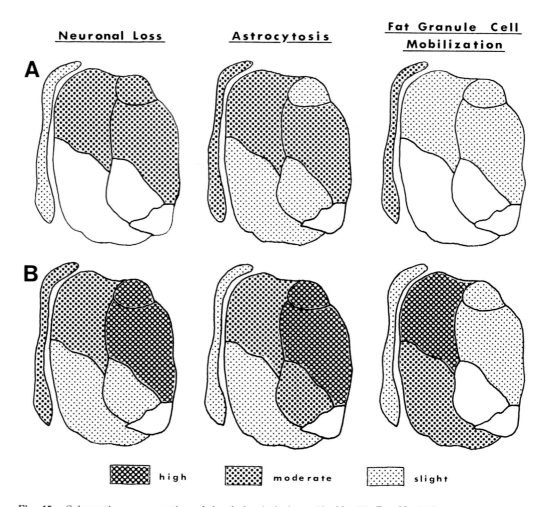

**Neuronal Loss**  **Astrocytosis**  **Fat Granule Cell Mobilization**

A

B

high    moderate    slight

**Fig. 15.** Schematic representation of the thalamic lesion. (A: *No. 76;* B: *No. 79.*)

**Fig. 16.** **A:** Substantia nigra. Severe loss of pigmented neurons and marked vacuolation of the remaining neurons (arrows), and conspicuous proliferation of astrocytes. × 80. *No. 87.* **B:** Marked vacuolation of the dendrite of pigmented neuron in the substantia nigra (arrow-head). × 400. *No. 117.* **C:** Marked vacuolation of the cytoplasm of pigmented neuron in the substantia nigra. × 500. *No. 117.* **D:** Subthalamus. Severe neuronal loss and marked astrocytosis. × 100. *No. 117.* **E:** Red nucleus. Marked loss of neurons and astrocytosis. × 250. *No. 117.* (A: H-E; B & C: Bodian; D & E: H-E)

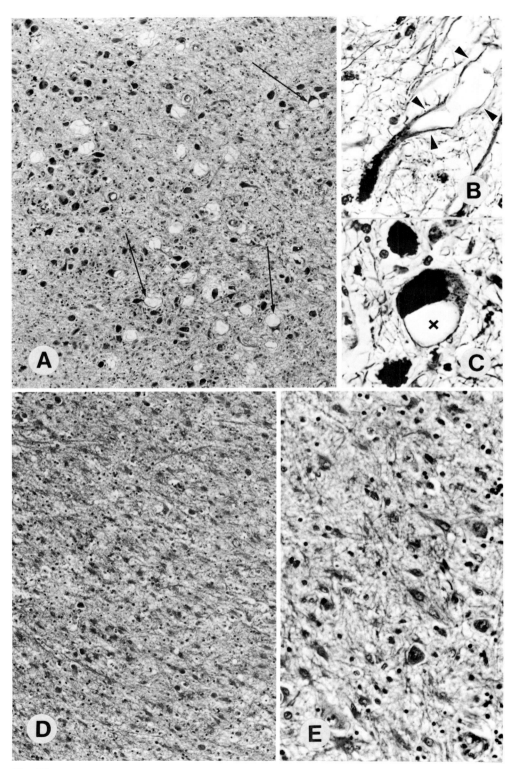

Fig. 16

146

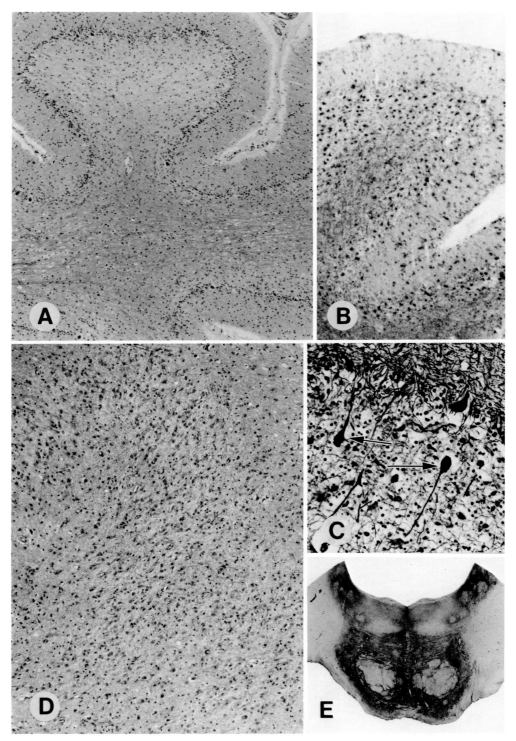

Fig. 17

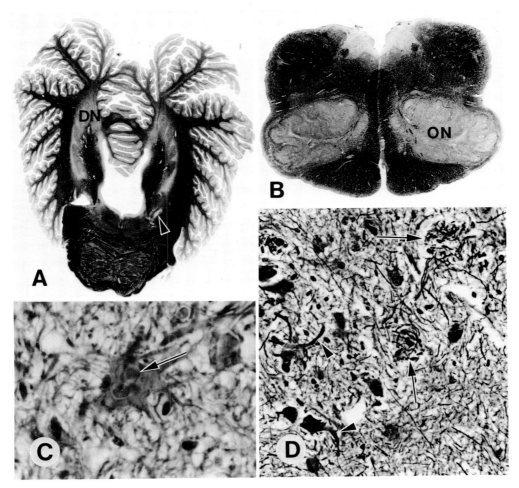

**Fig. 18.** Olivary hypertrophy (*No. 79*). **A:** Marked degeneration of the white matter just lateral to the dentate nucleus (DN) and restiform body (arrow-head). Severe degeneration of granule cell type in the entire cerebellar cortex. **B:** Marked olivary hypertrophy. Conspicuous loss of myelin in the fleece and hilus of the inferior olive. **C:** Giant and bizarre astrocyte with eosionphilic inclusions (arrow) in the inferior olive. × 800. **D:** Tangles of argyrophilic fibers (so-called glomerular structures, arrows) and thickened dendrites of neurons in the inferior olive. × 410. (A & B: K-B; C: H-E; D: Bodian)

**Fig. 17.** **A:** Severe loss of the granule cells with less severe loss of Purkinje cells, and marked proliferation of astrocytes in the cerebellar cortex. × 50. *No. 117.* **B:** Phagocytic cells laden with fat droplets scattered in the molecular, Purkinje and granular layers of the cerebellum. × 60. *No. 82.* **C:** Torpedo formation of Purkinje cells (arrows). × 240. *No. 79.* **D:** Conspicuous loss of neurons and proliferation of astrocytes in the dentate nucleus. × 100. *No. 87.* **E:** Marked fibrillary gliosis in the pontine base and restiform body and less severe in the pontine tegmentum. *No. 117.* (A: H-E; B: Sudan III; C: Bodian; D: H-E; E: Holzer)

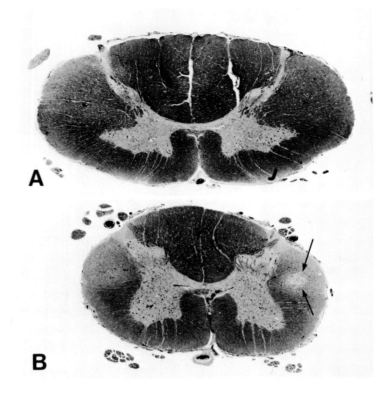

**Fig. 19.** Corticospinal tract degeneration of distal-dominant nature (*No. 76*). Circumscribed spongy focus superimposed on the degenerated corticospinal tract at the level of the lumbar cord (arrows). (A & B: K-B)

involvement far exceeded that in the ataxic form (Brownell & Oppenheimer, 1965). In the less severely affected cerebral cortex as well as in the hippocampus, astrocytosis predominated, while neuronal loss was less pronounced. Inflated neurons scattered in the deeper layers were found typically in the simple poliodystrophic type and also in SSE. However, inflated neurons in most cases of the panencephalopathic type were found exclusively in the cerebral cortex, while in the simple poliodystrophic type they were scattered extensively in the central nervous system (see Chapter III-2).

The cortical degeneration in the panencephalopathic type indicates that a rapid development of severely destructive process occurred even at the acute stage, and thereafter, there existed almost complete loss of nerve cells with fatty degradation, irrespective of the different length of the total clinical course, from 4.5 to 108 months. Serial CT surveys may support this view. It is also noticeable that a majority of cortical lesions were different from typical clustered and grape-like spongy state in SSE. Even in the case of SSE in which spongy degeneration fully developed in the cerebral cortex, the thickness of the cortical ribbon was not so reduced as the panencephalopathic type in which cleft-like tissue destruction resulted in conspicuous narrowing of the cortical ribbons. Furthermore, the cortical change in the panencephalopathic type was more pronounced in the walls and depths of the sulci, while in SSE spongy degeneration occurred in the cortex, irrespective of the gyral crowns and the sulcal depths, and never showed laminar pattern. It could be suggested that this pathological process brought about a marked decrease in brain weight.

Kirschbaum stated in his monograph that the degree of the brain atrophy was proportional to the length of the total duration of illness (1968). In the pancencephalo-pathic type this was true, while the other subtypes showed no obvious correlation (see Appendix). It, however, should be emphasized that most of the brain atrophy occurred mainly during the acute stage. It, therefore, is unlikely that the panencephalopathic type is a severe type of SSE.

Nevertheless, if there is a minor change in neurons in some cortical areas, in spite of diffusely proliferated astrocytes and spongy tissue loosening, it is not always possible to make a clear-cut distinction between this type and typical SSE.

An outstanding distinction of the panencephalopathic type to SSE as well as the other subtypes of CJD does exist in the widespread and severe degeneration of the cerebral white matter in this type. It is true that, although the secondary degeneration attributed to severe cortical deterioration overlapped in the white matter lesions, a great majority of them were regarded as results of the primary damage of the cerebral white matter for the following reasons: 1. The circumscribed spongy necrotic foci in the gyral subcortex with the well-preserved U-fibers but also in the internal capsule, cerebral peduncle and spinal cord is not explained as secondary degeneration; 2. The pyramidal tract and internal capsule themselves were never involved, while the centrum semiovale was strikingly deteriorated; 3. The pyramidal tract degeneration, if present, was clearly distal-dominant in character, and thus, could not simply be attributed to secondary degeneration alone; 4. The white matter lesion of Japanese brain with CJD similar to the panencephalopathic type has been successfully transmitted to experimental animals which will be discussed in Chapter V; 5. Review of the literatures shows the cases in which, in spite of severe cortical devastation, medullary degeneration was mild or even absent (Foley & Denny-Brown, 1955; Nevin, et al., 1960; Silberman, et al., 1961; Katzman, et al., 1961).

In recent autopsy cases of this type the white matter change was so severe and extensive that circumscribed necrotic foci were not found. Such cases showed a tendency to be protracted. Accidentally and/or secondarily superimposed changes may result in difficulty in identifying the antecedent circumscribed foci.

## 2) Review of foreign literatures simulating panencephalopathic type of CJD

There were seven reported cases up to date (Table 1), two of which are probable (Jacob, et al., 1958; Kirschbaum, 1968).

In the first case of Jacob's series, he pointed out a possibility in which the white matter lesion could not be attributed simply to secondary degeneration of cortical change. In this case there occurred diffuse loss of myelin in the centrum semiovale, cerebellar peduncles, pyramidal tracts and posterior columns, while neuronal changes in the cerebral

**Table 1.**

| Authors | Age at death/ Sex/Duration (months) | Clinical Features | Neuropathological Findings |
|---|---|---|---|
| Jacob, et al., (1958) | 57/F/16 | Weight loss, abdominal pain-Amnesia, aphasia, confusion, tremor, ataxia-Choreiform movement, myoclonus-Dementia | Brain weight ? Minor neuronal changes compared with marked spongy state, moderate astrocytic proliferation and some fat droplets in the cerebral cortex. Diffuse myelin pallor in the centrum semiovale, cerebellar peduncles, medial lemniscus, inferior longitudinal fasciculus, external arcuate fibers, pyramidal tracts and posterior columns. No involvement of the cerebellum. |
| Kirschbaum (1968) Selected Case XVII | 63/F/12 | Progressive amnestic-apractic mental disturbance, unsteady gait, parkinsonian posture, muscular rigidity, Babinski's sign, muscle atrophy, fasciculation, akinetic mutism, decorticate posture | Brain weight, 1250g. Moderate arteriosclerosis. Marked atrophy of the frontal, temporal and occipital lobes. Marked reduction of the cortical ribbons with widening of the sulci. Atrophy of the caudate and thalamus. Marked atrocytosis, neuronal loss, cleft-like tissue destruction in the cortex. Inflated neurons with weakly argentophilic inclusion-like structure in the cytoplasm. Focal necrosis in the subcortex. Diffuse loss of myelin, status spongiosus, isomorphic gliosis in the centrum semiovale. Severe depletion of neurons with astrocytosis in the caudate and thalamus. Granule cell loss with preservation of Purkinje cells. Slight loss of neurons in the anterior horn and the brainstem. Pyramidal tract degeneration. |
| Park. et al. (1980) | 77/F/12 | Progressive visual disturbance-Amnesia, speech disturbance, perseveration-Unresponsive-Vegetative state | Brain weight, 900g. Widening of the cerebral sulci. Marked ventricular dilatation. Almost total loss of neurons, marked astrocytosis, cleft-like tissue loosening of the cerebral cortex. Inflated neurons in the cortex. Marked loss of myelinated fibers, astrocytosis, foamy macrophages in the white matter. Severe loss of the granule cells and moderate loss of Purkinje cells in the cerebellar cortex. |
| Monreal. et al., (1981) | 16/M/28 | Amnesia, mental slowness-Startle reaction -Irregular jerks of the fingers-Marked disorientation-Unsteady gait, slurred speech -Paraplegia in flexion, myclonus-Agitation | Brain weight ? Moderate neuronal loss, astrocytosis and slight to moderate spongiform change. Pallor of myelin, large vacuolated areas around the blood vessels, marcrophages and marked astrocytosis in the cerebral white matter. Marked spongiform changes in the striatum. Marked neuronal loss with gliosis in the dorsomedial nucleus of the thalamus. Gliosis in the hypothalamus and mammillary body. Some neuronal degeneration and foci of astrocytosis in the pontine nuclei. Reduction of myelinated fibers in the pyramis. Severe loss of the granule cells, moderate to severe spongiform change in the molecular layer of the cerebellar cortex. Some myelin loss and gliosis in the cerebellar white matter. Patchy loss of neurons in the inferior olive. (Failure to transmitt to the experimental animals) |

| | | | |
|---|---|---|---|
| Schoene, et al. (1981) | 54/M/18 | Abnormal sleep pattern -Myoclonus-Paresthesia of the legs-Papular skin lesion-Unsteady gait, Romberg's sign-Skin biopsy (arteriolitis)-Immunosuppresant therapy-Vertigo, diplopia, cerebellar ataxia -Cushing's syndrome -Impaired cerebral function-Stupor | Obliterative endovasculitis limited to skin lesions and the anterior spinal artery at Th-5 (Köhlmeier-Degos syndrome). Brain weight, 1600g. Spongiform change, neuronal loss and astrocytosis in the cerebral cortex, striatum and thalamus. Kuru plaques in the cerebral cortex. Neuronal loss and gliosis in the dentate nucleus. Some loss of Purkinje cells. Cribriform change in the brachium, conjunctivum, basis pontis, corticospinal and spinocerebellar tracts and the posterior columns. (Successful transmission of spongy degeneration in the cortex of the animals) |
| Vallat, et al. (1983) | 56/M/60 | Familial case. Loss of memory, inability to concentrate, fine postural tremor with myoclonic jerks-Dysarthria, unsteady gait, apraxia-Akinetic mutism, marked spasticity, painful movement | Brain weight, 1100g. Marked atrophy of both prefrontal and left temporal lobes. Almost complete loss of neurons, marked astrocytosis and diffuse sponginess in the cerebral cortex. Loss of the granule cells in the cerebellar vermis. Diffuse loss of myelinated fibers and astrocytosis in the cerebral white matter. Demyelination and onionbulb formation in the peripheral nerves. |
| Macchi, et al., (1984) | 57/F/18 | Mental deterioration -Coma, decorticate posture, spasticity, myoclonus-Reduction of twitching movements | Brain weight, 800g. Severe cortical devastation with total loss of neurons and astrocytosis in the cerebrum, Marked loss of both myelin and axon, accompanied by fatty degradation and astrocytosis in the cerebral white matter. Severe deterioration of the basal ganglia. Astrocytosis in the thalamus. Sponginess in the granular layer and subcortical white matter of the cerebellum. Slight demyelination of the superior peduncle. No pyramidal tract degeneratiton |

cortex were minor in contrast with marked and widespread spongiform change. No circumscribed spongy foci were found. The white matter change was slight in comparison with the gross lesions of the cerebral gray matter, and thus, this may be secondary to the cortical degeneration. However, degeneration in the cerebellar peduncles and posterior columns and probably in the pyramidal tracts of the spinal cord is never secondary. The clinicopathological feature of this case as a whole is not always compatible with that of the panencephalopathic type. However, it should be noted that degeneration in the brainstem and spinal cord may be regarded as system degeneration.

On the other hand, the selected case XVII described by Kirschbaum is much more compatible with the panencephalopathic type. In this case there occurred focal necrosis in the subcortical white matter which could be considered not of vascular origin but primary. They were separated from a less pronounced degeneration in the deeper white matter. The centrum semiovale showed an isomorphic gliosis and spongy state. The cerebral cortex disclosed similar change to that in the panencephalopathic type. Inflated neurons with weakly argentophilic inclusion in the cytoplasm were scattered, while Alzheimer's neurofibrillary tangles were not frequent. Kirschbaum thought that this case

152

may be a variant of Pick's disease, since neuronal change of inflation was suggestive but the distribution of the process throughout the cortex including the occipital lobes was uncommon for Pick's disease. It, however, is likely that this case has many aspects of the common neuropathological changes of the panencephalopathic type.

The remaining four cases are considered within the spectrum of the panencephalopathic type. Two of them are the members of the same French family (Buge, et al., 1978; Vallat, et al., 1983). A similar family in Japan will be described in Chapter IV. Vallat's case disclosed mottled or ill-defined patchy pallor of myelin occurring in the occipital white matter, which was also found in one of our series (Mizutani, et al., 1981a). The authors also demonstrated peripheral neuropathy. Park's case had the shortest duration of illness among the cases listed in the Table 1. There occurred conspicuous cerebral atrophy (brain weight, 900 g) and marked destructive process in the cerebral cortex and white matter. Monreal's case is the youngest among the previously reported cases of CJD. This induced the authors to discuss a relationship to Alpers' disease and Kuru. They concluded that although spongy change observed in many of the cases of Alpers' disease failed to satisfy the criteria for a diagnosis of CJD (Masters & Richardson, 1978), it is not possible categorically to reject all of these cases on the basis of their histopathological findings alone. Schoene's case showed atypical clinical features and pathological finding suggestive of Koehlmeier-Degos syndrome. The white matter change occurred mainly in the brainstem and spinal cord in which obliterative endovasculitis was found, but could not be attributable to vascular disturbance.

Most authors considered the white matter lesion a primary involvement, while Monreal, et al. suggested its secondary degeneration due to extensive neuronal depletion in the cortex in the case with prolonged clinical course. It, however, is obvious that the white matter lesions were much too extensive to be explained solely on this basis (Park, et al., 1981). In addition, Monreal, et al. suggested that the panencephalopathic type represents either infection with variant strains of the CJD virus or unusual host response. In two cases attempts were made to transmit spongy degeneration to animals (Monreal, et al., 1981; Schoene, et al., 1981), and the latter showed successful transmission to the cortex of experimental animal. The experimental spongy degeneration in the white matter, however, was successful only in the Tateishi's laboratory up to date (1979, 1980).

### 3) White matter change and plaques

Kodama's (1981, *No. 111*) and Ohta's (*No. 89*) cases were remarked, since they showed both the changes compatible with that in the panencephalopathic type and those of the chronic spongiform encephalopathy with plaques characterized by antecedent and longlasting cerebellar ataxia which will be described in the next section (Chapter III-7).

**Fig. 20.** Schematic distribution of the lesions with emphasis on system degeneration. See text! Upper: *No. 79*; Lower: *No. 87*. (From: Neuropsychiatric Disorders of the Elderly, eds., Hirano. A. & Miyoshi, K., Igaku-Schoin, 1983, with permission)

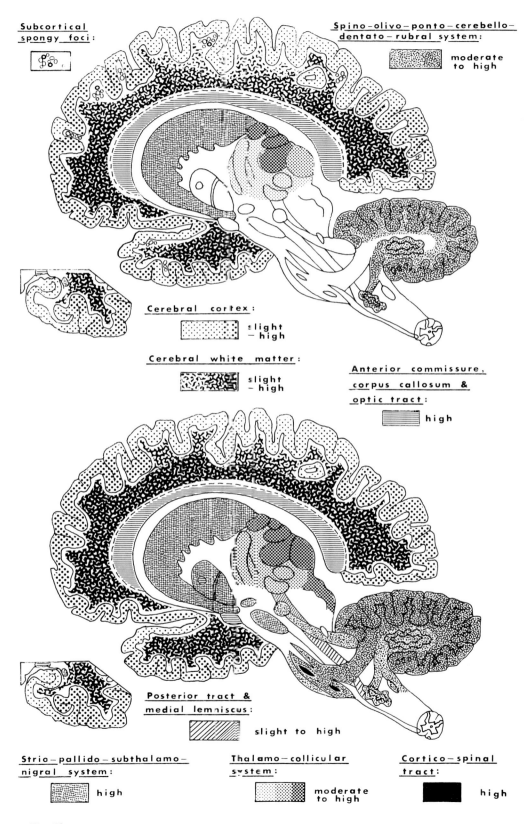

Fig. 20

In Kodama's case, there occurred a diffuse degeneration of the cerebral white matter (Fig. 22F), while the internal capsule was well preserved. No cystic cavitations were found. The cerebral cortex showed severe degeneration (Fig. 22A). Inflated neurons were disseminated in the deeper cortical layers (Figs. 22D & E). The thalamus disclosed a conspicuous degeneration with gliosis particularly predominant in the dorsomedial nucleus (Fig. 22G, and Fig. 5B in Chapter III-7). The cerebellar cortex showed typical degeneration of granule cell type (Fig. 22H). In addition, numerous plaques were disseminated in the cerebral cortex but not in the cerebellar cortex (Figs. 22B & C). The brainstem showed marked atrophy but no histopathological changes were found. The spinal cord was not examined. In the panencephalopathic type plaques were extremely rare, but only one typical kuru plaque was found in the thalamus of one case (*No, 79*), as mentioned before.

Ohta's case is the first one in which the spongy degeneration was successfuly transmitted to the white matter of the small rodents by Tateishi and his associates (see Chapter V). In this case there occurred numerous plaques in the cerebral and cerebellar cortex, basal ganglia and brainstem nuclei, thalamic degeneration and cerebello-cortical degeneration of granule cell type.

The degeneration of the cerebral white matter was more pronounced and thus, cystic cavitations were disseminated. An intense fibrillary gliosis occurred in the white matter, although it was not found in the cavities. Circumscribed spongy necrotic foci were not found. The striatum showed far less severe change, while the thalamus disclosed marked neuronal loss and fibrillary gliosis, partly accompanied by fat granule cells. In the brainstem there occurred degeneration of the pontine base and middle cerebellar peduncle, and neuronal depletion of the inferior olive and degeneration of the restiform body. The dentate nucleus disclosed marked neuronal loss. Some remaining neurons showed typical grumose alteration. Many axonal swellings were found in and around the dentate nucleus. Some of them were situated closely adjacent to the cytoplasm or dendritic processes of nerve cells. The brachium conjunctivum was conspicuously degenerated, and the red nucleus showed severe neuronal loss and gliosis. The substantia nigra also revealed marked neuronal depletion. In the spinal cord there occurred degeneration of the corticospinal and spinocerebellar tracts, and posterior columns. Furthermore, there were spongy microcavitations with axonal swellings and fat granule cells superimposed on these degenerated tracts.

Clinically, on the other hand, Kodama's case had about two-years' duration, while Ohta's case had about four-years' duration. Both cases showed a slowly progressive deterioration of mental state, unlike that seen in the panencephalopathic type. In Kodama's case no obvious symptoms and signs of cerebellar ataxia were found, while Ohta's case showed a distinct cerebellar ataxia at the initial stage which lasted for about one year. The clinical course in which longlasting cerebellar ataxia preceded mental deterioration, was also pointed out in the chronic spongiform encephalopathy (Fig. 1 in Chapter III-7).

Thus, Kodama's and Ohta's cases, particularly the latter had several common features to the panencephalopathic type, while they shared other aspects with the chronic spongiform encephalopathy. Therefore, both cases should be remarked in consideration of the interrelationship between the these two conditions.

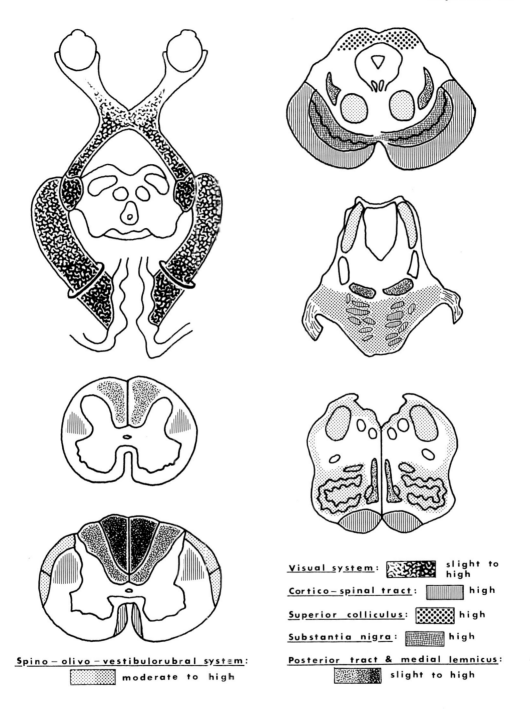

Spino – olivo – vestibulorubral system:
moderate to high

Visual system: slight to high

Cortico-spinal tract: high

Superior colliculus: high

Substantia nigra: high

Posterior tract & medial lemnicus: slight to high

**Fig. 21.** Schematic representation of system degeneration. See text ! (From: Neuropsychiatric Disorders of the Elderly, Hirano, A. & Miyoshi, K., Igaku-Schoin, 1983, with permission)

156

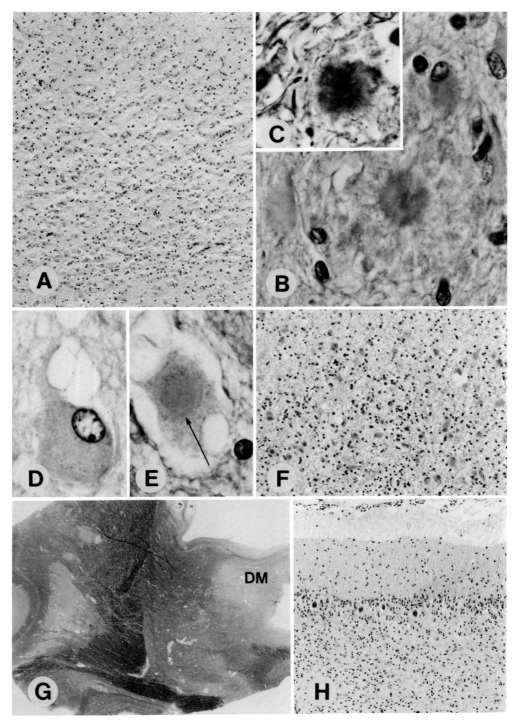

Fig. 22

## 4) System Degeneration in the panencephalopathic type

The pathological changes discussed here can be considered as system degeneration. They were restricted precisely to the anatomo-physiologically interrelated system symmetrically and bilaterally, accompanied by conspicuous fibrillalry gliosis. System degeneration could not be explained simply by extensive degeneration of the cerebral white matter, since not only the descending but also the ascending pathways were involved. They were found frequently in the panencephalopathic type, but also in the other subtypes, and thus, they can be considered to be one of the essential morphological features of CJD.

The dorsomedial (DM) nucleus of the thalamus was most severely damaged (Fig. 15). Since the DM nucleus is connected mainly with the frontal lobe, some overlapping process of the secondary degeneration attributed to both the cortical and white matter damages of the frontal lobes did exist in the thalamic lesion. Nevertheless, it must be considered as a primary degeneration for the following reasons: 1. It is particularly important that the topography of the characteristic lesions showed a complete symmetric bilaterality; 2. In spite of severe damage in the parieto-occipital lobes, the pulvinar thalami disclosed mild or equivocal loss of neurons and no fibrillary gliosis; 3. The severity of the thalamic involvement far exceeded that in the case with prefrontal lobotomy (Yokoi, 1957); 4. There existed no definite evidence for an interpretation of the lesions due to secondary degeneration of both ascending and descending tracts to the thalamic nucleus. These findings suggest an associated primary cerebro-thalamic degeneration in pairs (see Chapter III-4). Degeneration of the lateral geniculate body, on the other hand, has not been so remarked, but actually was not unusual.

Thalamic degeneration in the panencephalopathic type was frequently associated with degeneration of several other systems (inferior olivary nucleus - restiform body - cerebellar cortex, inferior olivary nucleus - pontine nuclei - brachium pontis - cerebellar cortex, dentate nucleus - brachium conjunctivum - red nucleus, globus pallidus - subthalmus - substantia nigra, optic tract - lateral geniculate body - optic radition, spinocerebellar tract, corticospinal tract) (Figs. 20 & 21). The changes in the spinal cord, brainstem and cerebellum are particularly remarked, since they strongly simulate olivo-ponto-cerebellar atrophy (OPCA). The similar aspect is pointed out in the chronic spongiform

---

**Fig. 22.** Panencephalopathic type of CJD with kuru plaques (*No. 111*). **A:** Severe neuronal loss, tissue loosening and proliferation of astrocytes in the frontal cortex. × 80. **B:** Kuru plaque with radition, surrounded by hypertrophic astrocytes in the occipital cortex. × 800. **C:** Kuru plaque with argentophilia and radition in the insular cortex. × 1000. **D:** Inflated neuron in the frontal cortex. × 1000. **E:** Inflated neuron with cytoplasmic vacuolation and eosinophilic inclusion-like structure (arrow) in the frontal cortex. × 1000. **F:** Severe degeneration of the occipital white matter accompanied by astrocytic proliferation and fat granule cell mobilization. × 100. **G:** Marked degeneration of the dorsomedial nucleus of the thalamus (DM). **H:** Cortical degeneration of granule cell type. No plaques in the cerebellum. × 80. (A & B: H-E; C: Bodian; D, E & F: H-E; G: LFB - H-E; H: H-E)

encephalopathy with plaques characterized by antecedent and longlasting cerebellar ataxia (see Chapter III-7), and Kuru itself. It, furthermore, is well known that OPCA is not infrequently combined with primary thalamic degeneration (see Chapter III-4). Degeneration in the dentate nucleus, brachium conjunctivum and red nucleus could be compatible with dentato-rubral degeneration and, extrapyramidal involvement could be regarded as pallido-luysian atrophy (Smith, et al., 1958), Therefore, various combinations of degeneration could be considered reasonably as multisystemic degeneration.

## 5) Clinicopathological Correlation

Rapid mental deterioration resulting in akinetic mutism or apallic state could be attributable to conspicuous destruction of both the cerebral cortex and white matter. Thalamic degeneration could also play an important role in its development. Myoclonus became apparent when akinetic mutism and muscular rigidity developed. This period was actually corresponded to that when a rapid skrinkage of the cerebrum was demonstrated by CT. However, CT was unable to demonstrate that the cortical, white matter and striatal lesions developed simultaneously or not. Para- or tetraplegia in flexion in the later stage could be due to severe damage of the cerebral hemispheres (Yakovlev, 1954).

Various neurological symptoms were observed during short period of the acute stage. Gait disturbance was the most common feature found in the initial stage. However, ataxic gait was found only in a few cases. Not only the involvement of the cerebellum but also striatum, frontal cortex and spinal cord may be taken into consideration. Cerebellar symptoms and signs were scanty, in spite of cerebello-cortical degeneration, while extrapyramidal symptoms predominated. One can speculate that clinical involvement of cerebellum became overshadowed by coexistence of extrapyramidal symptoms. In Brownell and Oppenheimer's cases characterized by predominant cerebellar symptoms and less severe rigidity, cerebello-cortical degeneration far exceeded degeneration of the extrapyramidal system. In this regard, it is remarked that cerebellar symptoms became obscure by subsequent or simultaneous development of extrapyramidal symptoms in cases of OPCA with striato-nigral degeneration (Hirayama, et al., 1977a & b). Choreo-athetoid involuntary movement observed in some cases may be due to degeneration of the dentato-rubral system and others.

The panencephalopathic type disclosed unique clinical course of rapid mental deterioration at the early stage followed by non-progressive and stationary course. The acute to subacute stage could be associated with the cortical shrinkage of the cerebrum demonstrated by CT surveys and corresponded to three to five months after the onset. Cerebral atrophy itself, on the other hand, appeared to be continued even until the terminal stage, but clinical condition was not always downhill. On the contrary, cerebral atrophy in both the simple poliodystrophic type and SSE appeared to remain in slight to moderate degree, in spite of steady progression of mental deterioration until death. Unfortunately, there has been no serial CT studies on these two subtypes of CJD.

## 6) Morphopathogenesis

Astrocytic reaction is considered to be most significant in morphopathogenesis, because it has a distinctly different aspect from that in various well-known diseases, such as anisomorphic gliosis in cerebrovascular disease and isomorphic gliosis in system degeneration. For Holzer's stained preparation in these diseases, one can easily find that astrocytes not only proliferate but also form numerous thin-calibered gliofibers, causing fibrillary gliosis.

Astrocytes in the panencephalopathic type, however, extended their foot processes but did not form a feltwork of thin-calibered gliofibers (Fig. 8). Thus, there existed a discrepancy of astrocytosis without fibrillary gliosis in this type. In addition activated microglial and gitter cells with fat droplets showed no obvious tendency in their perivascular accumulation, irrespective of the length of total duration of the illness. It, therefore, could be indicated that some normal functions of astrocytes and microglial cells were severely suppressed or insufficient. It is likely that such a glial dysfunction in this type played an important role in markedly destructive process in both the cortical and white matter lesions. This glial dysfunction was pointed out in all subtypes of CJD, but was most predominant in the panencephalopathic type.

The cortical change in the panencephalopathic type was more accentuated in the walls and depths of the sulci, although it was less distinct than in hypoxic encephalopathy. The laminar devastation of the cortex existed, irrespective of different clinical features, although hypoxia due to myoclonus and convulsion may play some part of role in the development of this finding.

It can be emphasized that a coexistence of glial dysfunction and laminar cortical deterioration in the panencephalopathic type is not unique, since it has already been pointed out in various types of hepatocerebral disease, particularly pseudoulegyric type (Oda, et al., 1964; Shiraki & Oda, 1968). There certainly exist several similarities between the two conditions: distribution pattern of the laminar cortical lesion of the cerebrum characterized by involvement of the association cortex and relative sparing of the hippocampus; the degeneration of the white matter of both circumscribed and diffuse nature; and glial dysfunction. However, Alzheimer type II glia with or without intranuclear glycogen granules was found only in the pseudoulegyric type but not in the panencephalopathic type.

The white matter change in the panencephalopathic type has been successfully transmitted to animals by Tateishi and his associates, and this will be discussed in the latter section (Chapter V).

Certain morphological similarities of the white matter changes of this type of CJD to some cases of sudanophilic leukodystrophy are pointed out. In the latter, the circumscribed spongy focus closely resembling that of panencephalopathic type scattered preferentially at the various levels of the corticospinal tract, such as the internal capsule, cerebral peduncle and lateral column of the spinal cord as well as subcortical white matter (Oda, et al., 1983; Suzuki, et al., 1983; Mizutani, et al., 1983). It is remarked that axonal swellings were found in the focus in both conditions, although far more numerous in the sudanophilic leukodystrophy. In addition sudanophilic leukodystrophy frequently showed thalamic degeneration of both primary and secondary natures, and glial insufficiency was occasionally demonstrated in some cases (Mizutani, et al., 1983).

Consequently morphopathogenetic aspect of the panencephalopathic type are summarized as follow: a close coexistence of glial dysfunction and some circulatory disturbance, and system degeneration. It could be emphasized that such combination of the morphopathogenesis were found in some toxic-metabolic disorders.

## Aknowledgement

We thank Professor Tateishi, Department of Neuropathology, Kyushu University, and Drs. Okamoto, Riku and Hashizume, Departments of Neurology and Pathology, Nagoya University, and Dr. Hayashi, Department of Pathology, Okayama University, for permission to study clinical data and necropsy materials. We also thank Dr. Yamada, Department of Neurology, Tokyo Metropolitan Neurological Hospital, for permission to study CT findings.

## REFERENCES

**Brownell, B. and Oppenheimer, D. R.**: An ataxic form of subacute presenile polioencephalopathy (Creutzfeldt-Jakob disease), J. Neurol. Neurosurg. Psychiat., 28: 350-361, 1965.

**Buge, A., Escourlle, R., Brion, S., Rancurel, G., Hauw, J. J., Mehaut, M., Gray, F. and Gajdusek, D. C.**: Maladie de Creutzfeldt-Jakob familiale - Étude clinique et anatomique de trois cas sur huit répartis sur trois générations. Transmission au singe écureuil, Rev. Neurol., 134: 165-181, 1978.

**Foley, J. M. and Denny-Brown, D.**: Subacute progressive encephalopathy with bulbar myoclonus, Excerpta Med., Sect. VIII, 8: 782-784, 1955.

**Hirayama, K., Saito, M., Chida, T., Iizuka, R. and Murofushi, K.**: A clinicopathological study on extrapyramidal components in cerebellar degeneration with special reference to olivo-ponto-cerebellar atrophy, Adv. Neurol. Sci. (Japan), 21: 37-54, 1977a.

**Hirayama, K., Saito, M., Chida, T., Iizuka, R., Murofushi, K. and Fukuda, Y.**: Olivo-ponto-cerebellar atrophy and striato-nigral degeneration - Clinico-patholoigical study, Adv. Neurol. Sci. (Japan), 21: 461-475, 1977b.

**Kashiwamura, K., Takasato, C., Kodama, K., Kusunose, Y. and Sakata, Y.**: Serial computed tomographic study on subacute spongiform encephalopathy, Clin. Neurol. (Japan), 21: 938-943, 1981.

**Kawai, M., Iwata, M., Takatsu, M., Toyokura, Y. and Nagashima, K.**: When does the brain atrophy in Creutzfeldt-Jakob disease ?, Clin. Neurol. (Japan), 20: 691-697, 1981.

**Katzman, R., Kagan, E. H. and Zimmerman, H. M.**: A case of Jakob-Creutzfeldt disease, J. Neuropathol. exp. Neurol., 20: 78-94, 1961.

**Kirschbaum, W. R.**: Jakob-Creutzfeldt Disease, American Elsevier, New York, 1968.

**Kishida, S., Yano, Y. and Muro, T.**: Creutzfeldt-Jakob disease and serial computerized tomography, Neurol. Med. (Japan), 15: 505-507, 1981.

**Kodama, R., Shibata, T., Mizutani, T. and Ishihara, Y.**: An autopsy case of spongiform encephalopathy with kuru plaques, Neuropathol. (Japan), 2: 53, 1981.

**Jacob, H., Eicke, W. and Orthner, H.**: Zur Klinik und Neuropathologie der subakuten praesenilen spongiösen Atrophien mit dyskinetischem Endstadium, Dtsch. Z. Nervenheilk., 178: 330-357, 1958.

**Macchi, G., Abbamondi, A. L. Di Trapani, G. and Sbriccoli, A.**: On the white matter lesions of the Creutzfeldt-Jakob disease.  Can a new subentity be recognized in man ?, J. Neurol. Sci., 63: 197-206, 1984.

**Masters, C. L. and Richardson, E. P. Jr.**: Subacute spongiform encephalopathy (Creutzfeldt-Jakob disease) - The nature and progression of spongiform change, Brain, 101: 333-344, 1978.

**Meyer, A., Leigh, D. and Barron, D. W.**: A rare presenile dementia associated with cortical blindness, J. Neurol. Neurosurg. Psychiat., 17: 129-133, 1954.

**Mizutani, T.**: Creutzfeldt-Jakob disease with cerebellar cortical degeneration - Special reference to a subtype of Creutzfeldt-Jakob disease with severe cerebrocerebellar atrophy. Adv. Neurol. Sci. (Japan), 21: 135-143, 1977; Excerpta med., Sect. VIII, 41: 542, 1977.

**Mizutani, T., Okumura, A., Oda, M. and Shiraki, H.**: Panencephalopathic type of Creutzfeldt-Jakob disease: Primary involvement of the cerebral white matter, 44: 103-115, 1981a.

**Mizutani, T.**: Neuropathology of Creutzfeldt-Jakob disease in Japan - With special reference to the panencephalopathic type, Acta Path. Jpn., 31: 903-922, 1981b.

**Mizutani, T., Hiraiwa, A., Satoh, J., Morimatsu, Y., Eguchi, H., Hirayama, K. and Suzuki, K.**: An autopsy case of leukoencephalopathy with thalamic and striatal degenerations, The 24th Annual Meeting of Japanese Neuropathological Society, Nagoya, 1983.

**Mizutani, T., Morimatsu, Y. and Shiraki, H.**: Clinical pictures of Creutzfeldt-Jakob disease based on 97 autopsy cases in Japan - With special reference to clinicopathological correlation of cerebellar symptoms, Clin. Neurol. (Japan), 24: 23-32, 1984.

**Monreal, J., Collins, G. H., Masters, C. L., Fisher, C. M., Kim, R. C., Gibbs, C. J. Jr. and Gajdusek, D. C.**: Creutzfeldt-Jakob disease in an adolescent, J. Neurol. Sci., 52: 341-350, 1981.

**Nagura, H., Tohgi, H., Yamanouchi, H. and Tomonaga, M.**: Neuropathological correlations with the computed tomograms in Creutzfeldt-Jakob disease, Neurol. Med. (Japan), 18: 252-262, 1983.

**Nevin, S., McMenemy, W. H., Behrman, S. and. Jones, D. P.**: Subacute spongiform encephalopathy - A subacute form of encephalopathy attributable to vascular dysfunction (spongiform cerebral atrophy), Brain, 83: 519-563, 1960.

**Oda, M.**: Ein Beitrag zu den klinischen und histopathologischen Problemen über die hepatozerebralen Erkrankungen, insbesondere über 'Pseudoulegyrie-Typ", Pschiat. Neurol. Jpn. (Japan), 66: 892-931, 1964.

**Oda, M., Ejima, H., Abe, H., Ariga, T., Myatake, T. and Totsuka, S.**: Familial sudanophilic leukodystrophy with multiple and semisystematic spongy foci: Autopsy report of three adult females, Neuropatholgy (Japan), Suppl. 1., 173-185, 1981.

**Ohta, M., Koga, K., Tateishi, J., Motomura, S., Yamashita, Y., Kawanami, S., Oda, K. and Kuroiwa, Y.**: An autopsy case of spong form encephalopathy associated with kuru plaques and leukomalacia, Adv. Neurol. Sci. (Japan). 22: 484-496, 1977.

**Park, T. S., Kleinman, G. M. and Richardson, E. P.**: Creutzfeldt-Jakob disease with extensive degeneration of white matter, Acta Neuropath., 52: 239-242, 1980.

**Rao, C. V. G. K., Brenman, T. G. and Garcia, J. H.**: Computed tomography in the diagnosis of Creutzfeldt-Jakob disease, J. Comput. Assist. Tomogr., 1: 211, 1977.

162

Riku, S., Okamoto, T., Hashizume, Y., Koike, Y. and Sobue, I: Panencephalopathic type of Creutzfeldt-Jakob disease and special reference to its pyramidal tract degeneration, Clin. Neurol. (Japan), 23: 147-151, 1983.

Schoene, W. C. Masters, C. L., Gibs, C. J., Gajdusek, D. C., Tyler, H. R., Moore, F. D. and Dammin, G. J.: Transmissible spongiform encephalopathy (Creutzfeldt-Jakob disease) - Atypical and pathological findings, Arch. Neurol., 38: 473-477, 1981.

Shiraki, H. and Oda, M.: Neuropathology of hepatocerebral disease with emphasis on comparative studies, In: Pathology of the nervous system, ed. Minckler, J., McMraw-Hill, New York, Vol. 1, pp. 1089-1103, 1968.

Shiraki, H. and Mizutani, T.: Neuropathologic characteristics of types of Creutzfeldt-Jakob disease with special reference to the panencephalopathic type prevalent among Japanese, In: Neuropsychiatric disorders in the elderly, eds. Hirano, A. and Miyoshi, K., Igaku-Shoin, Tokyo, New York, pp. 139-188, 1983.

Silverman, J., Cravioto, H. and Feigin, I.: Cortico-striatal degeneration of the Creutzfeldt-Jakob type, J. Neuropathol. exp. Neurol., 20: 105-118, 1961.

Smith, J. K., Gonda, V. E. and Malamud, N.: Unusual form of cerebellar ataxia. Combined dentato-rubral and pallidoluysian degeneration, Neurology, 8: 205-209, 1958.

Suzuki, S., Tabira, T., Goto, I., Kuroiwa, Y. and Anraku, S.: A simple form of adult onset familial sudanophilic leukodystrophy manifesting pyramidal tract involvement and presenile dementia, Clin. Neurol. (Japan), 23: 32-37, 1983.

Tateishi, J., Ohta, M., Koga, M., Sato, Y. and Kuroiwa, Y.: Transmission of chronic spongiform encephalopathy, Ann. Neurol., 5: 581-584, 1979.

Tateishi, J., Koga, M., Sato, Y. and Mori, R.: Properties of the transmissible agent derived from chronic spongiform encephalopathy, Ann. Neurol., 7: 390-391, 1980.

Ueno, U., Akioda, T., Hayashi, M., Kimura, F., Shinoda, K., Fukuda, I., Mozai, T., Shibayama, T. and Nakada, K.: CT findings in the panencephalopathic type of Creutzfeldt-Jakob disease, Clin. Neurol. (Japan), 23: 902, 1983.

Vallat, J-M., Dumas, M., Corvisier, N., Leboutet, M-J., Loubet, A., Dumas, P. and Cathala, F.: Familial Creutzfeldt-Jakob disease with extensive degeneration of white matter, Ultrastructure of peripheral nerve, J. Neuorl. Sci., 61: 261-275, 1983.

Yakovlve, P. I.: Paraplegia in flexion of cerebral origin, J. Neuropathol. exp. Neurol., 13: 267, 1954.

Yokoi, S.: Neuropathological study of prefrontal lobotomy, J. Neuropathol. exp. Neurol., 16: 254-260, 1957.

# Chronic Spongiform Encephalopathy with Plaques Characterized by Antecedent and Longlasting Cerebellar Ataxia

Toshio Mizutani, M. D.

Kuru, kuru-like and/or senile plaques were not infrequently found in the cases of SSE, the clinical features of which were, as a rule, not different from those of SSE without plaques. Some cases with plaques, on the other hand, showed outstanding characteristic clinical features which could be differentiated from the other subtypes of CJD. A definite question as to whether this group should be considered a distinct subtype of CJD or a different entity from CJD still remains, to some extent to be decided, in the future, since there are only seven cases up to date and their pathological change were variable from case to case, despite an exceeding uniformity of their clinical features.

Nevertheless the reason why we describe this subtype of CJD in some detail here is that this group may occupy a critical point in regard with some relationship among types of CJD, particularly of the panencephalopathic type and Ohta's case (see Chapter III-6), Kuru and Gerstmann-Sträussler-Scheinker disease (GSSD) (Masters, et al., 1981; Mizutani, 1981b; Tateishi, et al., 1983; Kuzuhara, et al., 1983; Mizutani, et al., 1984). At the present moment, we designate tentatively this group as "Chronic spongiform encephalopathy with plaques characterized by antecedent and longlasting cerebellar ataxia".

## 1. Clinical Features

The number of the cases was 7, they comprised 5 males and 2 females. Three cases had a family history of neuropsychiatric disorders: spinal progressive muscular atrophy (Nakashima, et al., 1976, *No. 121*); schizophrenia (Kuroda, et al., 1977, *No. 123*); cerebellar ataxia (Nakamura, et al., 1979, *No. 124*; Iwabuchi, et al., 1983, *No. 126*). Hirano's case (1977, *No. 122*) was a daughter of Yoshimura's case (1982, 1984, *No. 125*) which showed similar pathological findings.    The age at death ranged from 29 to 66 years with average age of 53.    The total duration of illness was from 4 to 11 years and the average was 6 years.

The clinical course of this group could be divided into two different stages (Fig. 1A). The early or the first stage comprized the greatest part of the total duration of the illness and lasted for several years.    The onset of the disease at the most initial stage was usually insidious, as a rule: paresthesia and/or dysesthesia of the distal part of the limbs, which afterwards spread to the upper limbs frequently, were the initial symptoms or found in many cases.    The most characteristic feature at the early stage, on the other hand, was a gradual development of cerebellar and/or ataxic symptoms and signs.    Initially they were found only in the lower limbs leading to unsteady gait, but at the advanced stage there occurred ataxia of trunk and upper limbs.    As a consequence of these neurological disabilities, the patient was admitted to the hospital within two or three years from the onset.    Neurological examination revealed muscle weakness and atrophy and sensory disturbance of the limbs consistently combined with marked cerebellar signs.    Hypotonia and hyporeflexia were observed in five cases, although some of the other cases showed spasticity.    However, rigidity was never encountered at this stage.    Organic mental

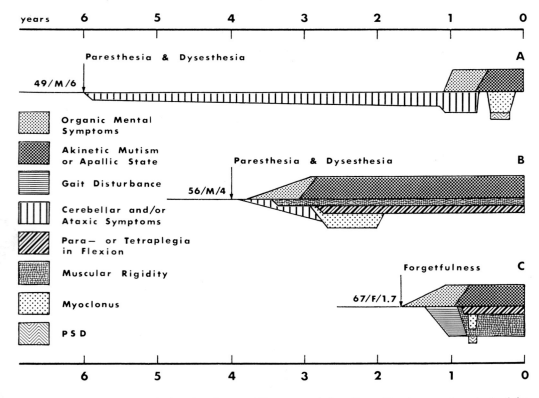

**Fig. 1.** Clinical courses of the chronic spongiform encephalopathy with plaques characterized by antecedent and longlasting cerebellar ataxia. Nakamura's case (A, *No. 124*), Ohta's case (B, *No. 89*) and Kodama's case (C, *No. 111*).    See Chapter III-6.

disturbance was occasionally found, but its degree was variable from case to case and, as a rule, to a lesser extent.    Thus, these clinical features resulted in a diagnosis of spinoce-rebellar degeneration (SCD), particularly when family history revealed hereditary degene-rative disorders.    As the disease progressed, the patient was gradually unable to stand or walk without assistance, and thus, became bedridden.    Simultaneously mental deteriora-tion also advanced, but its progress was different from case to case, although this was far less rapid than that in the other subtypes.    One or two years prior to death, cerebellar and/or ataxic symptoms were rapidly accelerated in most cases.

The terminal stage started with an appearance of rapid deterioration of mental state resulting in akinetic mutism or apallic state within a comparatively short period of time. Myoclonus also developed and PSD was recorded on EEG.    However, rigidity of muscles was not found in many cases.    At this terminal stage the diagnosis of CJD was first suspected or became definite later.    Akinetic mutism of this group was continued for one year or less and the patient died of intercurrent infection or generalized emaciation.

The marked cerebellar and/or ataxic disturbance of this group are compatible with those in the ataxic form of CJD and also in SCD, although the length of the total duration and the clinical evolution are quite different. At the early stage of the panencephalopathic type, on the other hand, ataxia was slight or absent even when the cerebellum of all cases was, as a rule, severely or most severely affected as revealed by postmortem examination (100% in the chronic spongiform encephalopathy with ataxia and plaques and 27% in the panencephalopathic type).    In the panencephalopathic type the precise nature of so-called gait disturbance was obscure, while most cases of this group distinctly showed ataxic gait. Rigidity was found only 2 out of 7 cases (29%) in this group, while 72% in all cases of CJD and 71% in the panencephalopathic type (see Appendix).    As mentioned before (see Chapter III-6), one can assume that because of slight or negative rigidity in this group, ataxia was apparently observed even at the later stage.    Rapid deterioration and nature of mental state at the terminal stage was similar or almost identical to that at the early stage of the panencephalopathic type.    Myoclonus with PSD on EEG, one of the most characteristic features of CJD, was frequently found.    Therefore, this group could reasonably be understood within the spectrum of CJD, although the main feature particu-larly at the early stage could be comparable with SCD.    Finally high frequencies of paresthesia and/or dysesthesia were frequently found at the initial stage, although they were occasionally noticed in the other subtypes.

## 2. Neuropathological Findings

Brain weight ranged from 1180 to 890 g and the average was 1068 g.    Cerebral atrophy was pronounced, but the cortical ribbon was not so reduced in width as that in the panencephalopathic type (Fig. 2A).    The thalamus became atrophic and the ventricular system was markedly dilated, while the striatum and globus pallidus showed less severe atrophy.    The cerebral white matter showed brownish discoloration, and cystic cavita-tions in various sizes were occasionally scattered, particularly pronounced in Hirano's case.    It was remarked that the brainstem and cerebellum showed no obvious atrophy in some cases, although they became conspicuously atrophic in other cases. In these cases with severe atrophy of the brainstem the pontine tegmentum also showed atrophy.

Kuru and/or kuru-like plaques were the consistent finding in this group. They were eosinophilic, PAS-positive, argentophilic and congophilic (Figs. 3, 6A & B). The central cores showed a single dot or often the clusters of coarse granules of various sizes but surrounding tissues never disclosed neuritic alterations nor reactive astrocyes (Fig. 3). Some single cores had clear-cut radiation (Fig. 3C). Ultrastructurally these plaques were composed of tubular filaments of 7 - 10 nm in diameter, which was considered to be amyloid filament. Coarse dense granule of 15 - 100 nm in diameter were scattered between the tubular filaments (Ohta, et al., 1978). Multiple kuru plaques were widespread in the central nervous system including the cerebral cortex, basal ganglia, thalamus (Fig. 4B), and even cerebral white matter, but most frequently in the cerebellar cortex, particularly in the molecular layer (Fig. 6A). In some cases they were found in the nuclei of the brainstem.

In the cerebral cortex spongy microcavities of small sizes were disseminated, irrespective of gyral crowns and depths of sulci (Fig. 2D). Spongy degeneration occurred mainly in the third or more deeper layers, but not infrequently in the lower part of the molecular layer and in the second layer. Astrocytes became conspicuously hypertrophic and proliferated, while fibrillary gliosis was not outstanding (Fig. 2E). Neuronal loss was obvious in the sponginously degenerated cortex, but less severe in contrast with marked spongy state in the neuropil (Fig. 2B). The remaining neurons, particularly in the deeper layers showed inflation (Figs. 2C & D). Fat granule cells were rather rare. The cortical lesion was more or less widespread, but never predominant in the visual cortex of the occipital lobe. The parahippocampal cortex was severely damaged, while the hippocampus showed only minor changes.

The change of the white matter ranged from slight loss of myelin to microcavitaion (Fig. 2A). The lesions occurred diffusely in the centrum semiovale and corpus callosum, but the internal capsule was seldom affected. There occurred loss of myelin and axon, hypertrophy and proliferation of astrocytes, and fatty degradation. Fibrillary gliosis was pronounced in the cases with involvement of the white matter (Fig. 2E), while it was absent or slight in the panencephalopathic type. In all cases of this group there was no evidence of circumscribed spongy necrotic foci in the digital white matter. Two cases showed no obvious changes in the cerebral white matter (*Nos. 123 and 127*).

The striatum showed slight or even absent change: mild neuronal loss with slight spongy state and astrocytic proliferation in the caudate and putamen in some cases; no obvious loss of nerve cells in the others (Fig. 4A). The thalamus, on the other hand, showed severe neuronal loss accompanied by fibrillary gliosis (Fig. 4B). The remaining

---

**Fig. 2. A:** Diffuse loss of myelin in the frontal white matter. **B:** Slight loss of cortical neurons and inflation of neurons (arrows) in the insular cortex. × 100. **C:** Inflated neuron with thickened axon (arrows). × 500. **D:** Diffuse and fine spongy state in the entire cortical layers except for the molecular layer, proliferation of astrocytes and plaques (arrows). Insular cortex. × 40. **E:** Fibrillary gliosis in the subcortical white matter, and in the molecular layer of the rectal cortex. (A: Woelke; B & C: Nissl; D: H-E; E: Holzer)

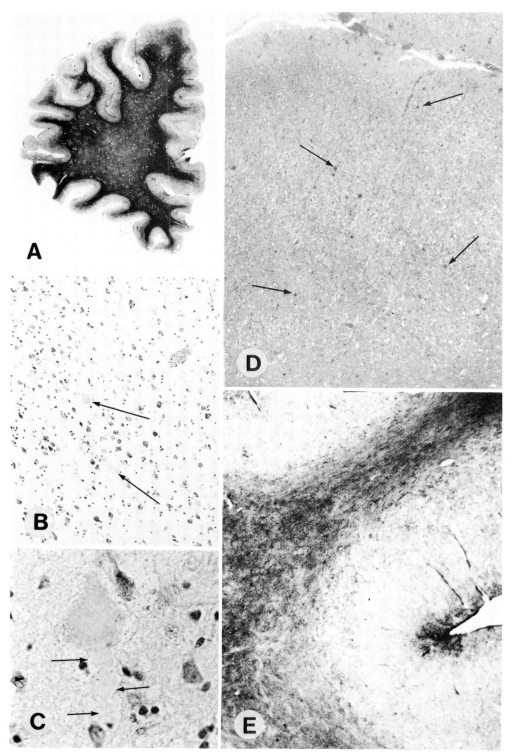

Fig. 2

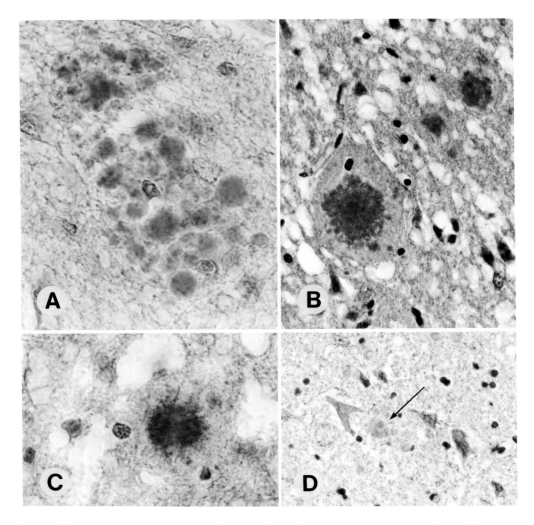

**Fig. 3.** Different aspects of plaques. **A:** Plaque with multiple cores in the molecular layer of the insular cortex. × 1000. **B:** Multicentric plaque in the insular cortex. **C:** Plaque with radiation in the insular cortex. × 1000. **D:** Multicentric plaque in the ventral postero-lateral nucleus of the thalamus. × 500. (A & C: Congo red; B & D: H-E)

neurons occasionally showed inflation. The changes were completely symmetrical and bilateral. The preferential localization of the lesion in the thalamic subnuclei was almost identical to that in the panencephalopathic type (Fig. 5A). In Nakamura's case there occurred axonal swellings in the ventral postero-lateral and postero-medial nuclei. The subthalamus occasionally showed conspicuous fibrillary gliosis, but neuronal loss was variable from case to case.

The substantia nigra and red nucleus frequently showed fibrillary gliosis with or without neuronal loss, but no neuronal vacuolation was found there. Severe degeneration in the pontine nuclei and transverse fibers was found in some cases, while not in the others. In the case with severe involvement of the pontine base, degeneration occurred in the middle cerebellar peduncle and cerebellar white matter. The pontine tegmentum disclosed marked atrophy with fibrillary gliosis in variable degrees. The inferior olivary nucleus revealed slight to severe loss of nerve cells with fibrillary gliosis. Inflated neurons were occasionally found, but a distinct olivary hypertrophy was not observed (Fig. 6E). The restiform body was degenerated in three cases.

In the cerebellum, typical cortical degeneration of granule cell type was found in Hirano's case. Nakashima's case showed conspicuous loss of Purkinje cells with proliferation of Bergmann's glia, while loss of the granule cells was less severe. The distribution of the lesion in these three cases was diffuse and symmetrical, irrespective of paleo- and neocerebellum. In Kuroda's and Nakamura's cases, on the other hand, no obvious loss of Purkinje cells was found and the granule cells were slightly depleted (Fig. 6A), while fibrillary gliosis occurred in the vermis and flocculus. The cerebellar white matter change ranged from slight gliosis in the subcortical white matter to marked degeneration

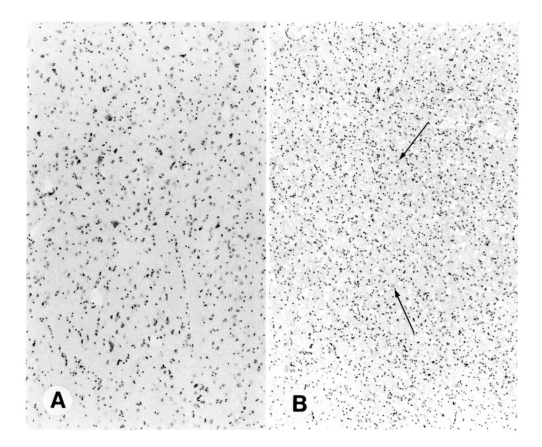

**Fig. 4.** **A:** No obvious loss of neurons with astrocytic proliferation in the putamen. × 100. **B:** Severe neuronal loss, marked proliferation of astrocytes and plaques (arrows) in the ventral lateral nucleus of the thalamus. × 100. (A: Nissl; B: H-E).

in the deeper white matter accompainied by fat granule cell mobilization and fibrillary gliosis. The cortical changes were roughly in parallel with the white matter change. The dentate nucleus disclosed slight to severe loss of neuron and fibrillary gliosis in three cases (Fig. 6C). Some of the remaining neurons showed grumose alteration which were identified in the H-E preparation (Fig. 6D). Degeneration was found in the brachium conjunctivum in one case.

The corticospinal tract degeneration occurred in three cases, while the spinocerebellar tract showed degeneration in four cases. The posterior column degeneration was found in three cases. Nakamura's case showed inflation of the anterior horn cells, while Iwabuchi's case disclosed widespread distribution of inflated cells in the brainstem motor nuclei and anterior horn. The posterior root ganglion was not examined.

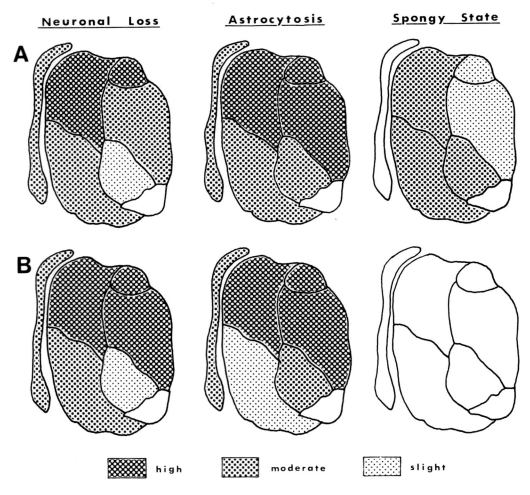

**Fig. 5.** Schematic distribution of the lesions in the thalamus. A: *No. 124*; B: *No. 111* (see Chapter III-6).

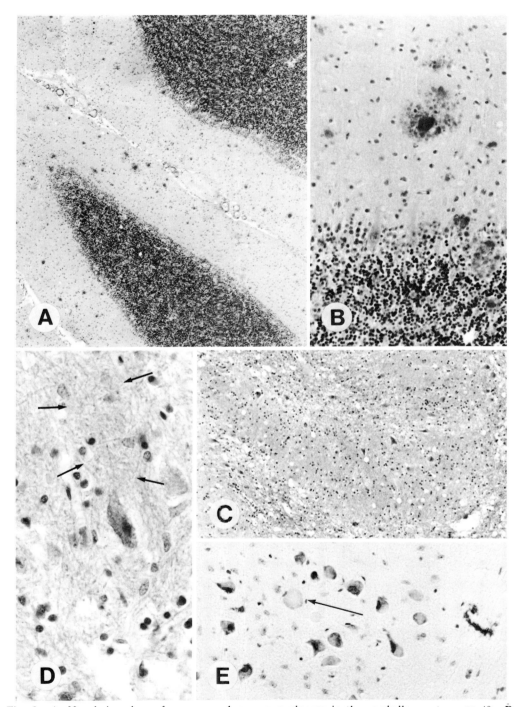

**Fig. 6.   A:** No obvious loss of neurons and numerous plaques in the cerebellar cortex.   × 40.   **B:** Multicentric plaques with or without central core in the molecular layer of the cerebellar cortex.   × 200. **C:** Slight to moderate loss of neurons in the dentate nucleus.   × 100.   **D:** Grumose alteration of neuron in the dentate nucleus.   × 500.   **E:** Inflated neuron in the inferior olive (arrow).   No obvious loss of neurons.   × 250.   (A, C & D: H-E;   B: Congo red;   E: Nissl)

# 3. Discussion

The chronic spongiform encephalopathy with plaques characterized by antecedent and longlasting cerebellar ataxia showed a relative uniformity of clinical features. It could be comparable with that of SCD in several aspects: very long duration lasting for seveal years; progressive cerebellar and/or ataxic symptoms and signs; slight or even absent rigidity; hereditary or familial tendency. In SCD and Kuru, on the other hand, mental deterioration resulting in apallic state or akinetic mutism was never found, even at the terminal stage. Myoclonus and PSD were not found in SCD.

The neuropathological findings, on the other hand, were not uniform, although there were the essential features of CJD, such as spongy state, neuronal loss and astrocytosis without any fibrillary gliosis. The nature of the white matter change in both cerebrum and cerebellum was variable from case to case. In Hirano's and Nakashima's cases the white matter lesion could be regarded as a primary change, while in Nakamura's case this was not so conspicuous, and Kuroda's case disclosed no change. Furthermore, the cortical damage in the cerebellum was not uniform in nature, degree and distribution in all cases. Nevertheless, multisystemic degeneration in the brainstem and spinal cord combined with thalamic degeneration were more consistently found out.

CJD with kuru or kuru-like plaques have been identified in various types of CJD, except for the simple poliodystrophic type. It is certain that the presence of kuru plaques comprizes one of the characteristics of Kuru, but the most essential feature of Kuru exists in a close combination of its clinical feature to its neuropathology. Kuru is a subacute progressive cerebellar ataxia, while dementia remains to be slight even at the terminal stage and apallic state is never found (Hornabrook, 1968). The main neuropathology is a combined system degeneration in the cerebellum, brainstem and spinal cord (Klatzo, et al., 1958). Shiraki emphasized that the most significant neuropathology of Kuru could be considered to be multisystemic degeneration comparable mainly with olivopontocerebellar atrophy (OPCA) (1974, see Chapter III-8). Unfortunately the significance of system degeneration has been overlooked or less evaluated in the essential neuropathology not only of Kuru but also of CJD. However, as mentioned before, it was convincing that system degeneration is one of the essential features of CJD (see Chapter III-6). This is also true in the group presented here. This group could be linked with Kuru by the clinicopathological similarites rather than by the presence of kuru plaques, except for a difference of age at the onset of the illness which will be discussed elsewhere (see Chapter III-8). Therefore, it is reasonable that Kuroda's and Tomi's cases are also in the spectrum of this group, despite that they showed no obvious lesion in the cerebral white matter.

The conspicuous deterioration of the cerebral cortex responsible for akinetic mutism of this group disclosed the most differential point from the absence of akinetic mutism in Kuru. This could also be pointed out in Gerstmann-Sträussler syndrome (GSS) including the cases with ataxia, dementia and massive multiform plaques in the brain with or without cerebral spongiform changes (Masters, et al., 1981). Prior to discussing GSS, the original Gerstmann-Sträussler-Scheinker's disease (GSSD) should be taken into considera-

tion (Gerstmann, et al., 1936).  The main features of the disorder included the disturbances reminiscent of OPCA and dementia, in which its neuropathology showed the
systemic atrophies involving mainly the spinal cord, brainstem and cerebellum together
with the massive, unusual plaque-like deposits of kuru-like, multicentric, senile and
primitive types widespread in both the cerebellum and cerebrum (Braunmühl, 1954;
Seitelberger, 1961).  It, however, should be emphasized that apallic state or akinetic
mutism, and pathological changes responsible for this clinical feature were never found in
GSSD.  Reviewing the original Austrian familial cases, Seitelberger concluded that GSSD
may be a heredodegenerative disease and that the clinical and neuropathological similarities of GSSD to Kuru and CJD are only superficial (1981).  In the Masters' series, on the
other hand, both Nakamura's case (1979, No. 124) and Matsuoka's case (1970, No. 27)
were included.  However, clinical and/or neuropathological features of both cases are
different obviously from GSSD (Matsuoka's case is discussed in Chapter III-3).  Moreover, the animal experiments so far failed to produce spongiform encephalopathy with
brain specimens from patients with GSSD (Masters, et al., 1981).  On the other hand,
Hirano's and Tateishi's cases were transmitted successfully to animals.  In the lack of
evidence that GSSD is a transmissible disorder, this unusual disease, in which no spongiform encephalopathy in true sense of words was identified, should clinicopathologically be
excluded from this group of CJD (Kuzuhara, et al., 1983; Mizutani, et al., 1984).

In most cases of this group multisystemic degeneration appeared to be more pronounced than cerebellar involvement.  In Nakamura's case, both spinocerebellar tract degeneration and cerebello-cortical degeneration were slight in degree, in spite of marked
cerebellar symptoms, and thus, ataxia may be rather attributable to multisystemic
degeneration in the spinal cord and brainstem.  It is still unknown what kind of role kuru
plaques in the cerebellum can play in cerebellar ataxia.

Although spongy degeneration in CJD and Kuru can be transmissible to experimental
animals, system degeneration, one of the most essential clinicopathological features of
Kuru and CJD, has not been reproduced at least up to date.

## Summary

1) The question as to whether the chronic spongiform encephalopathy could be a distinct
subtype of CJD or a different entity from CJD still remains in the future, since the
neuropathology of only seven cases varied from case to case, despite an exceeding
unformity of their clinical features.
2) It should be remarked that this group may occupy a critical point in regard with some
relationship among CJD, Kuru and Gerstmann-Sträussler-Scheinker disease.

## Acknowledgement

We wish to thank Prof.  Anraku, Kurume University for permission to study the
clinical data and necropsy materials.

# REFERENCES

**Braumühl, von A. V.**: Über eine eigenartige hereditär-familiäre Erkrankung des Zentralnerven-systems, Arch. Psychiatr. Z. Neurol., 191: 419-449, 1954.

**Gerstmann, J., Sträussler, E. and Scheinker, I.**: Über eine eigenartige hereditär-familiäre Erkrankung des Zentralnervensystems: zugleich ein Beitrag zur Frage des vorzeitigen lokalen Alterns, Z. Ges. Neurol. Psychiatr., 154: 736-762, 1936.

**Hirano, T., Tsuchiyama, H., Kawai, K. and Mori, K.**: An autopsy case of Creutzfeldt-Jakob disease with kuru-like neuropathological changes, Acta Path. Jpn., 27: 231-238, 1977.

**Hornabrook, R. W.**: Kuru - a subacute cerebellar degeneration. The natural history and clinical features, Brain, 91: 53-74, 1968.

**Iwabuchi, K., Nakano, T., Sakai, H., Yagishita, S., Amano, N. and Yokoi, S.**: An autopsy case of Creutzfeldt-Jakob disease with amyloid plaques, cell - protein dissociation in CSF and manifold findings on EEG, Neuropathol. (Japan), 4: 157, 1983.

**Klatzo, I., Gajdusek, D. C. and Zigas, V.**: Pathology of Kuru, Lab. invest., 8: 799-847, 1959.

**Kuroda, S., Morisada, A., Tateishi, J., Fukui, H. and Hosokawa, K.**: A necropsy case of progressive ataxia ending in apallic state with kuru plaques, Brain & Nerves (Japan), 29: 301-306, 1977.

**Kuzuhara, S., Kanazawa, I., Sasaki, H., Nakanishi, T. and Shimamura, K.**: Gerstmann-Sträussler-Scheinker's disease, Ann. Neurol., 14: 216-225, 1983.

**Masters, C. L., Gajdusek, D. C., and Gibbs, C. J. Jr.**: Creutzfeldt-Jakob disease virus isolations from the Gerstmann-Sträussler syndrome with an analysis of the various forms of amyloid plaque deposition in the virus-induced spongiform encephalopthies, Brain, 104: 559-588, 1981.

**Matsuoka, T., Hamanaka, T., Taii, S., Tatebayashi, Y., Kijima, S. and Nishikawa, T.**: Subacute spongiform encephalopathy as a subtype of Creutzfeldt-Jakob disease - Report of two cases, Psychiat. Neurol. Jpn., 72: 669-680, 1970.

**Mizutani, T.**: Neuropathology of Creutzfeldt-Jakob disease in Japan: With special reference to the panencephalopathic type, Acta Path. Jpn., 31: 903-922, 1981.

**Mizutani, T., Morimatsu, Y. and Shiraki, H.**: Clinical pictures of Creutzfeldt-Jakob disease based on 97 autopsy cases in Japan - With special reference to clinicopathological correlation of cerebellar symptoms, Clin. Neurol. (Japan), 24: 23-32, 1984.

**Nakamura, T., Takamatsu, I., Shida, K., Kotorii, K., Anraku, S. and Kida, H.**: A case of subacute spongiform encephalopathy with numerous kuru-plaques in the cerebral and cerebellar cortices, Adv. Neurol. Sci. (Japan), 23: 484-492, 1979.

**Nakashima, K., Makino, T., Kinoshita, J. and Yagishita, S.**: A peculiar case of panen-cephalopathy with widespread distribution of plaques, status spongiosus and demyelination, Adv. Neurol. Sci. (Japan), 20: 362-371, 1976.

**Ohta, M., Koga, M., Tateishi, J., Motomura, S., Yamashita, Y., Kawanami, S., Oda, K, and Kuroiwa, Y.**: An autopsy report of spongiform encephalopathy associated with kuru plaque and leukomalacia, Adv. Neurol. Sci. (Japan), 22: 487-496, 1978.

**Seitelberger, F.**: Eigenartige familiär-hereditäre Krankheit des Zentralnervensystems in einer niederösterreichischen Sippe, Wien Klin. Wochenschr., 41/42: 687-691, 1961.

**Seitelberger, F.**: Sträussler's disease, Acta Neuropathol. (Suppl), 7: 341-343, 1981.

**Shiraki, H.**: The neuropathological background of Creutzfeldt-Jakob disease (Creutzfeldt-Jakob syndrome), Adv. Neurol. Sci. (Japan), 18: 4-30, 1974.

**Tateishi, J., Sato, Y. and Ohta, M.**: Creutzfeldt-Jakob disease in humans and laboratory animals, In: Progress in Neuropathology, ed. Zimmerman, H. M., Raven Press, New York, Vol. 5, pp. 195-221, 1983.

**Tomi, H., Haruhara, N., Mukoyama, M., Ando, K. and Satoyoshi, E.**: An autopsy case of spongiform encephalopathy with longlasting cerebellar signs, Clin. Neurol. (Japan), 23: 617, 1983.

**Yoshimura, T., Muro, T., Sato, S., Ide, Y., Mori, M., Tsujihata, M., Takamori, M., Nagataki, S. and Tateishi, J.**: A case of Creutzfeldt-Jakob disease in a family, Clin. Neurol. (Japan), 22: 89, 1982.

**Yoshimura, T., Tateishi, J., Tsujihata, M., Muro, T., Mameya, G. and Nagataki, S.**: A case of spongiform encephalopathy with ataxia and amyloid plaques, Brain & Nerves (Japan), 36: 789-795, 1984.

# Kuru in New Guinea

Hirotsugu Shiraki, M. D.

In the occasion in which one of the authors (Shiraki) was the Chairman of the Session of Amyotrophic Lateral Sclerosis, Dementia-Parkinsonism Complex and Kuru in Western Pacific Islands at the Fifth International Congress of Neuropathology, Zürich, 1965, the author had had an opportunity to examine the original slides of kuru in New Guinea. The author is particularly grateful to Dr. Klatzo, Department of Neuropathology, NINDB, Bethesda, for permission to examine his materials on kuru.

Although the clinicoepidemiologic characteristics of kuru, for example, incidence, age distribution, sex ratio, clinical appearance and prognosis, have changed during the past decade, the disease is still showing some trends away from its current status in this regards.

## 1. Clinical and Epidemiological Features

The basic clinicoepidemiologic characteristics as determined at the initial stage of investigations (Klatzo, et al., 1961) could be summarized as follows:

The disease originally affected only the Fore natives, who lived in an isolated region located in the highlands of the northeastern part of New Guinea. Kuru began during chilhood, at about five years of age, and developed gradually through adolescence until early adult years.

The sex ratio among affected native who had a high familial incidence of the disease was almost equal before adolescence; thereafter, cases were much more common among women than among men. The course of the illness was short, and affected persons usually died six to nine months after the onset of symptoms.

The illness ran afebrile course, beginning invariably with insidious onset of ataxia, which progressively worsened, and a distinctive tremor, involving the trunk, limbs and head, developed. Then, ataxia and tremor became outstanding, usually within one month after the onset of symptoms. These manifestations rapidly became more severe, and within a few months, victims of illness were no longer able to walk or even stand. Subsequently, dysarthria, incontinence, convergent strabismus, hyperactive or hypoactive (or both grades of) deep-tendon reflexes pathological reflexes, dysphagia, decubiti and other signs and symptoms appeared one after another, but the cerebellar signs and symptoms were most pronounced until death. Affected persons usually died in a cachectic state, mainly as a result of dysphagic impairment.

During the clinical course of the illness, psychiatric disturbances, on the other hand, were restricted to marked emotionalism and frequently a tendency toward euphoria.

## 2. Neuropathological Features

Although the neuropathological characteristics of kuru varied from case to case, the following findings were most prominent:

Disintegration of nerve cells was most pronounced in the inferior olivary and pontine nuclei (Figs. 2c & 2d), followed by the cerebellar granular layer (Fig. 1a & 1b), dentate nucleus (Fig. 1e), striatum (Fig. 4b), certain thalamic subnuclei (Fig. 4c), substantia nigra and red nucleus. In addition, the surviving nerve cells in these nuclei occasionally contained one or several vacuoles in their cytoplasm (Figs. 1f, 3c, 4b & 4e). Nerve cells in the cerebral cortex, however, either did not show vacuoles or their presence was questionable (Fig. 5a).

Fine, sieve-like tissue disruption, mainly of an isolated character, was severe in the striatum and thalamic subnuclei (Figs. 4b & 4c) and was less marked in the substantia nigra (Fig. 4a) and cerebellar molecular layer (Fig. 1c), in which torpedoes were clustered or sporadically disseminated (Fig. 1b). Sponginess in the cerebral cortex, however, was only of slight to at least moderate severity (Fig. 5a).

Astrocytosis and fibrillary gliosis with thin gliofibers was most pronounced in the inferior olivary nucleus and bases of the pontine nuclei (Figs. 2a & 2e), followed by the anterior horn of the spinal cord (Fig. 3b) striatum (Fig. 4b), thalamus (Figs. 4c and 4d), cerebellar granular layer and vestibular (Fig. 2e) and dentate nuclei (Fig. 1e), and reticular formation of the brainstem (Fig. 3c). There was a mild astrocytosis in the cerebral cortex in which thin gliofibers were absent (Fig. 5b).

Typical kuru plaques, on the other hand, were most commonly seen in the paleocerebellar and neocerebellar cortex (Figs. 1c and 1d), followed by the striatum and thalamus; these plaques were rarely found in the cerebral cortex (Fig. 5b).

Certain forms of systemic degeneration, for example, distal-dominant degeneration with myelin pallor without fibrillary gliosis, occurred in the corticospinal, posterior and dorsal and ventral spinocerebellar tracts at the level of the spinal cord as well (Figs. 3a & 3b). In most cases, the degeneration of the corticospinal tract at the spinal level could be traced up to the level of the medulla oblongata (Fig. 2c). Moreover, these changes were in most cases symmetric and occurred bilaterally.

178

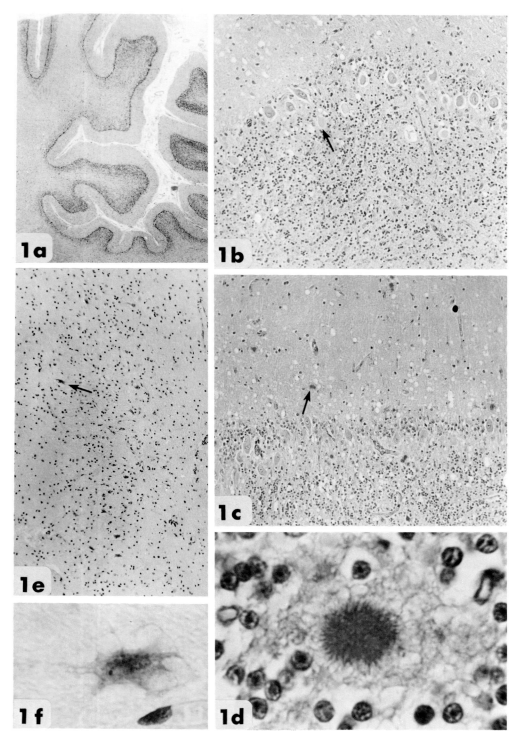

**Fig. 1** (Legend in page 183)

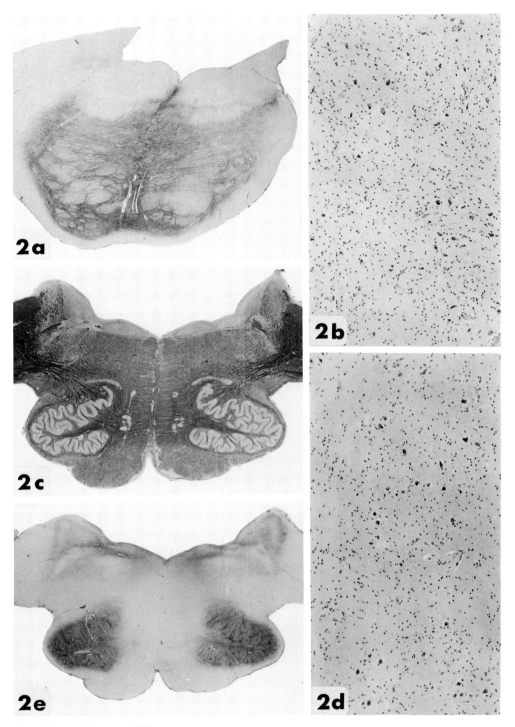

**Fig. 2** (Legend in page 183)

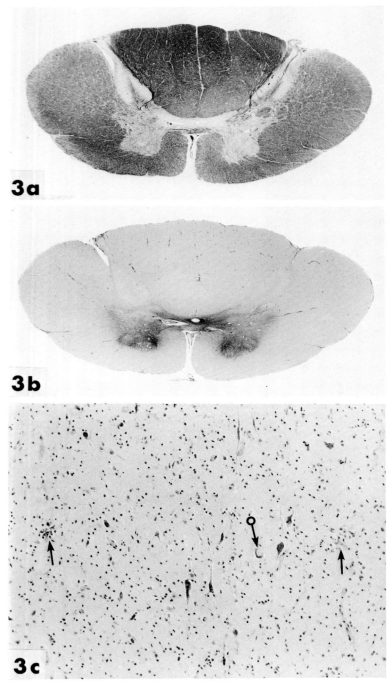

**Fig. 3** (Legend in page 183)

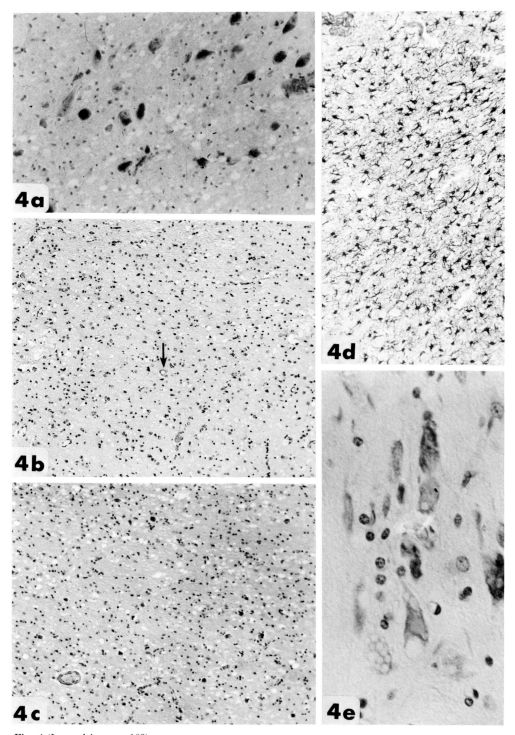

**Fig. 4** (Legend in page 183)

182

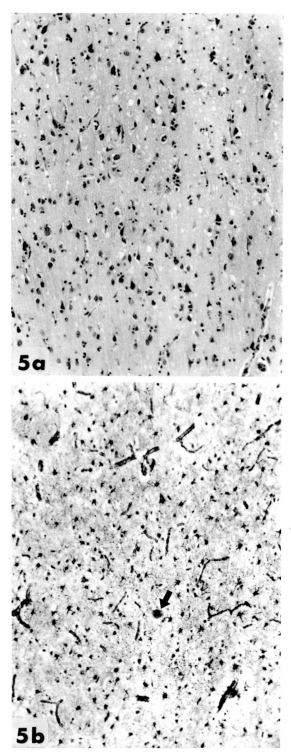

Fig. 5 (Legend in page 183)

**Fig. 1.** Kuru in New Guinea.  a, e and f: case NA-39-58;   b, c and d: case NA-145-57.

**(a)** Neocerebellum; slight to high disintegration of the granular layer in all foliae and comparatively good preservation of Purkinje cells.   × 11.5.   **(b)** Magnified neocerebellum; moderately disintegrated granule cells, good preservation of Purkinje cells accompanied by a proliferation of the Bergmann's glial nuclei and a number of the torpedos, one example indicated by the arrow.   × 130.   **(c)** Magnified neocerebellum; similar to (b); a number of the kuru plaques in both the granular and molecular layers, one example indicated by the arrow; fine, sieve-like tissue disruption in both the molecular and granular layers.   × 175.   **(d)** Highly magnified kuru plaque in the molecular layer in (c).   × 1300.   **(e)** Cerebellar dentate nucleus; severely disintegrated nerve cells and diffusely proliferated glial nuclei in the parenchyma.   × 89.   **(f)** Magnified nerve cell indicated by the arrow in (e); multiple vacuoles in the cytoplasm of the darkly shrunken nerve cell.   × 1100.   [(a), (e) & (f): Thionine;   (b), (c) & (d): PAS]

---

**Fig. 2.** Kuru in New Guinea.  a: case NA-185-57;   b: case NA-186-57;   c and e: case NA-27-58;   d: case NA-39-58.

**(a)** Pons; moderate to intense gliosis symmetrically and bilaterally, and restricted to the pontine basis and median raphe.   × 3.5.   **(b)** Magnified pontine nuclei; moderately to highly disintegrated nerve cells and widespread activation of glial nuclei.   × 89.   **(c)** Middle portion of the medulla oblongata; slight pallor symmetrically and bilaterally in the pyramidal tract.   × 6.0.   **(d)** Magnified inferior olivary nucleus; moderately to highly disintegrated nerve cells and widespread activation of glial nuclei.   × 86.   **(e)** Same section as in (c); slight to intense gliosis symmetrically and bilaterally in the inferior olivary nucleus and adjacent white matter, cuneate nucleus, fourth ventricular base and elsewhere.   × 5.0.   [(a) & (e): Holzer;   (b) & (d): Thionine;   (c): Woelcke myelin]

---

**Fig. 3.** Kuru in New Guinea.  a and b: case NA-27-58;   c: case NA-39-58.

**(a)** Cervical cord; ill-defined, slight pallor symmetrically and bilaterally in the lateral and anterior corticospinal tracts, dorsal and ventral spinocerebellar tracts, and the deep portion of the posterior tracts.   × 9.0.   **(b)** Same section as in (a); moderate to intense gliosis restricted to the bilateral anterior and lateral horns, and commissure.   × 9.0.   **(c)** Magnified reticular formation of the midbrain; two tiny glial nodules indicated by the arrows and diffuse activation of glial nuclei in the parenchyma; the arrow with zero indicates intracytoplasmic vacuolar formation of the pyramidal cell.   × 120.   [(a): Woelcke myelin;   (b): Holzer;   (c): Thionine]

---

**Fig. 4.** Kuru in New Guinea.  a: case NA-39-58;   b and e: case NA-27-58;   c: case NA-145-57;   d: case NA-185-57.

**(a)** Magnified compact zone of the substantia nigra; good preservation of the pigmented cells and fine, sieve-like tissue disruption in the parenchyma.   × 200.   **(b)** Middle portion of the putamen; more or less disintegrated nerve cells of both small and large types, pronounced astrocytosis in the parenchyma and fine, sieve-like tissue disruption; the arrow indicates a single large vacuole in the cytopalsm of the nerve cell of large type.   × 115.   **(c)** Dorsal portion of the lateral nucleus of the thalamus; pronounced, fine, sieve-like tissue disruption, proliferation of glial nuclei in the parenchyma, and comparatively good preservation of nerve cells.   × 115.   **(d)** Magnified anterior nucleus of the thalamus; conspicuous astrocytosis with a coarse gliofiber formation.   × 97.   **(e)** Magnified intralaminar nucleus of the thalamus; single or multiple vacuoles in the cytoplasm of a great majority of the nerve cells; activated astrocytic nuclei in the adjacent parenchyma.   × 600.   [(a), (b) & (c): H-E;   (d): Cajal's gold sublimate; (e): Thionine]

---

**Fig. 5.** Kuru in New Guinea.  a: case NA-145-57;   b: case NA-1-58.

**(a)** Deep layers of the insular cortex; fine, sieve-like tissue disruption only in slight degree and good preservation of the nerve cells.   × 130.   **(b)** Almost same region as in (a); far less pronounced astrocytosis; the arrow indicates an argentophilic kuru plaque.   × 97.   [(a): H-E;   (b): Cajal's gold sublimate]

# 3. Discussion

As a consequence, the typical clinical pictures and course of kuru consisted of cerebellar degeneration with a progressively downhill course. Psychiatric disturbances did not progress beyond marked emotionalism or euphoria. Thus, the neurologic disturbances overshadowed their psychiatric counterparts.

The most basic neuropathologic abnormality in kuru, on the other hand, was olivopontocerebellar atrophy more or less complicated with some systemic degeneration of spinal cord, coexisting with spongy tissue disruption, astrocytosis, kuru plaques and intracytoplasmic vacuolar formation of neurons. The foci of these changes, however, were preferentially localized in the thalamus, basal ganglia, brainstem and cerebellum. Among them, the cerebellar lesions were most pronounced, whereas the pallidonigral system in some cases showed no foci and in other cases foci of only mild severity. Thus, involvement of the extrapyramidal system and cerebral cortex were never severe enough to overshadow the cerebellar signs and symptoms, as just seen in the ataxic type of CJD. Moreover, the cerebral cortex and white matter in cases of kuru was unaffected or affected only slightly, even when thalamic subnuclei of ontogenetically recent origin were involved. Thus, severe psychiatric disturbances, such as an apallic state or akinetic mutism, never occurred, and more marked emotionalism or euphoria remained the most severe psychiatric disturbance.

Microscopic examination of each lesion from the different cases of kuru, however, revealed an appearance identical to those of the other types of CJD, namely, the subacute spongiform encephalopathy, ataxic type, panencephalopathic type and others. On the other hand, comparison of the distributions of the foci in various types of CJD demonstrated distinct differences between kuru and other types of CJD in regard of distribution of major foci.

For instance, the major foci in kuru were severe and extensive, but in general were restricted to the diencephalon, brainstem and cerebellum, whereas foci were less severe in the cerebral cortex, and none were found in the cerebral white matter. In the subacute spongiform encephalopathy, ataxic type and others, on the other hand, the major foci were most severe or usually severe in the cerebral cortex in every case that were studied, whereas the foci were also most severe in the cerebral white matter in the panencephalopathic type of CJD.

On the surface, therefore, it might appear that the underlying disease process in kuru could be differentiated from the underlying process in Creutzfeldt-Jakob disease, particularly on the basis of the difference in age at onset of each disease; kuru most often beginning during childhood and affecting all age groups until young adulthood, whereas Creutzfeldt-Jakob disease primary affecting middle-aged and older persons.

Nevertheless, in fact, experiments, in which spongy tissue disruption and astrocytosis accompanied by neuronal disintegration in kuru as well as in Creutzfeldt-Jakob disease could be transmitted from human being to animals and from animals to animals (Gibbs, et al., 1968; Tateishi, et al., 1979), demonstrated the probability of a common underlying process in kuru and different types of Creutzfeldt-Jakob disease.

In other words, kuru could be interpreted as an infantile, childhood and young adult form of Creutzfeldt-Jakob disease, and the different type of the latter could correspond to the adult, presenile and senile stages of the disease.  In any case, it can reasonably be assumed that these different diseases comprized all forms of Creutzfeldt-Jakob disease group (Fig. 6).

This assumption was actually based on other observations from, for example, cases of Japanese encephalitis and complications after vaccination against smallpox and neuroaxonal dystrophies, in which, regardless of the nature of the disease and the age at onset, preferential localization and shifts of major foci in general ran parallel to the progression of maturation of the central nervous system from spinal cord to cerebrum with age (Flechsig, 1920; Yakovlev & Lecour, 1967).  This observation and explanation have been discussed in greater detail elsewhere (Shiraki, 1981).

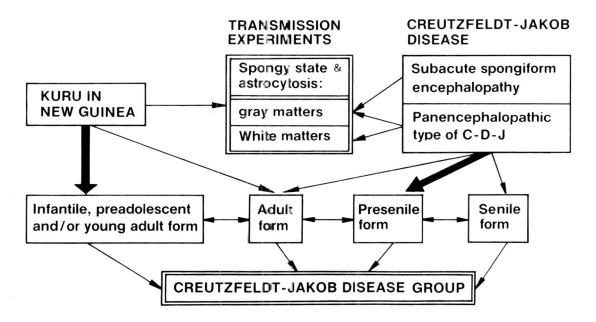

**Fig. 6.** Schematic diagrams of the relationship of kuru in New Guinea to the different types of Creutzfeldt-Jakob disease in human beings as determined from the results of transmission experiments in animals.
(From: Neuropsychiatric Disorders in the Elderly, eds., Hirano, A. & Miyoshi, K., Igaku-Shoin, 1983, with permission)

# REFERENCES

**Flechsig, P.**: Rindenfelder-Gliederung des menschlichen Gehirns auf myelogenetischer Grundlage, Georg Thieme, Leipzig, 1920.

**Gibbs, C. J. Jr., Gajdusek, D. C., Asher, D. M., Alpers, M. P., Beck, E., Daniel, P. M. and Matthews, W. B.**: Creutzfeldt-Jakob disease (subacute spongiform encephalopathy): Transmission to the chimpanzee, Science, 161: 388-389, 1968.

**Klatzo, I., Gajdusek, D. C. and Zigas, V.**: Evaluation of pathological findings in twelve cases of kuru, In: Encephalitides, eds. Van Bogaert, L., et al., Elsevier, Amsterdam, London, New York, Princeton, pp. 172-190, 1961.

**Shiraki, H.**: The complications of nervous system following various vaccinations, Immunol. Dis. (Japan), 2: 351-370, 1981.

**Tateishi, J., Ohta, M., Koga, M., Sato, Y. and Kuroiwa, Y.**: Transmission of chronic spongiform encephalopathy with kuru plaques from humans to small rodents, Ann. Neurol., 5: 581-584, 1979.

**Yakovlev, P. I. and Lecour, A. R.**: Myelogenetic cycles of regional maturation of brain, In: Regional Development of the Brain in Early Life, ed. Minkowsski, A., Blackwell, Oxford, Edinburgh, pp. 3-70, 1967.

# Discussion Particularly with Emphasis on Interrelationship of Each Type of Creutzfeldt-Jakob Disease

Hirotsugu Shiraki, M. D. and Toshio Mizutani, M. D.

*From a clinicopathologic point of view, it is true that there are definite similarities and dissimilarities among the various types of Creutzfeldt-Jakob disease.* First of all, the major dissimilarity between every case of the panencephalopathic type, including some cases of the chronic spongiform encephalopathy with plaques characterized by antecedent and longlasting cerebellar ataxia, and other types of the disease should be noted at this point. *The widespread and severe degeneration of the cerebral white matter in the former two types,* which in most cases is of a primary nature, has never been encountered in any type of Creutzfeldt-Jakob disease, except for the former two types, which, so far, can clearly demonstrate a panencephalopathic character but not only a polioencephalopathic character.

Although some overlapping process of the secondary degeneration attributed to the severe motor cortical and associated medullary damages, particularly in longstanding cases of the disease, did occur in the cerebral white matter in the former two types, particularly of the panencephalopathic type, much of it could be regarded as primary in character. The reasons, however, have already been discussed in greater detail previously (Chapter III-6).

It can tentatively be postulated here that the cases of the panencephalopathic type originated mainly from central and northern Japan, whereas those of the chronic spongiform encephalopathy with plaques characterized by antecedent and longlasting cerebellar ataxia originated mainly from southern Japan. In the cases from southern Japan, numerous kuru plaques and/or senile plaques were also found, whereas there were few plaques or none in the cases from central and northern Japan at least up to date. In the cases from southern Japan, the clinical course was, as a rule, very protracted, ranging from 4 to 11 years. Moreover, cerebellar disturbances at the initial stage preceded for a long period of time and thus, at this stage the patients were often diagnosed as cerebellar ataxia, whereas, when akinetic mutism once occurred, the patients were ended so soon. As a consequence, the brain weight was markedly decreased from 1,180 to 890 g. Brain atrophy in the cases from central and northern Japan, on the other hand, was also severe, but the clinical course was progressive and the duration of the illness was less than one year in most cases. Thus, the clinical manifestations and the duration of the illness were qualitatively and quantatively different in the two groups of the disease.

In other words, clinicopathologically, there are both similarities and dissimilarities among both groups of the disease, although the cerebromedullary foci of a primary character are common in both groups. A final evalution of interrelationship of both groups of the disease together with different types of Creutzfeldt-Jakob disease and kuru will be discussed later. In any case, from a viewpoint of clinical course, both groups of the disease can be divided into two subtypes; subacute and subchronic to chronic.

The present authors are unaware of any reports from the West of the chronic spongiform encephalopathy with kuru plaques and senile plaques characterized by antecedent and longlasting cerebellar ataxia. A very few autopsy cases of the panencephalopathic type of Creutzfeldt-Jakob disease, on the other hand, have recently been reported in the foreign references (Buge, et al., 1978; Park, et al., 1981; Valat, et al., 1983). Whereas, the autopsy cases of this type of the disease in the Japanese ranged approximately one third of all types of Creutzfeldt-Jakob disease. However, it still is not clear whether the panencephalopathic type and the chronic spongiform encephalopathy with plaques characterized by antecedent and longlasting cerebellar ataxia occur predominantly among the Japanese.

The neuropathologic characteristics of different types of Creutzfeldt-Jakob disease is that *systemic or multisystemic degeneration* was frequently a well-established, coexisting condition, even though the pattern of the degeneration varied from case to case and from type to type. Among them, this was particularly predominant in the panencephalopathic type and followed by the chronic spongiform encephalopathy with plaques characterized by antecedent and longlasting cerebellar ataxia.

Among them, thalamic or thalamo-collicular degeneration (or both) was a consistent feature in every case of two types of the disease that was studied.

In the panencephalopathic type of the disease, increasing order of frequency, other combinations of systemic degeneration were spinoolivopontodentatocerebellar degeneration occasionally with olivary hypertrophy, corticospinal and somatosensory pathway degeneration at the level of the spinal cord, primary and secondary visual pathway degeneration with disintegration of the lateral geniculate body and striopallidosubthalamorubronigral degeneration.

In the chronic spongiform encephalopathy of the disease, on the other hand, the cerebellar degeneration varied from case to case, although antecedent and longlasting cerebellar signs and symptoms were most outstanding; some degeneration was clearly of granule cell type; some cases showed conspicuous loss of Purkinje cells; others showed no particular alteration of the cerebellum in which, however, numerous plaques were distributed. The degeneration of both the ventral and dorsal spinocerebellar tracts were rather consistent in most cases and thus, it may be assumed that the clinical features of ataxia in this type can be attributed mainly to this degeneration of the spinal cord. The frequency of the degeneration of the corticospinal tract, anterior horn and posterior column was rather low. Severe degeneration of the pontine basis occurred in some cases, whereas not in the others. The pontine tegmentum disclosed marked atrophy in variable degrees. The inferior olivary nucleus revealed slight to severe loss of nerve cells. The striatum was, as a rule, only slightly involved, however.

The various patterns of degeneration mentioned above affected systems that are interrelated anatomically and physiologically. The foci of degeneration were symmetric, occurred bilaterally and in general were of a distal-dominant character. Not only pathways but also related gray matter was degenerated, and the degeneration was characterized by fibrillary gliosis with thin gliofibers. This characteristic was, thus, a distinct contrast to the spongy degeneration of the cerebral cortex and white matter. In these cerebral regions, there was a marked astrocytosis, but it was exclusively characterized by a coarse gliofiber formation.

On the other hand, in the case reported by Krücke et al. (1973), multisystemic degeneration coexisting closely with subacute spongiform encephalopathy and numerous kuru plaques was clearly identified; examples of the combinations demonstrated were thalamic, striopallidal and olivodentatocerebellorubral degeneration with olivary pseudohypertrophy as well as corticospinal and somatosensory tract degeneration at the level of the spinal cord. Further, other cases of subacute spongiform encephalopathy showed similar combinations with systemic and/or multisystemic degeneration.

In the ataxic type of Creutzfeldt-Jakob disease, one case in a Japanese demonstrated a distal-dominant degeneration of the corticospinal and postrior tracts, and dorsal and ventral spinocerebellar tracts as well.

Even in the simple poliodystrophic type of the disease in which spongy tissue disruption in a true sense of words was absent, both Japanese and western references indicated that degeneration of both the upper and lower motor neuron systems simulating amyotrophic lateral sclerosis was also found.

Further, as described in greater detail previously (Chapter III-8), a basic clinicopathologic feature of kuru in New Guinea was, in fact, multisystemic degeneration of the olivopontodentatocerebellar system, and, to a lesser degree, of the corticospinal, posterior and spinocerebellar tracts at the level of the spinal cord.

It, therefore, can precisely be concluded that the coexistense of single or multisystemic degeneration with Creutzfeldt-Jakob disease is not merely a coincidence. It actually is one of the most important manifestations of the disease.

Thalamic degeneration in different types of Creutzfeldt-Jakob disease has important implications because the severe psychiatric disturbances, such as the apallic syndrome or akinetic mutism, could be attributed not only to the severe deterioration of the cerebral cortex and white matter but also, and possibly exclusively, to the extremely severe involvement of the thalamic subnuclei, particularly those of ontogenetically recent origin.

In this connection, the so-called Stern-Garcin (thalamic) type of Creutzfeldt-Jakob can play a most significant role in an understanding of the different types of Creutzfeldt-Jakob disease, although the clinical criteria of the thalamic type of the disease cannot always coincide well with the major clinical features of Creutzfeldt-Jakob disease which have been discussed previously in detail (Chapter III-4). In any case, in this type of the disease, thalamic degeneration, regardless of a secondary and primary nature, was always combined with the other systemic degeneration; in one of the subtypes, the secondary thalamic degeneration was consistently combined with the corticomedullary degeneration and occasionally with the corticospinal and nigral degeneration; in another subtype, the primary thalamic degeneration was also consistently combined with the spinoolivopontocerebellar and less markdly with the striopallidonigrosubthalamic degeneration, and exceptionally with the rubroolivary and tegmental degeneration including that of the reticular formation of the brainstem.

*Kuru plaques,* which were consistently found in all cases of kuru in New Guinea as well as in almost all cases of the chronic spongiform encephalopathy with plaques characterized by antecedent and longlasting cerebellar ataxia, were occasionally encountered in different types of Creutzfeldt-Jakob disease. As mentioned before, kuru plaques were abundant particularly in the two cases of the subacute spongiform encephalopathy reported by Krücke, et al. (1973) and very few in one case of the panencephalopathic type. As mentioned before, senile plaque-like bodies, on the other hand, were also in one of the subacute spongiform encephalopathy in spite of the younger age of this patient at death, e. g., 35-year-old (Chapter III-3).

The fundamental question as to whether kuru plaques and senile plaques are identical has not yet been answered definitely. In our experience, both types of plaque have similarities and dissimilarities. The central core of each type of plaque has a similar chemical composition, which is amyloid nature, but the morphological structure of each, as studied with light and electron microscopy, more or less differs. Most senile plaques originate from blood vassels, whereas kuru plaques in most cases showed no obvious spatial relationship to blood vessels. There were frequent axonal as well as astrocytic and microglial responses around senile plaques, whereas the latter rarely occurred or were quentionable around kuru plaques.

Even though there were dissimilarities between the types of plaques, it is still conceivable that both showed a common phenotype of senile or precociously senile plaques. In this regard, it is interesting that, in a great majority of cases of the chronic spongiform encephalopathy with plaques characterized by antecedent and longlasting cerebellar ataxia, kuru plaques and senile plaques are concomitantly identified in the same areas or different areas of the same cerebrum and cerebellum.

An important question in this regard is why systemic or multisystemic degeneration in Creutzfeldt-Jakob disease was sometimes closely associated with kuru plaques or senile plaques. Similarities to other disease entities, on the other hand, have been reported. For example, in both the Mariana Islands in the southwestern Pacific and the Kii Peninsula in Japan, there is as extremely high incidence of amyotrophic lateral sclerosis. Neuropathologic studies from these areas, on the other hand, have demonstrated that all cases were accompanied by Alzheimer's neurofibrillary tangles in varying degrees of severity and in one case there actually occurred schizophrenia-like disturbances just prior to the development of amyotrophic lateral sclerosis. Whereas, most cases from more advanced countries do not or only rarely showe these tangles (Shiraki & Yase, 1975). Our interpretation is that this combination of amyotrophic lateral sclerosis with Alzheimer's neurofibrillary tangles is not concidental and thus, the latter could contribute to an understanding of how this sclerosis developed from senile or precociously senile changes in the motor neuron system. Consequently, the similar possibility could be speculated in regard to a coexistence of single and/or multisystemic degeneration and plaques in

Creutzfeldt-Jakob disease.

*Inflated nerve cells,* a few of which had inclusion body-like structures in their cytoplasm, were found in every case of the subacute spongiform encephalopathy and simple poliodystrophic, ataxic and the panencephalopathic type of Creutzfeldt-Jakob disease, and chronic spongiform encephalopathy with plaques characterized by antecedent and longlasting cerebellar ataxia, although their severity varied from case to case and from stage to stage.   Thus, inflation of nerve cells comprized an essential and consistent neuropathologic feature in every case that was studied.

On the other hand, in the simple poliodystrophic type of the disease, which showed almost complete agreement with other types of the disease in regard to clinical criteria, the inflated nerve cells were distributed widely from the cerebrum, diencephalon and brainstem to the spinal cord, whereas in the other types of Creutzfeldt-Jakob disease, inflated nerve cells were, as a rule, restricted to the cerebrum, except for one case of the panencephalopathic type of the disease reported recently by Riku, et al., as mentioned before (Chapter III-6).   In the different types of the disease, they demonstrated, to some extent, a preferential localization of certain cerebral gyri, but determination of their exact distribution was almost impossible because the most severely disintegrated neurons were in the same cerebral gyri.

Whether cytoplasmic inflation has a retrograde origin or whether it has a primary nature being the direct effect of some unknown metabolic abnormality in the affected neurons, remains unknown.   The cerebral white matter, particularly in the panencephalopathic type of the disease, was severely involved.   The possibility that this inflation has a retrograde origin cannot be excluded.   In most cases of other types of the disease, however, degeneration of the cerebral white matter was either not observed or was very questionable.   Thus, this possibility seems unlikely.

As mentioned before, the distribution of the inflated nerve cells along with other neuropathologic finding in the simple poliodystrophic type were almost identical to those of other disease, such as pellagra neuropsychosis, collagen disease and some neurotoxic disorders.   The latter disease groups, therefore, may provide some clue to an understanding of how the inflated nerve cells, actually one of the most important neuropathologic features of the disease, develop in Creutzfeldt-Jakob disease.

*Spongy tissue disruption of the gray matter,* which was in general severe and extensive, particularly in the neocerebral cortex, followed by other parts of the cerebral cortex, the putamen, claustrum and cerebellar molecular layer, to a lesser degree in the thalamus and substantia nigra and to a far lesser degree or even negative in the hippocampus, uncus and amygdala, was seen in all types of the disease, except for the simple poliodystrophic type.

Generally speaking, spongy degeneration was predominant in both the subacute spongiform encephalopathy and the panencephalopathic type and was less marked in the ataxic form, in which the infragranular layers were more severely affected than the supragranular layers.   The similar tendency and severity of the cortical sponginess as seen in the ataxic type of the disease was again identified in a majority of the cases of chronic spongiform encephalopathy with plaques characterized by antecedent and longlasting cerebellar ataxia.

In the simple poliodystrophic type, on the other hand, spongy tissue disruption was also observed sporadically in the cerebral cortex, but because of its nature it could primarily be attributed to an edematous process originating from a hemodynamic disturbance, and its topographic pattern was quite different from that of the other types of the disease.

Clusters of grape-like sponginess were more predominant in the subacute spongiform encephalopathy, whereas fine, sieve-like sponginess of an isolated character was more frequent in both the ataxic type and chronic spongiform encephalopathy with plaques characterized by antecedent and longlasting cerebellar ataxia. However, both types of sponginess occurred concomitantly in the same brain, particularly in cases of the subacute spongiform encephalopathy. Therefore, it may be not unreasonable to conclude that there is no fundamental difference between the two types of sponginess.

The spongy degeneration in the panencephalopathic type of the disease, on the other hand, was more or less different from that in the subacute spongiform encephalopathy, the ataxic type and chronic spongiform encephalopathy with plaques characterized by antecedent and longlasting cerebellar ataxia, because the cortical sponginess in the panencephalopathic type was distributed in a laminar manner and was more marked and widespread at the depths and between the walls than at the crowns of the gyri. By contrast, the sponginess in the subacute spongiform encephalopathy, ataxic type and chronic spongiform encephalopathy with plaques characterized by antecedent and longlasting cerebellar ataxia occurred to the same degree in all parts of the gyri. However, in the panencephalopathic type, careful examination revealed that a fine, sieve-like sponginess was also present, particularly in areas of the cortex in which no nerve cells were lost from these areas.

Interesting enough, in all types of Creutzfeldt-Jakob disease, despite the conspicuous spongy degeneration, the nerve cells, myelin sheaths and axons were comparatively well preserved in the septal regions, particularly near the initial foci, and further, they developed no remarkable abnormalities. Therefore, there was a precise dissociation of marked sponginess from well-preserved neuronal structures.

In all types of Creutzfeldt-Jakob disease, except for the simple poliodystrophic type, it, however, should be noted that the nerve cells in the severely degenerated areas were severely disintegrated. Hypertrophic and, to a lesser degree, gemistocytic astrocytes proliferated, but there was no fibrillary gliosis with thin gliofibers; only a coarse gliofiber formation was seen. This finding confirmed the observation that astrocytosis and fibrillary gliosis were not always parallel in this disease. However, this observation has received little attention. The phagocytes laden with byproducts of myelin breakdown, on the other hand, were mobilized in these severely degenerated areas, but they were exclusively of a fixed type, never showing an obvious tendency toward perivascular accumulation.

*Therefore, the above findings clearly indicate that both astrocytes and microglia showed dysfunctions, and they are important to an understanding of etiologic variable because certain exogeneous or endogeneous neurotoxic agents could cause such glial dysfunction.*

Similar glial dysfunctions were identified in the foci of the cerebral white matter in the panencephalopathic type was well. *Circumscribed, spongy foci,* showing a strong resemblance to the subcortical spongy foci in various hepatocerebral disease, including Wilson's disease, never demonstrated fibrillary gliosis, displaying only mobilization of phagocytes of a fixed type, regardless of the duration of the clinical course.

These two characteristics of glial dysfunctions have also been demonstrated beautifully in various hepatocerebral disease, such as Wilson's disease, portosystemic encephalopathy (Inose type), the pseudoulegyric type of the disease and hereditary hyperammonemia and they are important neuropathologic characteristics of hepatocerebral disease (Oda, 1964; Shiraki, 1968a, 1968b; Shiraki & Oda, 1968; Oda, 1979).   The pseudoulegyric type of the disease, which is prevailing among the Japanese, was accompanied by marked atrophy of the cerebral cortex and white matter, in which the topographic pattern of involvement was almost identical to that in the panencephalopathic type of Creutzfeldt-Jakob disease.   No fibrillary gliosis, nor mobile type of phagocytosis, which might be caused by an endogeneous toxic condition (e.g., hyperammonemia), occurred in this type of hepatocerebral disease, regardless of the duration of the illness.   The classification as pseudoulegyric derives from this characteristic of the illness.

It is true that the spongy tissue disruption of the gray matter in different types of Creutzfeldt-Jakob disease occurred in the neuropil, but whether this sponginess actually developed in the astrocytes or oligodendroglia, in the axon terminals or in the vicinity of these terminals, or in the dendritic processes of nerve cells has not yet fully been answered as far as we know.   The same is true of the mechanism causing the development of the sponginess of the cerebral white matter in the panencephalopathic type of the disease in human beings and laboratory animals.

*Transmission experiments* in kuru from New Guinea and in Creutzfeldt-Jakob disease from developed parts of the world have successfully been reproduced spongy tissue disruption as well as astrocytosis accompanied by neuronal disintegration in the gray matter (and in the panencephalopathic type, the white matter as well) from human beings to animals and from animals to animals.   These important results lend much support to the assumption that kuru and other types of Creutzfeldt-Jakob disease belong to the same category of the disease group.   This assumption, however, has been discussed in greater detail in the Chapter III-8, Fig. 6.

However, it should be borne in mind that transmission experiments have so far not been successful enough in reproducing typical and widespread inflated neurons, kuru or senile plaques and single or multisystemic degeneration in the combination mentioned, and these changes are basic neuropathologic features of this disease group as well.   Tateishi, et al. (1984), on the other hand, have recently been successful in reproducing kuru plaques and allied plaques in small animals.   In any case, for this reason, the term experimental kuru or experimental Creutzfeldt-Jakob disease should be replaced by the term experimental spongiform degeneration.

The reasons for our belief that the term spongiform degeneration should be used related to the results of transmission experiments are summarized as follows:

As mentioned in detail before, the neuropathologic characteristics of Creutzfeldt-Jakob disease and kuru in human beings were never simple or uniform.   The basic neuropathologic changes in the former consisted not only of spongiform degeneration but also of typical and widespread inflation of neurons, systemic or multisystemic degeneration and kuru plaques or senile plaques.   In each type of Creutzfeldt-Jakob disease, kuru plaques, or senile plaques were the most pronounced changes in some cases, followed by spongiform degeneration; in other cases of each type, however, the converse was true.   Further, one of the most important characteristics of the disease was a close combination with single or multisystemic degeneration.

Therefore, it is not unreasonable to conclude that Creutzfeldt-Jakob disease cannot merely be a collection of well-established combinations of several underlying neuropathologic syndrome, and that each neuropathologic syndrome or cellular pathology has a more or less different pathogenetic basis. In this connection, transmission experiments have so far been successful in reproducing only spongiform degeneration at least up to date.

It also is convincing that there is a transmissible agent in the Creutzfeldt-Jakob disease and kuru. So far, however, there is no evidence that the transmissible agent, if only exists, is a virus. For this reason, the term slow-virus infection should be replaced by the term slow transmissible disease in regard to the degeneration seen in the disease.

In all cases of all types of Creutzfeldt-Jakob disease and kuru that have been studied, there was no clear-cut indication of an inflammatory tissue response or resultant tissue damage occurring in reaction to a conventional viral infection or multiplication. In the rare cases of Creutzfeldt-Jakob disease in which mild inflammatory tissue damage was encountered, it was merely of a symptomatic nature or could be attributed to some intercurrent or coincidental infection and usually occurred during a state of cachexia near or at the terminal stage of the illness.

By contrast, the neuropathologic characteristics of slow-virus infections due to conventional viruses, for example, Japanese and tick-borne encephalomyelitides, subacute sclerosing panencephalitis, herpes simplex and cytomegalovirus encephalitides and progressive multifocal leukoencephalopathy, are completely different from those of Creutzfeldt-Jakob disease (Shiraki, 1975). For this reason, the term slow-virus infection and/or slow-unconventional-virus infection in regard to Creutzfeldt-Jakob disease are actually confusing and should be discarded.

Considering that Creutzfeldt-Jakob disease represents a collection of well-established combinations of neuropathologic syndromes or cellular pathologies, it should be remembered that even there are different etiologic basis, the same pathogenetic mechanism can occur, whereas different pathogenetic mechanism can in general be attributed to different etiologic bases.

*In summary* on the basis of these observation as well as neuropathologic findings, it can be postulated that there exist a series of different types of Creutzfeldt-Jakob disease, such as the simple poliodystrophic, ataxic and panencephalopathic types and subacute spongiform encephalopathy that are closely interrelated morphologically and clinically (Chapter III-1, Fig. 1). Although the major clinical features of the Stern-Garcin type of CJD are more or less different from those of CJD among which those of the panencephalopathic type of the disease are most typical, it is no doubt that this type can contribute a great deal in an understanding of morphopathogenesis of other different types of the disease.

The panencephalopathic type of the disease, on the other hand, demonstrated the most unusual combinations of neuropathologic involvement, such as spongiform degeneration in both the gray and the white matter, multisystemic degeneration and inflated neuron. As has been discussed in greater detail (Chapter III-6), Kodama's and Ohta's cases, particularly the latter, had several common features to the panencephalopathic type, whereas they shared common features to the chronic spongiform encephalopathy with plaques characterized by antecedent and longlasting cerebellar ataxia. Therefore, both cases should be

remarked in consideration of a more or less close interrelationship of the panencephalopathic type to the chronic spongiform encephalopathy.

As mentioned before (Chapter III-7), the common clinicopathologic characteristics, on
the other hand, are observed in kuru and chronic spongiform encephalopathy with plaques
characterized by antecedent and longlasting cerebellar ataxia, although some clinicopathological differences exist in the two types of the disease. Besides, as has also been
discussed in greater detail (Chapter III-8), it can be concluded that kuru demonstrate an
infantile, preadolescent and/or young adult form of Creutzfeldt-Jakob disease (Fig. 6 in
the same chapter and section).

Inasmuch, it is not unreasonable to concluded that all types of Creutzfeldt-Jakob
disease including kuru in New Guinea have a close interrelationship with each other and
thus, can belong to a category of the Creutzfeldt-Jakob disease group.

# REFERENCES

**Krücke, W., Beck, E. and Vitzum, K. G.**: Creutzfeldt-Jakob disease; Some unusual features
reminiscent of kuru, J. Neurol., 206: 1-24, 1973.
**Oda, M.**: Ein Beitrag zu den klinischen und histopathologischen Problem über den "Pseudoule-
gyrie-type", Psychiat. Neurol. Jpn., 66: 892-931, 1964.
**Oda, M.**: Hepatocerebral disease, In: Psychiatry at Present Stage. eds. Kaketa, K., Ohkuma, T.,
Shimazono, Y., Takahashi, R. and Hosaki, H., Vol. 19C, Neuropathology II, Nakayama Shoten,
Tokyo, pp. 73-112, 1979
**Riku, S., Okamoto, T., Hashizume, Y., Koike, Y. and Sobue, I.**: Panencephalopathic type of
Creutzfeldt-Jakob disease and special reference to its pyramidal tract degeneration, Clin. Neurol.
(Japan), 23: 147-151, 1983.
**Shiraki, H.**: The comparative study of various types of hepatocerebral disease, In: The Central
Nervous System, eds. Bailey, O. T. and Smith, D. E., Willams and Wilkins, Baltimore, pp. 252-272,
1968a.
**Shiraki, H.**: Comparative neuropathologic study of Wilson's disease and other types of hepato-
cerebral disease, In: Wilson's disease, Birth Defects Original Article Series, ed. Bergsma, D., Vol.
IV, No. 2, National Foundation - March of Dimes, New York, pp. 64-76, 1968b.
**Shiraki, H. and Oda, M.**: Neuropathology of hepatocerebral disease with emphasis on compara-
tive studies, In: Pathology of the Nervous System, ed. Minckler, J., Vol. 1, McGraw-Hill, New
York, pp. 1089-1103, 1968.
**Shiraki, H.**: Slow virus infections of nervous system in humans mainly from neuropathological
viewpoint - With special reference to comparison of so-called transmissible disease group to
encephalomyelitides with conventional virus infections, Adv. Neurol. Sci. (Japan), 19: 109-147,
1975.
**Shiraki, H. and Yase, Y.**: Amyotrophic lateral sclerosis in Japan, In: Handbook of Clinical
Neurology, eds. Vinken, P. J. and Bruyn, G. W., Vol. 22, Part II, North-Holland, Amsterdam, pp.
353-419, 1975.
**Tateishi, J., Nagara, H., Hikita, K. and Sato, Y.**: Amyloid plaques in the brains of mice with
Creutzfeldt-Jakob disease, Ann. Neurol., 15: 278-280, 1984.

# Chapter IV

# Familial Creutzfeldt-Jakob Disease in Japan

Junichiro Akai, M. D.

A systemic study for Creutzfeldt-Jakob disease (CJD) occurring between 1975 and 1977 was done throughout all of Japan to discuss chiefly epidemiological problems (Tsuji, et al., 1980).

Though 75 cases of CJD were collected in this study, it included some possible cases. To investigate accurately, 63 cases of definite and probable CJD were reconfirmed by the following study.  Tsujii, et al., reported 4 cases of familial occurrence in these 63 cases. This represents 6% of the total number of cases.  It consists of 2 cases of brother, one case of mother and one case of cousin.  But in their report, only case numbers of familial occurrence are described and neither familial history nor pedigree were reported.

According to the author's investigation based on the diagnostic criteria of CJD by Masters (Masters, et al., 1979), in Japan there are only three families, which had definite and probable cases of CJD.  One family of them is found in Fukuoka Prefecture in Kyushu Island and other two families in Yamanashi Prefecture in Honshu Island.

In this chapter, the author describes these families and discusses their various aspects.

## 1. Family M

Their clinical courses were reported in the form of brief communication (Koga, et al., 1973) and one of them who was verified was detailed later (Ishii, et al., 1978).

Table 1 indicates genealogical tree of this family.  In regard to the members of 1st generation, there is no precise record.  For 2nd generation, three died at 80 years old, two died in a coal mine accident.  II-6 died after her labor at 23 years old.  The cause of sudden death of II-7 at 60 years old is unkown.  II-8 died of acute pneumonia at 59 years old.  III-1 aged 65 years died of lung cancer.  The cause of sudden death of III-2 at 23 years old is unknown.    III-3 died of cardiac failure.

**Case 1. (III-4)**    Former elementary school teacher.    She was treated for hypertension since 62 years old.    No other remarkable past history.    64 years old in 1976.    In June, 1975, she complained of forgetfulness and insomnia.    Neurasthenic state was observed.    In July, she came for psychiatric consultation.    At that time, only an apathetic state was observed but no neurological deficit.    EEG showed normal recording pattern. In August, memory disturbance and insomnia increased and she had to be admitted to the psychiatric division.    She could no longer walk by herself.    Muscle tone in the extremities was hypotonic.    There was no pathological reflex.    Snout and grasping reflex were positive.    EEG showed irregular slow wave pattern.    In September, hyperreflexia with Babinski sign, muscle rigidity, aphonia and various involuntary movements including myclonus and choreatic movement appeared.    And then tetraplegia in flexion and decerebrated rigidity occurred.    EEG showed typical periodic synchronus discharge (PSD).    In November, she fell into a state of akinetic mutism.    After January 1976, myoclonus decreased and pattern of EEG became flat.    She expired due to bronchopneumonia in the middle of March.    Total duration of her illness was 9 months.

At autopsy, her brain weighed 940 gr.    The widening of cerebral sulci and atrophic feature of cerebral gyri were observed.    Cerebellar folia also were severely atrophic. Vertico-frontal sections showed remarkable atrophy of cerebral cortex, basal ganglia and severe ventricular dilatation.    Histologically, the cortical layer was completely destroyed and severe neuronal loss and conspicuous hypertrophic astrocyte were noticed (Figs. 1A & B).

Basal ganglia and thalamus showed moderate degenerative changes.    Cerebral white

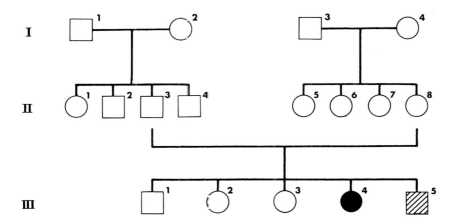

**Table 1.**    Genealogical tree of the Family M
Black circle indicates definite CJD.
Cross hatching represents probable CJD.
(For this family tree, the author thanks for Dr. T. Suzuki, Depertment of Psychiatry, Iizuka Hospital, Fukuoka Prefecture.)

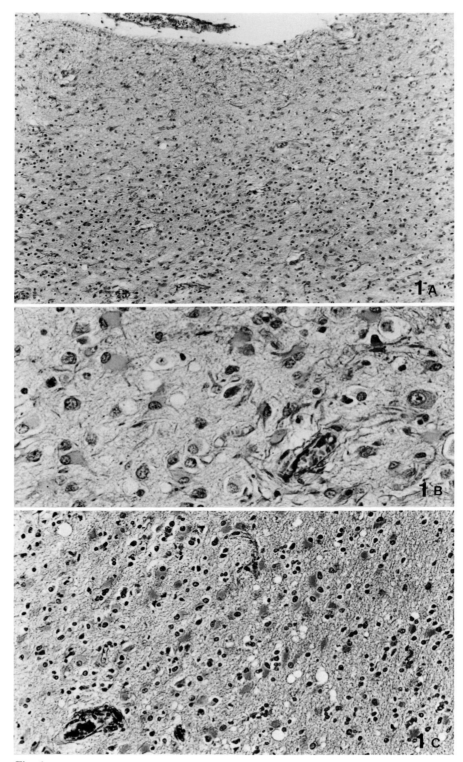

Fig. 1

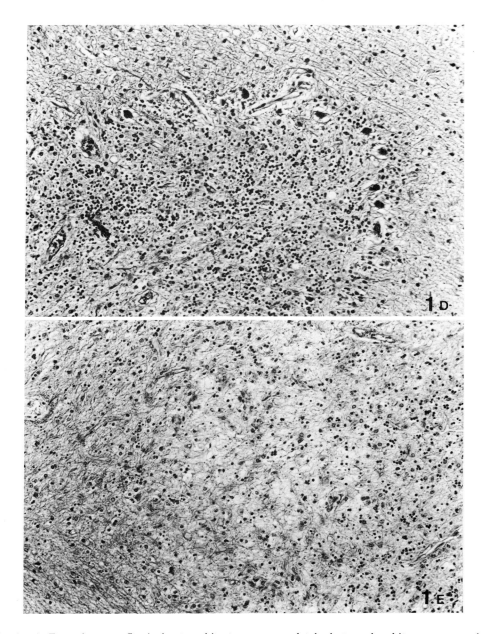

**Fig. 1.** **A.** Frontal cortex: Cortical cytoarchitecture are completely destroyed and its appearance shows pseudolaminar state. × 25. **B.** Frontal cortex: Magnified area in A. Severe neuronal loss, diffuse astrocytic proliferation with spongy disruption. × 100. **C.** White matter in frontal lobe: Moderate demyelination with gemistocytic astrocyte and spongy formation. × 50. **D.** Cerebellum: Preserved but shrunken Purkinje cell and severe loss of neuron in granular cell layer. × 40 **E.** Cerebellum: Highly devastated area with fibrous astrocyte in granular cell layer. × 40. (A, B, C & E: Mallory; D: Bodian)

matter had diffuse demyelination and decrease of axon and contained numerous lipid macrophages (Fig. 1C). No remarkable change in brainstem. In upper cervical cord, there was discrete demyelination of the pyramidal tract. No loss of neuron in anterior horn. In cerebellum, Purkinje cell was moderately preserved, but diminished neuron in granular cell layer and diffuse astrocytic proliferation were observed (Figs. 1D & E).

**Case 2. (III-5)** 56 years old. His record is very poor, but he manifested same clinical course and EEG showed also PSD. Total duration of his illness was 7 months. He had no anatomical verification. This case is considered to be probable CJD.

## 2. Family H

Family tree is shown in Table 2. I-2 was probable senile dementia. II-6 was 70 years in 1974. Since 67 years old, she complained of headache, insomnia and muscle twitching of extremities and for several months she was admitted to a psychiatric clinic. EEG showed irregular slow wave pattern. After discharge, dysesthesia of whole body and muscle twitching were observed. No dementia. She died three years after onset of her complaint. As she had no autopsied verification, the cause of her death was obscure.

II-7 is 85 years old. At 50 years of age, he had tremor of whole body and seven years later tetraparesis and blindness occurred. Since then he is obliged to live in bed lying. No dementia. As for his present state, the author cannot give an accurate diagnosis.

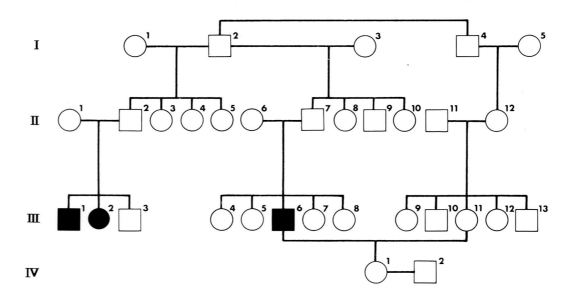

**Table 2.** Genealogical tree of the Family H
Black circle or square indicates definite CJD.

**Case 1 (III-1).**  Was reported in the form of brief communication (Oikawa, et al., 1969).  56 year in 1967, dentist.  At 20 years of age, neurasthenic state.  In April 1966, he began to complain of forgetfulness  In August, he could not continue to work due to twitching of his left hand.  This involuntary movement increased and he was admitted to department of psychiatry in December.  At this time, he was alert, but apathetic and a poor mimic.  Slurred and slow speech and impaired comprehension were noticed.  Neurologically, myoclonus, choreatic movements of upper extremities with slight rigidity were observed.  EEG showed bilateral synchronous high voltage slow discharge in parieto-occipital region.  After admission, mental deterioration progressed.  Urinary incontinence, dysphagia, confabulation and disorientation occurred.  And then startle response, primitive reflex and moderate muscle rigidity of extremities were observed.  EEG in February showed typical PSD.  After 14 months of onset, he fell in apallic state and involuntary movement decreased.  In EEG, interval of PSD prolonged.  He became gradually weaker due to emaciation and died of bronchopneumonia.  Duration of illness was approximately 18 months.

At autopsy, brain weighed 1,000 gr.  Macroscopically, diffuse cerebral atrophy.  Histologically, in fronto-temporo-occipital region, insula and caudate nucleus, there are spongiform changes, astrocytic proliferation and neuronal loss (Fig. 2A).  Solitary spongiform change accompanied coalescent spongy state (Fig. 2B).  In the severe region, there is moderate swelling of oligodendroglia.  In white matter, amoeboid degeneration macroglia.  Well preserved Purkinje and granular cell in cerebellum (Fig. 2C).  There are neither senile nor inflammatory changes.

**Case 2 (III-2).**  69 year in 1983.  At 68 years of age, diabetes mellitus.  In August 1982, depressive and inactive state was noticed.  In September, weakness of arm, unsteadiness of gait.  In October, she was admitted to neurological division.  At that time, alert, impairment of calculation, right hemiparesis.  Neither pathological reflex nor sensory change.  EEG showed 8-9 Hz background activity accompanying a synchronized 4-6 Hz slow wave.  In November, disturbance of coordination increased.  She could no longer walk and stand up by herself.  Tendency to drowsy state and myoclonic movement appeared.  In December, she fell to apallic state and EEG showed typical PSD.  In 24 December, sudden respiratory arrest and in 25 January 1983, she died of cardiac arrest.  Total duration was approximately 6 months.

At autopsy, brain weighed 1,070 gr.  Gyral atrophy and sulcal widening of the frontal, parietal and occipital lobes.  Severe neuronal loss with marked astrocytic proliferation in fronto-parietal and occipital lobes (Figs. 3A & B).  Spongy state in frontal lobe and basal ganglia and spongiform change in temporal lobe (Figs. 3C & D) and cerebellar vermis (Fig. 3F) were observed.  A patchy white matter lesion in subcortical region of the parietal lobe (Fig. 3E).  Well preserved brainstem and spinal cord.

**Case 3 (III-6).**  This case was reported as familial CJD (Akai, et al., 1979).  40 year in 1977.  Agricultural engineer.  In the beginning of 1975, he suffered from gastric disturbance and had intervention of gastric ulcer.  In July 1976, transient visual impairment.  Then he began to complain of forgetfulness and apathy, inactivity were observed.  He was able to work until the end of year.  In January 1977, he was admitted to

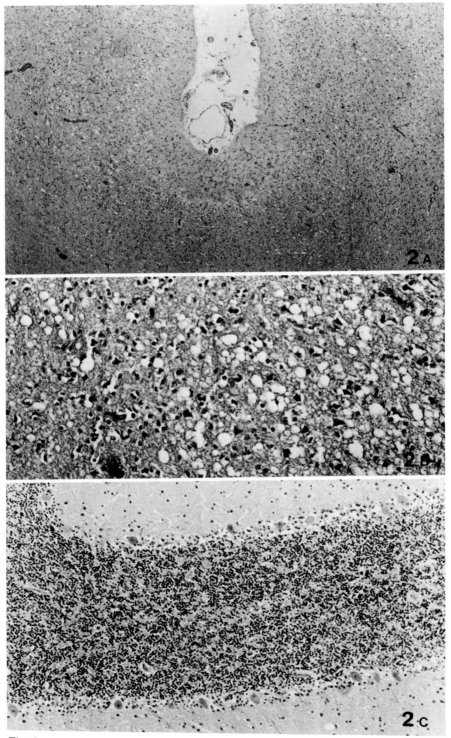

Fig. 2

neurological division.  At that time, alert, poor mimic, amnestic, apathetic state. Neurologically, unsteadiness of gait, paratonic rigidity of extremities were observed.   No pathological reflex.   EEG showed irregular diffuse 6-7 Hz slow wave with high voltage 1. 5-3 Hz wave in fronto-central region.   No treatable effect of amantadine hydrochloride. Involuntary movement, pathological reflex gradually appeared.  In June, myoclonus extended to whole body and he had paraplegic posture.  EEG showed typical PSD.   In August, mental deterioration progressed and he fell to mutism with various involuntary movement and transferred to apallic state.   In September, myoclonic movement decreased.   Under the condition of general marasmus, his emaciation progressed and in November expired after 17 months of evolution of symptom.

At autopsy, 1,065 gr. weighed brain had neither arteriosclerotic nor inflammatory change.  In fronto-antero-temporal region, moderate widening of sulci and atrophy of convolutions were visible.   Vertico-frontal sections also showed same atrophic change and moderate ventricular dilatation (Fig. 4A).   Macroscopic appearance of cerebellum was slightly atrophic.   Histopathologically, in fronto-temporo-occipital lobe, cytoarchitectural layers were completely destroyed with neuronal loss, variable gemistocytic astroglial proliferation and coalescent spongy disruption (Figs. 4B & D).   White matter had moderate hypertrophic astrocytes and pallor myelin sheath (Fig. 4C).   Basal ganglia, especially in caudate nucleus manifested disintegration of nerve cell, proliferated astrocyte and spongy state.   There were coalescent, rough gross spongy formation in subcortical region adjacent deep layer of occipital cortex (Figs. 4E & F).   Median nucleus of thalamus and midbrain showed shrunken and disintegrated nerve cell with pronounced spongy state and astrogliosis.   In cerebellum, diffuse loss of granular cell in granular layer was conspicuous (Fig. 4H).   White matter of cerebellum had moderate disintegration of myelin sheath.   In spinal cord, well preserved neuron in anterior horn.   There were rough and gross spongy formation in pyramidal tracts, fasciculus cuneatus and spinocerebellar tracts (Fig. 4G).

For clinical manifestation, initial symptom of these 3 cases started, by psychiatric disturbance, another neurological symptoms occurred subsequently.   Case 2 and 3 had unsteadiness of gait but case 1 had no symptom such as at initial stage.

Various neuropsychiatric disturbances which each case manifested in the course of illness were almost common feature of CJD.

## 3. Family K

This familial CJD was reported as cousin case (Kawai, et al., 1981).   Table 3 indicated genealogical tree of this family.  I-1 died of gastric cancer.  I-2 died at 40.  The

---

**Fig. 2.**   (8489-285)  **A.** Occipital cortex: Spongy tissue disruption with moderate disintegration of neuron in deep layer.   × 40.  **B.** Occipital cortex: Magnified area in A.   Spongiform change accompanied by coalescent spongy state.   × 200.  **C.** Cerebellum: Well preserved Purkinje and granular cell.   No spongy formation.   × 30   (A, B & C: H-E.)

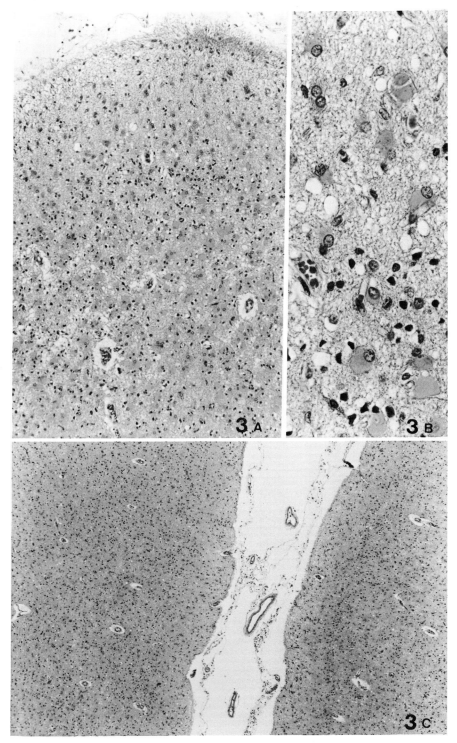

**Fig. 3**

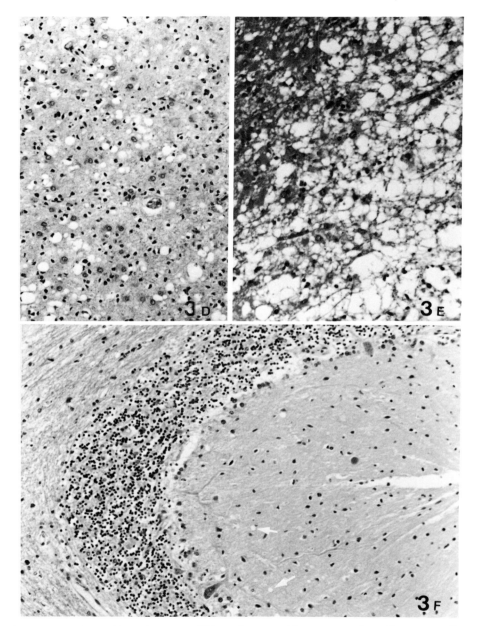

**Fig. 3.** (TP30313) **A.** Frontal cortex: Diffuse hypertrophic astrocytosis with spongy disruption. Complete loss of neuron in all layers.  × 25.  **B.** Frontal cortex: Magnified area in A.  Gemistocytic astrocyte with spongy formation.  × 100.  **C.** Temporal cortex: Diffuse disintegration of cortical architecture.  × 10.  **D.** Temporal cortex: Magnified area in C.  Spongiform change with still-remaining, shrunken neuron and proliferative astrocyte.  × 100.  **E.** Parietal lobe: A patchy white matter lesion in subcortical portion.  × 100.  **F.** Cerebellum: Discrete spongiform change in molecular layer (arrows).  No depletion of Purkinje cell.  × 40.  (A, B, C, D, & F: H-E; E: K-B.)

206

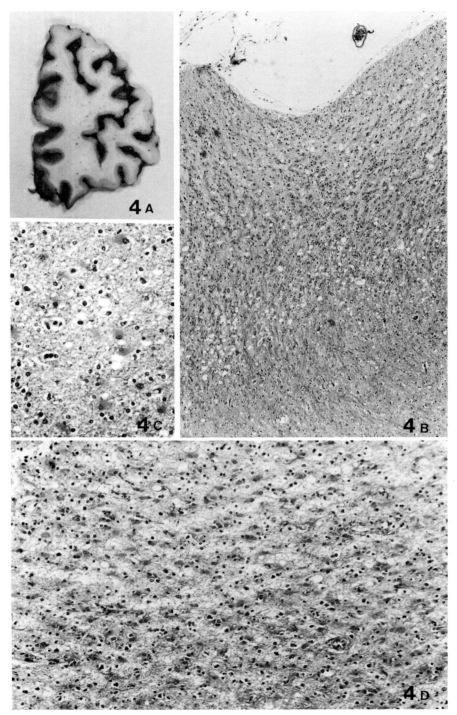

**Fig. 4** (Legend in page 208)

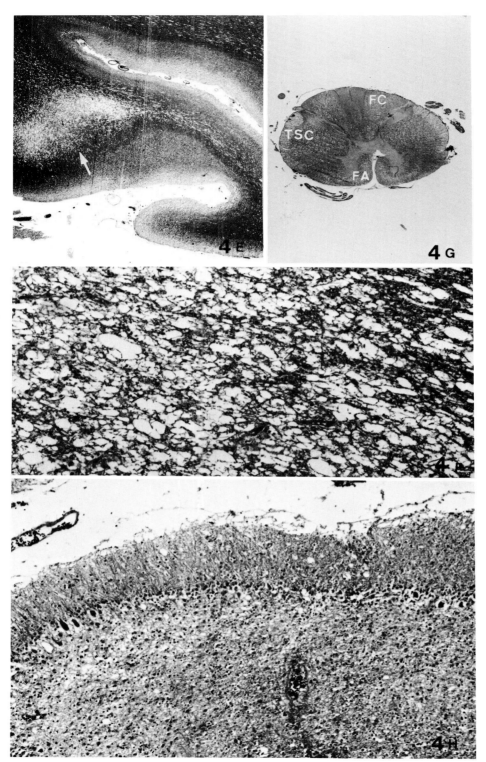

**Fig. 4** (Legend in page 208)

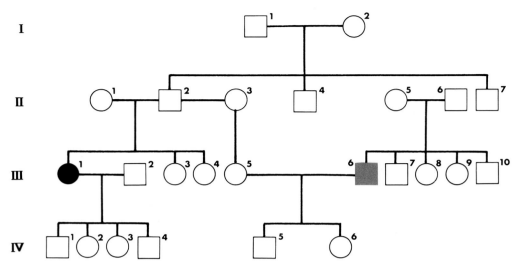

**Table 3.** Genealogical tree of the Family K
Black circle indicates definite CJD.
Square hatching indicates probable CJD.

cause of his death is obscure. II-2 died at 60 due to hepatic disease. II-3 died a sudden death at 40.

**Case 1 (III-1).** 57 year in 1980. Past history: Schistosomiasis japonica in her youth. At 55, intervention of upper mandibular cancer. In March 1980, unsteadiness of gait. In May, inactive and apathetic state. In June, disorientation, visual impairment. She was admitted to neurological division in the middle of July. At that time, tendency to drowsy state, slurred speech and decrease of visual acuity were noticed. Neither pathological reflex nor sensory change. EEG showed 3-5 Hz high voltage slow wave in frontal region accompanied sporadic spike discharge in occipital region. After 1 months of admission, pyramidal sign, paratonic rigidity, myoclonic movement, startle response appeared and then she fell rapidly to apallic state. EEG showed PSD. In August, she died suddenly of cardiac arrest. Total duration of disease was 5 months.

**Fig. 4.** (YSN 539) **A.** Frontal lobe: Vertico-frontal section shows narrowing of cortical ribbon and widening of sulci. **B.** Frontal cortex: Destroyed cytoarchitectural layer with gemistocytic proliferative astrocyte and isolate and coalescent spongy disruption. × 16. **C.** White matter in frontal lobe: Disintegration of myelin sheath and moderate hypertrophic astrocyte. × 100. **D.** Occipital cortex: Pseudolaminar appearance with remarkable hypertrophic astrocyte in whole layer. × 33. **E.** White matter in occipital lobe: Patchy lesion in subcortical portion (arrow). **F.** Magnified area in E. Coalescent, rough and gross spongy state. × 100. **G.** Cervical cord: Funiculus anterior (FA), Tractus spinocerebellaris (TSC) and Fasciculus cuneatus (FC) showing spongy formation. **H.** Cerebellum: Severe destruction of granular cell layer and still-remaining, shrunken Purkinje cell. × 100. (B-H: LFB-H-E.)

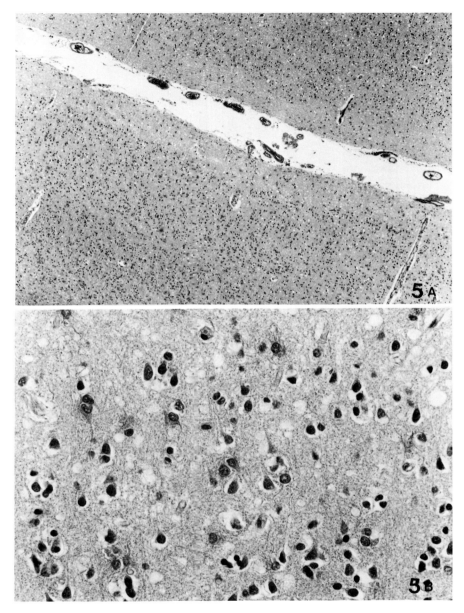

**Fig. 5.**   (TP 29663)   **A.** Occipital cortex: Discrete disintegration of cytoarchitectural layer.   × 14.4.   **B.** Magnified area in A: Spongiform change with well preserved neuron and slightly astrocytotic proliferation.   × 100.   (A & B: H-E.)

At autopsy, brain weighed 1,028 gr.  Macroscopic appearance showed no atrophic features.  Histopathologically, in cerebral cortex, thalamus, basal ganglia and cerebellum, diffuse spongiform change were noticed.  Neuronal loss and astrocytosis were slight (Figs. 5A & B).  Well preserved white matter.  No senile change.

**Case 2 (III-6).**  59 in 1981.  He had also past history of Schistosomiasis japonica.  In June, he caused a traffic accident due to transient diplopia.  In July, dysarthria and unsteadiness of gait appeared.  Admission in the middle of July.  At that time, discrete disorientation, dysphagia, dysarthria, hyperreflexia with pyramidal sign, paratonic rigidity, cerebellar ataxic gait were noticed.  EEG showed continuous irregular slow wave activity.  In August, he fell into apallic state and myoclonus appeared.  EEG showed PSD.  Serial CT scan showed progressive atrophic process of whole brain.  He became gradually emaciated and died on March 1981.  Total duration was about 8 months.

Though the autopsy was not permitted this case is thought as probable CJD on the basis of clinical course and finding of examination.

## Epidemiological, clinical and neuropathological aspects of Family M

As mentioned above, Family M was reported from Fukuoka Prefecture in Kyushu Island.  It is sure that place of residence through life of members of this family was in same Prefecture.  The cause of death of others of these CJD affected members is variable.  There might be no degenerative disease.  Both cases (III-4, III-5) manifested almost same clinical symptoms of CJD.  As for III-4 who was reported as "CJD with extensive white matter involvement, Ishii, et al., discussed the possibility of primary degeneration for severe white matter lesion.  According to criteria by Mizutani (1979), this case belongs to panencephalopathic type.  It is impossible to compare clinicopathological aspect of this family with the sporadic form of CJD in same Prefecture, as the data is very poor.

## Familial CJD in Yamanashi Prefecture (Akai, 1984)

For Family H and Family K whose dwelling is in Yamanashi Prefecture in Honshu, it was throughly investigated and the findings were studied from various points.

Yamanashi Prefecture situated in the central part of Honshu Island has total area of approximately 4,400 square kilometers and census population of 807,000 in 1981.  This Prefecture is surrounded by many mountains and has no sea-side.  It takes only two hours by train from Tokyo.  There is little industrial area and it belongs to agricultural administrative district.  Census population in this ten years is almost same.  Moreover, Kofu City, the capital is situated in the core of the Prefecture.  As there are main administrative bureau including hospitals and medical centers in this city, it seems to be easy to conduct epidemiological research.

## Onset and duration of illness in two families (Table 4)

III-1 in Family H suffered in 1966 and died after 18 months.    The interval between III-1 and onset of III-6, who suffered 17 months is about ten years.    The interval between III-6 and III-2, who suffered 5 month in 5 years.    The duration of III-1 and III-6 is almost same and the duration of III-2 is shorter than both of them.

The onset of affected members in Family K began within same year: III-1 in March, III-6 in June 1981.    The duration of III-1 is shorter than III-6.

## Life history and place of residence throughout life of affected members in two families

Place of residence of Family H situated in the valley of the eastern slope of Akaishi mountains in Minamikoma-gun.    Though this district belongs to administrative town, Nakatomicho which has 5,665 inhabitants in 1981, it is bordered by deep valley and isolated from the center of Nakatomicho.    In this small community, there are about 30 families which consists of 150 inhabitants.    Their main occupation is timber work, agriculture.    Relationship of inhabitants is very close and they preserve and practice many traditional ceremonies.

III-1 was born in 1911 in this community and grew until 12 years old.    After he graduated from dental school in Tokyo in 1941, he married and made his residence in Tokyo until his death in 1967.    There was little opportunity to return to his native place.

III-2 was born in 1913 in same house and grew up with her sibling.    In 1936, she

| case \ year | | 66 | 67 | 68-75 | 76 | 77 | 78 | 79 | 80 | 81 | 82 | 83 |
|---|---|---|---|---|---|---|---|---|---|---|---|---|
| **Family H** | case 1 III – 1 | ▆▆ | | | | | | | | | | |
| | case 2 III – 6 | | | | ▆▆ | | | | | | | |
| | case 3 III – 2 | | | | | | | | | | | ■ |
| **Family K** | case 1 III – 1 | | | | | | | | ■ | | | |
| | case 2 III – 6 | | | | | | | | | ▆ | | |

Table 4.    Onset and duration of illness in two families

married a man in same community and lived in Kofu until 1945. After the 2nd world war, they moved to Tokyo and lived there 38 years until her death.

They were living in Tokyo at the onset of illness. The distance of their dwelling in Tokyo between III-1 and III-2 is only 10 km. It seems that they had subsequently the possibility of family contact. When III-2 began to complain of forgetfulness, she said that she might have the same illness as her brother.

III-6 was born in 1928 in same community. The distance of the dwelling of his cousin is only 300 m. He married with his cousin (III-11) who lived also in same community and stayed in the house of his birth until his death in 1977. When he was admitted to the hospital, the author had the chance to listen to his history from III-2 who suffered from CJD later. It might be little, but surely possible that there is the possibility of contact between III-6 and his cousin in his childhood and later by the chance of wedding or funeral among their relatives.

As for Family K, their place of residence is in Nirasaki City with 27,490 inhabitants in 1981, which is 10 km distant from Kofu City. They lived in same small community in the western part of this city where there is an agricultural administrative center.

III-1 was born in 1923 and lived, married in same district until her death.

III-6 was born in 1923 and lived there also.

It is very interesting that the distance of their dwelling is only 10 m and they lived really on another side of the community road where they used to go and return. It seems that they had frequent opportunities to meet in not only ceremonies, but also daily life.


## Relation to the sporadic CJD in Yamanashi Prefecture (Teble 5)

The author studied the incidence of the disease and geographical clustering during 1972-1983. As the Table 6 shows, population census in Yamanashi Prefecture is almost stable at 800,000 inhabitants between 10 years. As mentioned above, the movement of population is really little, because there is little industrial zone. Table 7 showed also onset and death of CJD in each year. This includes also familial case in Yamanashi Prefecture. It is almost the same as the annual death rate in Japan. There is no evidence of increase of CJD in the past several years in this Prefecture. Between 1972 and 1983 there are 9 patients of CJD and 7 of them had histological confirmation and other 2 patients were diagnosed on clinical grounds. Place of residence of each case is shown in Table 5. There is no community aggregation except familial case. Each sporadic case is scattered throughout the whole region of the Prefecture. By the author's investigation, in each sporadic case there was no definitive possibilty of contact, though the distance of their dwelling is only 5-15 km. Their occupation were different and no particular sex distribution. There is no special relation between familial and sporadic cases.

For the occurrence of CJD including familial case, there is no point source of contamination. In Kofu City, there were 2 patients who might have no possibility of contact, because the distance of their dwelling was ca 5 km and they did not belong to same community. As for familial case, the author's investigation revealed that people in each community had no similar disorder including degenerative disease. This suggests

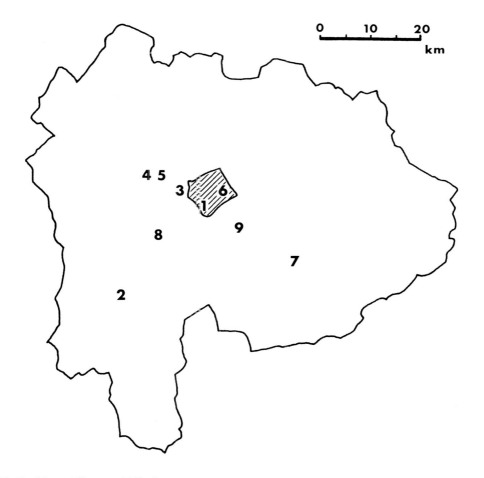

**Table 5.**  Map of Yamanashi Prefecture
Hatched cross represents Kofu City, the capital of the prefecture.
Number indicates the place of residence of CJD patient (Number is the same as case number of Table 7).

little possibility of subclinical patients.

## Neuropathological aspect

As for sporadic case, each showed a feature consisted with SSE diagnosis.  The case 1 in Table 6 was categorized as panencephalopathic type by Mizutani (1981).

As for Family H, III-1 was diagnosed as SSE by Oikawa, et al. (1969), and other 2 patients (III-2, III-6) also were diagnosed as SSE.  Each brain weighted about 1,000 grams and atrophic process was dominant in frontal lobe.  According to the criteria by Mizutani (1981), each case in Family H might belong to panencephalopathic type, because there are white matter lesions including subgyral lesion.  Cerebellar lesion in III-2 and III-6 might

214

| year | onset | death | total poplation |
|------|-------|-------|-----------------|
| 1972 | 1 | 1 | 765,782 |
| 1973 | | | 770,222 |
| 1974 | | | 775,171 |
| 1975 | | | 783,050 |
| 1976 | 1 | | 786,979 |
| 1977 | | 1 | 791,449 |
| 1978 | 1 | | 794,854 |
| 1979 | | 1 | 798,991 |
| 1980 | 2 | 1 | 804,256 |
| 1981 | 1 | 1 | 807,676 |
| 1982 | 2 | 2 | |
| 1983 | 1 | 2 | |

**Table 6.** Annual onset and death of CJD in Yamanashi Prefecture

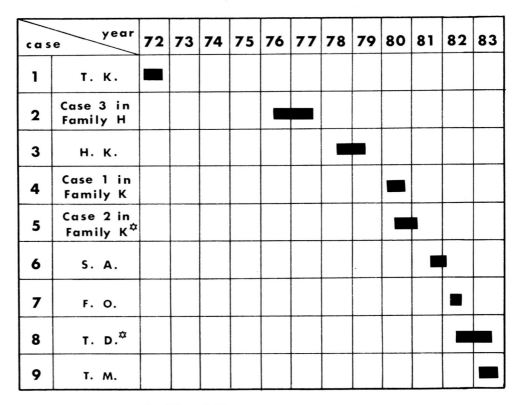

**☆: probable CJD**

**Table 7.** Duration of illness which has its onset in Yamanashi Prefecture

reflect clinical manifestation (unsteadiness of gait, etc.) in these cases. There was no pathological change in cerebellum of III-1 which had no cerebellar symptom.

As for case in Family K, it belongs to SSE. With these results, the author revealed that there is no specific finding in familials case including feature suggested as belong of possible meaning in the aetiology of the disease. Relation between familial and sporadic case did not show any significant correspondence.

## Summary

Three familial CJD in Japan, particularly two families in Yamanashi Prefecture were discussed in a point of view of many aspects. The clinical and neuropathological finding and epidemiological facts of CJD affected members were compared to those patients with the sporadic form of CJD. Possibility of contact between familial and sporadic case might be negative. There was no familial consanguinity between the two families. Though subclinical case in each geographical clustering might be set, this hypothesis cannot be proven. There is no infectious evidence in each cases. As for familial case, it might be necessary to approach and investigate such as metabolic disintegration and so on.

## REFERENCES

**Akai, J., Kato, Y. and Oyanagi, S.:** Familial Creutzfeldt-Jakob disease. Clinicopathological observation on cousins. Adv. Neurol. Sci. (Japan), 23: 472-483, 1979.

**Akai, J.:** Creutzfeldt-Jakob Disease, pp 99-101, pp 106-108, Seiwa Shoten, Tokyo, 1984.

**Ishii, N., Suzuki, T., Nishi, E., Koga, Y. and Takeda, T.:** Two cases of Creutzfeldt-Jakob disease with extensive white matter involvement. Neurol. Psychiat. Kyushu (Japan), 24: 227-233, 1978.

**Kawai, M., Takatsu, M., Mamiya, Y., Yamaoka, M., Toyokura, Y. and Ishihara, O.:** Creutzfeldt-Jakob disease in cousins. Neurol. Med. (Japan), 15: 165-171, 1981.

**Koga, Y., Suzuki, T., Nakamura, S., Cyara, S. and Ishii, N.:** Two cases of probable Creutzfeldt-Jakob disease (Kindred cases). Neurol. Psychiat. Kyushu (Japan), 22: 273, 1973.

**Masters, C. L., Harris, J. O., Gajdusek, D. C., Gibbs, C. J. Jr., Bernoulli, C. and Asher, D.M.:** Creutzfeldt-Jakob disease; Patterns of worldwide occurrence and significance of familial sporadic clustering. Ann. Neurol., 5: 177-188, 1979.

**Mizutani, T.:** Neuropathology of Creutzfeldt-Jakob disease in Japan with special reference to the panencephalopathic type. Acta Pathol., Jpn., 31: 903-922, 1981.

**Oikawa, K., Fukazawa, K., Hasegawa, K., Sasaki, M. and Shimpuku, H.:** An autopsy case of subacute spongiform cerebral atrophy. Adv. Neurol. Sci. (Japan), 13: 392, 1969.

**Tsujii, S., Kuroiwa, Y. and Ishida, N.:** The epidemiological and clinical studies of Creutzfeldt-Jakob disease in Japan. Clin. Neurol. (Japan), 20: 1161, 1980.

# Chapter V

# Spongiform Encephalopathy Induced in Rodents

Jun Tateishi, M. D. and Yuji Sato, M. D.

After the successful experimental transmisson of Kuru (Gajdusek, et al., 1966), Creutzfeldt-Jakob disease (CJD) was transmitted to chimpanzees and other primates (Gibbs, et al., 1968). The transmission, however, required incubation periods measured in years and was not successful in small laboratory animals. Manuelidis and Manuelidis (1979) and Tateishi et al. (1979) succeeded in the serial transmission of CJD into small rodents. The acquired data will aid in studies both of the nature of the causative agent and pathogenesis of this disease. Some of our studies on the latter are summarized herein.

## 1. Transmission Experiments

Brain and other tissue from more than 25 autopsied patients with CJD were homogenized in saline and inoculated into several species, through various routes, as described previously (Tateishi, et al., 1983).

Up to early 1984, animals receiving tissues from 19 patients have been observed for more than 2 years after intracerebral inoculations. Fourteen transmissions of the spongiform encephalopathy were given to rodents (Table). The incidence of positive transmission and length of incubation periods were peculiar to each inoculated material and animal species. In the first passage, the incidence was not high and the periods were extremely long, in some cases. In the second passage, however, the incidence became high and incubation periods were reduced approximately to 4 months in mice after intracerebral inoculation of the brain tissue. Various inoculated materials other than the brain and inoculation routes other than intracerebral injection enabled transmission of the

**Table**  CJD patients and results of experimental transmisson

| | CJD patients | | | | | | | Animals in the 1st passage | | | |
|---|---|---|---|---|---|---|---|---|---|---|---|
| No. | Age | Sex | Duration of illness | Myo-clonus | PSD | Amyloid plaques | Pathol. diagnosis | Total No. examined | No.with disease | No.with plaques | Incubation periods (days) |
| 1 | 70 | M | 3m | (+) | (+) | (−) | SSE | 6 | 6 | 5 | 764±102 |
| 2 | 71 | M | 5m | (+) | (+) | (−) | SSE | 33 | 6 | | 318± 92 |
| 3 | 75 | F | 7m | (+) | (+) | (+) | SSE | 19 | 7 | 3 | 683± 82 |
| 4 | 70 | M | 8m | (+) | (+) | (−) | SSE | 14 | 10 | 3 | 735±103 |
| 5 | 49 | M | 8m | (+) | (+) | (−) | SSE | 15 | 7 | 3 | 701±119 |
| 6 | 69 | M | 8m | (+) | (+) | (−) | SSE | 37 | 11 | 4 | 665±122 |
| 7 | 72 | F | 10m | (+) | (+) | (−) | SSE | 9 | 6 | 3 | 739± 70 |
| 8 | 59 | M | 12m | (+) | (+) | (+) | SSE | | | | |
| 9 | 61 | F | 1y 1m | (+) | (+) | (−) | SSE | 4* | 2 | | 382±  1 |
| 10 | 56 | F | 1y 3m | (+) | (+) | (−) | SSE | | | | |
| 11 | 56 | F | 1y 8m | (+) | (+) | (−) | SSE | 32 | 7 | 4 | 477±191 |
| 12 | 66 | F | 1y 9m | (+) | (+) | (−) | SSE | | | | |
| 13 | 48 | F | 2y 3m | (+) | (+) | (−) | SSE | 37 | 4 | 2 | 705± 53 |
| 14 | 62 | M | 2y10m | (+) | (+) | (−) | SSE | 41 | 5 | | 423± 53 |
| 15 | 62 | M | 3y 7m | (−) | (−) | (−) | SSE | | | | |
| 16 | 52 | M | 3y10m | (+) | (−) | (+) | atypical | 3 | 2 | | 320± 15 |
| 17 | 59 | M | 4y 2m | (−) | (−) | (+) | GSS | 15 | 13 | | 255± 53 |
| 18 | 58 | M | 7y | (−) | (−) | (+) | GSS | | | | |
| 19 | 37 | F | 9y | (+) | (+) | (−) | SSE | 44 | 16 | 4 | 377±105 |

*: Mice were used, except for guinea pigs in one case.

disease, but only after longer incubation periods (Tateishi, et al., 1983).  The diseased animals shared clinicopathological features in common but each species shared definite aspects in common.  Spongiform change and proliferation of astrocytes were common to all the animal species used (Fig. 1).  The predominant site of lesions in mice inoculated with material from case 16 in Table was seen in the white matter, while in monkeys, guinea pigs and gerbils the site was in the gray matter, and in rats and hamsters, in both areas.  In addition, the distribution of the lesions in mice differed with each material from the patient.  The mice inoculated with tissues from cases 2 and 16 showed severe lesions in the white matter of the cerebrum, brainstem, cerebellum, spinal cord, internal capsule, and optic and olfactory tracts.  The mice infected from case 11 showed maximal lesions in the cerebral cortices (Fig. 2) and in the group transmitted from cases 17 to 19, the thalamus and basal ganglia were also severely affected.  These particular distributions remained the same throughout the serial propagations in mice.  Degeneration and loss of nerve cells were minimal, in comparison with the marked spongy state and gliosis.  A few phagocytes containing degeneration products and which stained positively with Sudan III were seen in the white matter.

Amyloid plaques seen in 5 patients were also reproduced in mice inoculated with tissues from 9 patients (Table).  The plaques were spherical with diameters of up to 30 $\mu$m, and stained weakly eosinophilic with H-E, green with Masson's trichrome, and were less argyrophilic and strongly positive with PAS staining (Fig. 3).  With Congo red and thioflavin S stainings, the birefringent and fluorescent nature of amyloid protein was observed.  Some plaques were associated with a few glial cells and phagocytes containing inoculation materials, but with no particular change in the surrounding neuropils (Tateishi, et al., 1984a).  These were located mostly in the cerebral white matter close to the lateral ventricles, such as the corpus callosum, hippocampus and parietal white matter. The plaques were more numerous on the right, injected side but sometimes the incidence was equal in both hemispheres.

## 2. Electron Microscopic Studies

Ultrastructural findings in the diseased animals were all but identical, in all species (Sato, et al., 1980).  The spongiform change of the gray matter corresponded to numerous vacuoles located in the neuropils (Fig. 4).  Some were identified as intradendritic oraxonal vacuoles bounded by single or double membranes (Fig. 5) and others were regarded as swelling and clearing of the neuronal processes.  The nuclei and parikarya of the nerve cells appeared normal.  Ultrastructurally, various degrees of the spongiform change were observed in the white matter of all diseased animals, especially in mice (Fig. 6).  Vacuoles

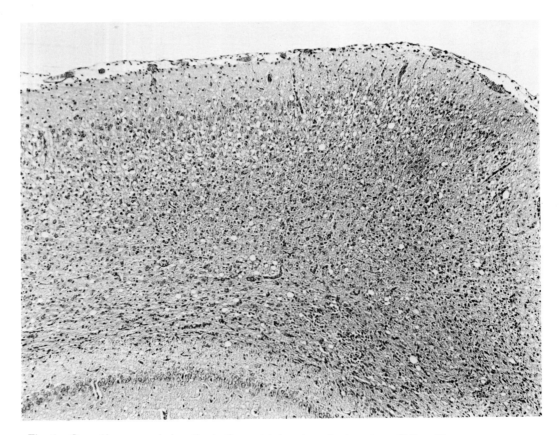

**Fig. 1.**  Spongiform encephalopathy in the parietal cortex of a hamster.  H-E × 85.

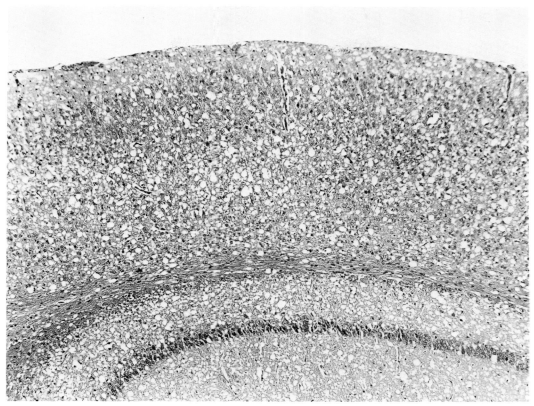

**Fig. 2.**   Lesion in a mouse inoculated with tissue from case 11.   H-E × 95.

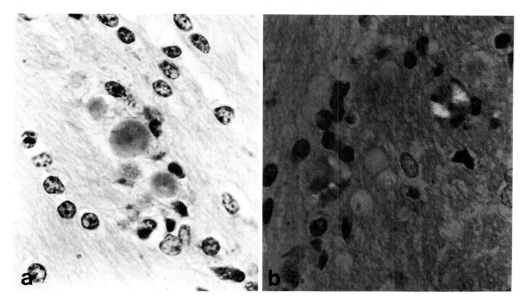

**Fig. 3.**   Amyloid plaques in the parietal white matter of a mouse.   **a)** PAS staining.   × 800.
**b)** Birefringency with Congo red staining.   × 800.

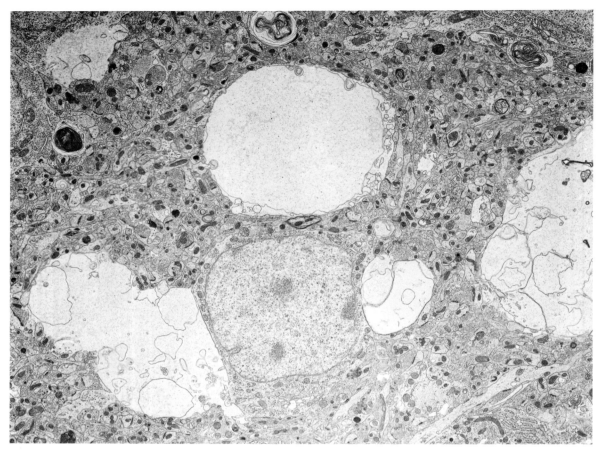

**Fig. 4.** Vacuoles in the neuropil of a mouse parietal cortex, containing floccular materials and membranous structures.  × 4,500.

developed between the myelin layers by splitting of the major dense line (Fig. 7) and swelling of the inner loop, indicating vacuolation in the oligodendroglial processes.  Most axons with vacuolated myelin sheaths were preserved but a few myelinated and unmyelinated axons were markedly expanded by large vacuoles in the axoplasm.  These vacuoles usually contained various amounts of floccular or granular materials, irregular membranous structures and vesicles.  The extracellular space was dilated in severely affected animals but the vessel walls showed no obvious change.  Reactive astrocytes and macrophages were scattered throughout the white matter.

Electron microscopic observation of the plaques in mice revealed amyloid filaments, 70-100 Å in diameter and a small amount of vesicular and dense granular structures (Tateishi, et al., 1984a).  These were surrounded by the processes of astrocytes and of macrophages, although degenerative changes in the surrounding neuronal processes were rare or absent.  Neither viral particles nor spiroplasma-like structures were found in our materials.

## 3. CJD in Humans and Animals

Of the 19 patients from whom inoculation materials were taken, 16 were classified as cases of subacute spongiform encephalopathy (SSE).  Many of them, however, had a protracted clinical course and might be classed as "chronic spongiform encephalopathy". Two (cases 17 and 18) were diagnosed as Gerstmann-Sträussler-Scheinker's disease or syndrom (GSS).   One (case 17) belonged to German family "Sch" (Schumm, et al., 1981) and the other to a Japanese family (Yoshimura, et al., 1984, *No. 125*).   One atypical patient (case 16) showed spongiform change associated with severe white matter change, pontocerebellar degeneration and numerous amyloid plaques (Tateishi, et al., 1979). Distinctive clinical features such as myoclonus and periodic synchronous discharge (PSD) on the electroencephalogram were not detected in some of the chronic cases.

Pathological features of these patients were not uniform and were with or without

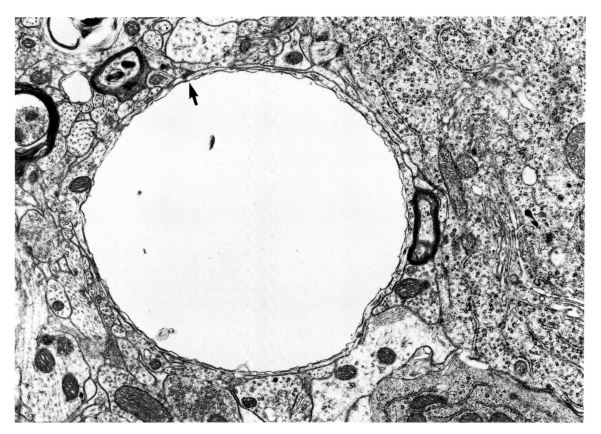

**Fig. 5.**   A large vacuole bounded by double membranes in a dendrite.   An arrow indicates a synapse. Rat parietal cortex.   × 15,000.

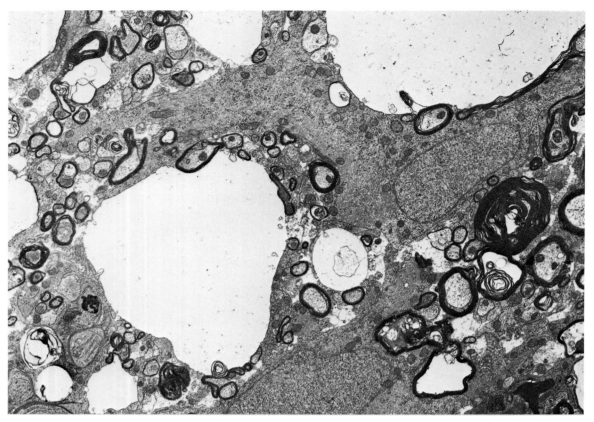

**Fig. 6.** There are various sizes of vacuoles bounded with thin myelin sheaths, degenerated myelinated fibers and reactive astrocytes in the cerebral white matter of a mouse. × 6,000.

severe spongiform change, neuronal loss, white matter change and amyloid plaques. Differences in the positive transmission to laboratory animals, length of incubation periods, distribution of spongiform changes in mice, and incidence of amyloid plaques may suggest strain differences in the causative agents in these patients, although definite correlations between the features in the patients and animals were not determined.

Various degrees of change in the white matter were seen in many patients and laboratory animals, light microscopically. Ultrastructurally, there were spongiform changes in the white matter as well as in the gray matter, in all the laboratory animals. Therefore, white matter change may occur primarily in CJD. Spongiform change was not detected in case 17 with typical GSS, while a severe sponginess was present in the sister (Schumm, et al., 1981). Mice infected from the brother developed severe spongiform change (Tateishi, et al., 1984b). Therefore, spongiform change in GSS is rather concomitant and the disease is transmissible, regardless of the spongiform change. The other GSS patient (case 18) showed spongiform change and the disease was not transmissible to rodents, while in tissues from his daughter the disease was transmitted to monkeys (Masters, et al., 1981). Cases 16 and 18 shared common clinico-pathological features with some reported cases in Japan (Nakashima, et al., 1976, *No. 121*; Hirano, et al., 1977, *No. 122*; Nakamura, et al., 1979, *No. 124*).    There was a long clinical course with progressive cerebellar symptoms, and pathologically spongiform change, profound white matter lesion, amyloid plaques and often systemic degeneration resembling olivo-ponto-cerebellar atrophy.    This type may constitute a transitional type between SSE and GSS.

Production of amyloid plaques in mice did not correlate with the presence of the plaques in patients but rather with an adequate length of incubation periods in the first passage (Tateishi, et al., 1984a).    The plaques were produced neither within short incubation periods after the second passage, nor in species other than mice.    The amyloid plaques in mice were the same as cores of the senile plaques in Alzheimer's disease, albeit without changes in the surrounding neuropils.    This difference may relate to ground structures; senile plaques appear mostly in the gray matter and amyloid plaques of mice in the white matter.    The latter plaques may serve as an animal model of the former.

The question is raised as to why CJD was transmitted from so many patients to

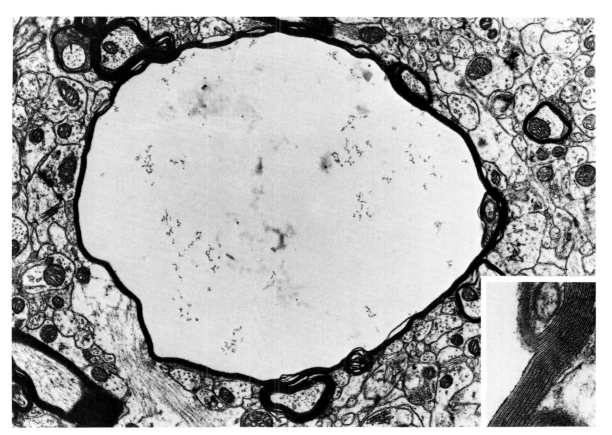

**Fig. 7.**   An intramyelinic vacuole in a rat parietal cortex.   × 15,000.   Inset: The myelin splitting developed at the major dense line.   × 75,000.

rodents in our experiments and why amyloid plaques occurred only in our mice. Some-one suggested a peculiar character of CJD patients in Japan (Kingsbury, et al., 1982). Characterization of causative agents in our two patients; one with typical SSE (case 11) and the other atypical case (case 16) showed the same unconventional properties found in scrapie, kuru and CJD in other countries (Tateishi, et al., 1980; Kingsbury, et al., 1982). Clinicopathological difference among these disease and patients may be due to the strain differences of the causative agents. The successful transmission into rodents suggests that the pathogenesis among these disease is fundamentally the same.

## Summary

We successfully transmitted CJD to rodents from 19 patients with different clinico-pathological features. From 14 patients including a typical case of GSS, spongiform encephalopathy was transmitted to rodents and amyloid plaques were produced in mice given tissues from 9 patients. Incidence of positive transmission, length of incubation periods, distribution of lesions and production of amyloid plaques in mice differed with each patient, suggesting strain differences of the causative agents. Characterization of the agent from two patients showed the same unconventional properties found in scrapie, kuru and CJD in countries other than Japan. Further elucidation of the CJD agent can be expected using this animal model.

The authors are grateful to Drs. M. Ohta and H. Nagara for electron microscopical studies, to Misses K. Hatanaka, K. Beppu, and Y. Sakurai for excellent technical and secretarial assistance, and to M. Ohara for critical reading of the manuscript. This work was supported by grants from the Ministry of Education, and of Health and Welfare of Japan.

## REFERENCES

**Gajdusek, D. C., Gibbs, C. J. Jr. and Alpers, M. P.**: Experimental transmission of a kuru-like syndrome to chimpanzees, Nature, 209: 794-796, 1966.
**Gibbs, C. J. Jr., Gajdusek, D. C., Asher, D. M., Alpers, M. P., Beck, E., Daniel, P. M. and Mathews, W. B.**: Creutzfeldt-Jakob disease (subacute spongiform encephalopathy): Trans-mission to the chimpanzee, Science, 161: 388-389, 1968.
**Hirano, T., Tsuchiya, H., Kawai, K. and Mori, K.**: An autopsy case of Creutzfeldt-Jakob disease with kuru-like neuropathological changes, Acta Pathol. Jpn., 27: 231-238, 1977.
**Kingsbury, D. T., Smeltzer, D. A., Amyx, H. L., Gibbs, C. J. Jr. and Gajdusek, D. C.**: Evidence for an unconventional virus in mouse adapted Creutzfeldt-Jakob disease, Infect. Immun., 37: 1050-1053, 1982.
**Manuelidis, E. E. and Manuelidis, L.**: Clinical and morphological aspects of transmissible Creutzfeldt-Jakob disease. In: Zimmerman, H. M. ed. Progress in Neuropathology, Vol. 4. 1979;

1-26, New York, Raven Press.

**Masters, C. L., Gajdusek, D. C. and Gibbs, C. J. Jr.:** Creutzfeldt-Jakob disease virus isolations from the Gerstmann-Sträussler Syndrome: With an analysis of the various forms of amyloid plaque deposition in the virus-induced spongiform excephalopathies, Brain, 104: 559-588, 1981.

**Nakamura, T., Takamatsu, I., Shida, K., Kotorii, K., Anraku, S. and Kida, H.:** A case of subacute spongiform encephalopathy with numerous Kuru-plaques in the cerebral and cerebellar cortices, Adv. Neurol. Sci. (Japan), 23: 484-492, 1979.

**Nakashima, K., Makino, T., Kinoshita, J. and Yagishita, S.:** A peculiar case of panencephalopathy with widespread distribution of plaques, status spongiosus and demyelination, Adv. Neurol. Sci. (Japan), 20: 362-371, 1976.

**Sato, Y., Ohta, M. and Tateishi, J.:** Experimental transmission of human subacute spongiform encephalopathy to small rodents. II. Ultrastructural study of spongy state in the gray and white matter, Acta Neuropathol., 51: 135-140, 1980.

**Schumm, F., Boellaard, J. W., Schlote, W. and Stöhr, M.:** Morbus Gerstmann-Sträussler-Scheinker. Familie Sch.-Ein Bericht über drei Kranke, Arch Psychiatr. Nervenkr., 230: 179-196, 1981.

**Tateishi, J., Koga, M., Sato, Y. and Mori R.:** Properities of the transmissible agent derived from chronic spongiform encephalopathy, Ann. Neurol., 7: 390-391, 1980.

**Tateishi, J., Nagara, H., Hikita, K. and Sato, Y.:** Amyloid plaques in the brains of mice with Creutzfeldt-Jakob disease, Ann. Neurol., 15 278-280, 1984a.

**Tateishi, J., Ohta, M., Koga, M., Sato, Y. and Kuroiwa, Y.:** Transmission of chronic spongiform encephalopathy with kuru plaques from humans to small rodents, Ann. Neurol., 5: 581-584, 1979.

**Tateishi, J., Sato, Y., Nagara, H. and Boellaard, J. W.:** Experimental transmission of human subacute spongiform encephalopathy to small rodents. IV. Positive transmission from a typical case of Gerstmann-Sträussler-Scheinker's disease. Acta Neuropathol. (Berl), 64: 85-88, 1984b.

**Tateishi, J., Sato, Y., and Ohta, M.:** Creutzfeldt-Jakob disease in humans and laboratory animals. In: Zimmerman, H. M. ed Progress in Neuropathology, Vol. 5, 1983: 195-221, New York, Raven Press.

**Yoshimura, T., Tateishi, J., Tsujihata, M., Muro, T., Mameya, G. and Nagataki, S.:** A case of spongiform encephalopathy with ataxia and amyloid plaques, Brain and Nerves (Japan), 36: 789-795, 1984.

Chapter VI

# Status Spongiosus in the Gray Matter of Human Disease and Experimental Toxic Encephalopathies

Naoki Horita, M. D.

Status spongiosus or spongy state is a descriptive term for the fine and/or coarse vacuolation of the neuropil and white matter.   This change is heterogenous and composed of swelling of astrocytic cytoplasm and processes, vacuolation and distension in the neuronal perikaryon, swelling of neurites including presynaptic terminals and post-synaptic dendrites, dilatation of the extracellular space, bleb formation in myelin sheaths, etc.   The main thema is pathogenesis of the spongy state in the gray matter of Creutzfeldt-Jakob disease (CJD).   In this chapter, therefore, the ultrastructure of status spongiosus in the gray matter will be observed in human cerebral disease and in experimental toxic encephalopathies, in which this change is a prominent feature, and then status spongiosus in CJD will be discussed in relation to that of other disease and induced by toxic substances especially 6-aminonicotinamide (6-AN).   Status spongiosus in the white matter and induced by slow transmissible viral infections should be referred to the chapter and other reviews (Gonantas, 1970; Lampert, et al., 1972).

## 1. Status Spongiosus in Human Cerebral Disease

With the light microscope, this change is composed of the presence or conglomeration of empty vacuoles of spherules in the neuropil, and observed in CJD, acquired chronic hepatocerebral disease including Inose and pseudoulegyric types, Wilson's disease, disease of kuru, Huntington's chorea, Pick's disease, Lissauer's dementia paralytica, Alpers' disease (poliodystrophia cerebri progressiva), etc.

CJD is neuropathologically characteristic of status spongiosus in the neuropil, loss of neuronal cells and proliferation and hypertrophy of astrcytes.   These changes are obser-

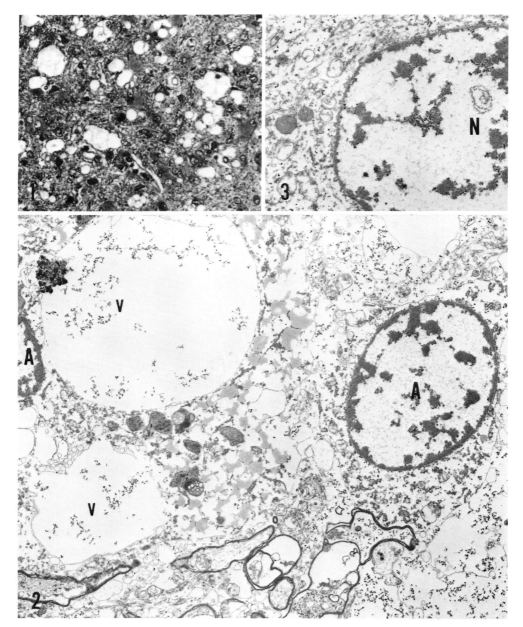

**Fig. 1.** 57-years-old female. Creutzfeldt-Jakob disease. Occipital cortex. One micron Araldite section stained with toluidine blue. Status spongiosus and many hypertrophic astrocytes in the cortical layers. × 240.

**Fig. 2.** CJD. Occipital cortex. Membrane-bounded vacuoles in the cytoplasm of astrocyte. They contained glycogen granules, fragmented membranous structures and vesicles. There were lipofuscin granules and rough endoplasmic reticulum in the cytoplasm of astrocyte. A: nucleus of astrocyte. v: vacuole. × 6,300.

**Fig. 3.** CJD. Occipital cortex. Hypertrophic astrocyte contained nuclear body in the nucleus and gliofilaments and glycogen granules in the cytoplasm. N: nuclear body (simple type) in the nucleus of astrocyte. × 10,400.

ved in the cerebral cortex and, in some cases, in basal ganglia, thalamus, brainstem, cerebellum and spinal cord. The ultrastructure of this disease has been reported by several authors. Some found that the spongy change was composed of swelling of astrocyte and its processes (Marin, et al., 1964; Sluga, et al., 1967; Foncin, 1967; Torack, 1969), while the others described swelling of neuronal components such as neuronal perikaryon (Gonatas, et al., 1965), neurites (Lampert, et al., 1972; Hirano, et al., 1972), dendrites (Kidd, 1967) and presynaptic endings and preterminal axons (Brion, et al., 1969; Bignami, et al., 1970; Gonatas, 1970), in addition to swelling of astrocytes. Lampert et al. (1972) and Hirano et al. (1972) insisted that neuronal changes were primary, while swelling of astrocytic components and hypertrophy and hyperplasia of astrocytes were secondary.

The ultrastructure of status spongiosus (Fig. 1) in our material taken at autopsy exhibited electron-lucent swelling of the astrocytic cytoplasm and its processes (Figs. 2 & 4). The swollen cytoplasm contained membrane-bound vacuoles, probably derived from expansion of the endoplasmic reticulum (Fig. 2) and/or was separated into a few vacuoles by membranes (Fig. 4). They included often fragmented or folded membranes, vesicles and glycogen granules. The cytoplasm surrounding vacuoles was frequently filled with gliofilaments, glycogen granules and dense bodies. There was no dilatation of the extracellular space. However, the origin of cells with affected processes could not always be identified, because the material was taken at autopsy and specimens for electron microscope showed artefacts resulting from the autolysis. The nucleus of hypertrophic astrocytes filled with gliofilaments contained frequently nuclear bodies of simple or complex type (Fig. 3) (Grunnet, 1975; Payne, et al., 1975). It will be concluded that spongy state observable under the light microscope is mainly composed of swelling of astrocytic components, whether it is primary or not.

The cardinal neuropathologic findings in Inose type of acquired chronic hepato-cerebral disease (Inose, 1952) are diffuse in the size and number of protoplasmic astrocytes (Alzheimer type II glia) frequently containing intranuclear PAS-positive inclusion, and diffuse but patchy degeneration of neurons and myelins which is associated with pronoun-ced status spongiosus in the pseudolaminar or laminar pattern.

According to our observation (Horita, et al., 1979), Inose type of hepatocerebral disease exhibited status spongiosus in the 2nd layer of the frontal cortex (Fig. 5). It was composed of swelling of astrocytic cytoplasm and its processes, in which vacuoles probably derived from the endoplasmic reticulum, hypertrophied mitochondria and glyco-gen granules were observed (Fig. 6). The cells, thought to be comparable to Alzheimer

---

**Fig. 4.** Occipital cortex. Polycystic vacuoles separated by a few membranous structures, probably derived from endoplasmic reticulum. They contained glycogen granules and a few vesicles. × 5,100.

**Fig. 5.** 67-years old male. Inose type of hepatocerebral disease. Temporal cortex. One micron Epon section stained with toluidine blue. Stauts spongiosus in the second layer of temporal cortex. × 240.

**Fig. 6.** Inose type of hepatocerebral disease. Temporal cortex. Astrocytic processes were swollen and electron-lucent, and contained a few fragmented or vesiculated membranous structures and glycogen granules. × 5,100.

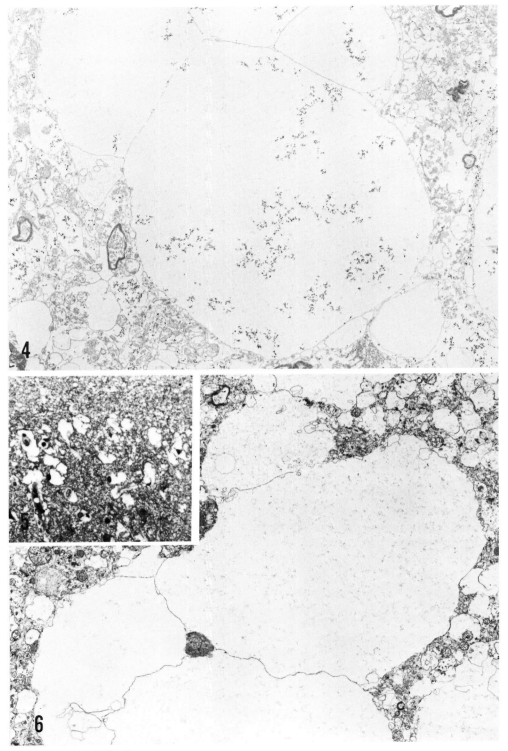

Fig. 4, Fig. 5 and Fig. 6

type II glia under the light microscope, had also swollen electron-lucent cytoplasm, containing glycogen granules and focal aggregates of lipofuscin granules of irregular lines with internal area of low density and foamy appearance. But they did not include gliofilaments in the cytoplasm. Their nuclei contained nuclear bodies with or without aggregates of glycogen granules in the central portion and conglomerates of glycogen granules without any surrounding capsule (Horita, et al., 1979 & 1981b; Kida, 1980; Miyakawa, et al., 1982). The simple type of nuclear bodies was also observed in the nuclei of endothelial cells.

## 2. Status Spongiosus in Experimental Toxic Encephalopathies

Ouabain, an inhibitor of $Na^+$, $K^+$-ATPase, produced distension of dendrites at the initial stage and secondarily swelling of astrocytes, when it was topically applied to the cerebral cortex (Towfighi, et al., 1973; Tanaka, et al., 1977). Some authors reported swelling of presynaptic terminals (Cornog, et al., 1967; Wolff, et al., 1975) or of presynaptic endings and apical dendrites (Lowe, 1978), in addition to that of astrocytes. These discrepancies might be due to severity of lesions, different methods of tissue fixation and various intervals after application of this drug. An acute penicillin-induced epileptogenic lesion showed swelling of dendrites before cortical paroxysm and during convulsive seizure. After sustained convulsive activity, astrocytic swelling was observed (Okada, et al., 1972). The epileptic lesion induced by ionic or metallic cobalt was composed of dendritic swelling at the initial stage, and then astrocytic swelling and dilatation of the extracellular space (Fischer, 1969; Butler, et al., 1976; Nakamura, et al., 1981).

Although the transmembrane ion homeostasis is normally regulated by the activity of cation-activated ATPase, the application of ouabain, penicillin and ionic or metallic cobalt will induce a direct effect on the excitatory function of membrane, such as resting potential and active transport of cations through the membrane, and cause disequilibrium of intra- and extracellular cation concetrations, especially $K^+$ ions. Astrocytes play an important role in maintaining the correct concentrations of $K^+$ ions in the extracellular space and cause neuronal electrical transmission to take place (Kuffler, et al., 1966). The above physiological changes, therefore, might produce swelling of dendrites at the initial stage and, after that astrocytic swelling.

When pyrithiamine, a thiamine antagonist, was administered daily on the condition of thiamine deficiency at adult animals, initial changes in the parenchyma were swelling of

**Fig. 7.** Pyrithiamine-induced thiamine deficient encephalopathy. Six daily injections of pyrithiamine 10 mg/kg on thiamine deficient diet after administration of the same thiamine deficient diet for 18 days. Mammillary nucleus of 3-month-old rat. Postsynaptic dendrites were swollen and electron-lucent, and contained mitochondria, microtubules and hypolemmal cisterna. Arrow: synaptic junction. × 10,200.

**Fig. 8.** Pyrithiamine-induced thiamine deficient encephalopathy. Mammillary nucleus of 34-day-old rat. The postsynaptic dendrite was swollen. The perivascular dendrites were also slightly swollen and contained glycogen granules. × 17,000.

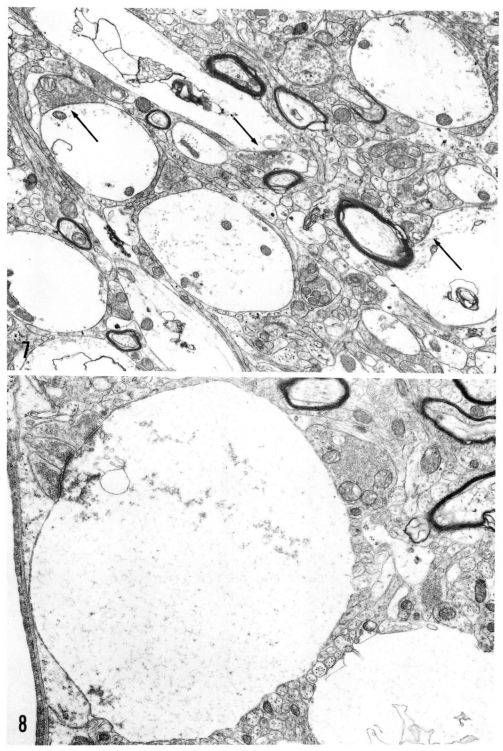

**Fig. 7** and **Fig. 8**

postsynaptic dendrites (Figs. 7 & 8) (Ule, et al., 1968; Horita, et al., 1983) and dilatation of the adaxonal space of myelinated fibers (Watanabe, et al., 1978 & 1981; Horita, et al., 1983). Thiamine is involved in the function of the excitable membrane (Itokawa, et al., 1970), in addition to the action as a coenzyme of oxidative decarboxylation of pyruvate and alpha-ketoglutarate and transketolation steps of hexose monophoshate shunt. Pyrithiamine inhibits catalysis of the voltage-dependent changes in sodium-permeable membrane (Barchi, 1976). Therefore, the administration of pyrithiamine to thiamine-deficient animals may induce swelling of postsynaptic dendrites, as ouabain which inhibits $Na^+$, $K^+$-ATPase and promotes the release of thiamine from the nerve membrane (Itokawa, et al., 1970) does.

The neuroexcitatory amino acids, monosodium glutamate or DL-glutamic acid, DL-aspartic acid, L-cysteine sulfinic acid, L-cysteic acid and L-cysteine, produced spongy state at the initial stage and neuronal degeneration in the retina and hypothalamus, particularly in arcuate nucleus, when administered subcutaneously in the infant animals (Olney, 1969 & 1971; Lemkey-Johnston, et al., 1974). These lesions showed reversible swelling of astrocytic cytoplasm, and severe swelling of neuronal perikaryon and postsynaptic dendrites. The latter was followed by irreversible degeneration and phagocytosis by macrophages. The derivatives of the above amino acids, N-methyl DL-glutamic acid, N-methyl DL-aspartic acid and DL-homocysteic acid, showed more potent neurotoxic activity than monosodium glutamate in necrotizing neurons. On the other hand, the other derivatives of DL-glutamic acid and DL-aspartic acid such as DL-alpha aminoadipic acid, alpha methyl DL-glutamic acid, alpha methyl DL-aspartic acid, 2-amino-3-phosphonopropionic acid and 2-amino-4-phosphonobutylic acid, produced swelling of astrocytes and their processes in the retina and arcuate nucleus, when administered subcutaneously in the infant animals (Olney, et al., 1971).

Kainic acid, a rigid analogue of the putative neurotransmitter glutamic acid, showed the same cytopatholgic change (mainly dendritic swelling) in olfactory system, amygdaloid complex, hippocampal formation, thalamus and neocortex when administered parenterally to adult rats (Olney, et al., 1979; Schwob, et al., 1980; Sperk, et al., 1983). The injection into the cerebellum and striatum showed also similar changes (Lovell, et al., 1980; Krammer, 1980). The folic acid, consisting of pteridine, para-aminobenzoic acid and glutamic acid, and its derivatives, such as methyl tetrahydrofolate (MTHF) and N-5-formyltetrahydrofolate (FTHF), are derivatives of glutamic acid and have kainic acid-like neurotoxic activities. The injection into the amygdala induced pathological changes similar to kainic acid treatment, but the lesions were restricted largely to the piriform cortex and hippocampus (Olney, et al., 1981). Folic acid injections into substantia innominata produced degeneration of many GABAergic neurons in the distant area but spared relatively cholinergic ones (McGeer, et al., 1983).

The intravenous injection of bicuculline, a gamma-aminobutyric acid (GABA) receptor blocking agent, induced status epilepticus and exhibits nerve cell abnormalities of two kinds and status spongiosus in the cerebral cortex and hippocampal formation. The status spongiosus was composed of swelling of astrocytes and their processes resulting in both perivascular and perineuronal vacuolation (Soederfeldt, et al., 1981; Atillo, et al., 1983). Allylglycine showed also similar cytopathologic changes and to a more severe degree; watery swelling of astrocytes particularly surrounding blood vessels and pyramidal neurons, and neuronal changes (Meldrum, et al., 1973; Griffiths, et al., 1982). This substance is an inhibitor of glutamic acid decaboxylase, the cerebral enzyme synthesizing the inhibitory transmitter substance GABA.

Glutamate, aspartate, L-cysteine and their analogues are neuroexcitatory and possess the neurotoxic activity which causes convulsion and morphologic change. The sustained high concentrations around the synaptic clefts can lead to persistent depolarization and altered ionic permeability of neuronal membranes resulting in neuronal necrosis in some restricted regions. Astrocytic cytoplasm and processes might also show pathologic spongy change, because they wrap synaptic cleft region and are associated with the reuptake of the putative neurotransmitter glutamate and the maintenance of ionic equilibrium in the extracellular space. The preponderance of astroglial swelling epecially in DL-alpha aminoadipic acid remains to be solved. Bicuculline and allylglycine affect the action of GABA, a putative inhibitory neurotransmitter. When the release of GABA acting on exciting neurons is continuously reduced, excitatory neurons might increase the probability of multiple discharges in response to a constant stimulus and lead to neuropathologic changes. Penicillin application, of which pathologic change was discussed above, reduces also inhibitory action of GABA through the recurrent synapses (Dingledine, et al., 1980).

Pentylenetetrazole, a convulsant agent, induced a considerable swelling of astroglial cells around the capillaries and neurons at the time of convulsion (2-5 minutes after injection) (DeRobertis, et al., 1969). But this change might be, in part, artefactual, because histological preparation was taken from materials by immersion fixation.

Oral administration of Cupurizone, a chelater used as a reagent for copper analysis, produced severe status spongiosus in the central nervous system of mouse, and enlargement of mitochondria and proliferation of smooth endoplasmic reticulum in hepatocytes. Status spongiosus was composed of vacuole formation in the myelin sheath and vacuolation in the swollen cytoplasm of glial cells (Suzuki, et al., 1969). It is worthwhile to note that pathologic changes in the nervous system and liver appear simultaneously, although their relationship is not clear. The spongy state in the gray matter consisting of the swelling of astrocytic cytoplasm and processes, has been reported in experimental hepatic encephalopathy (Cavanagh, et al., 1972; Zamora, et al., 1973; Norenberg, et al., 1974). This encephalopathy is produced by hyperammonaemia after total hepatectomy, portocaval anastomosis, ammonia infusions, urease injections, etc. The ammonium ions function as an almost similar hydrated ionic radius, so that they pass through the membrane in the same manner as potassium ions. The incorporated $NH_4^+$ ions are metabolized to glutamine by glutamate dehydrogenase catalysing the amination of alpha-ketoglutarate to glutamate and glutamine synthetase catalyzing the amination of glutamate to glutamine, both localized in a small glutamate synthetic compartment of astroglia (Balázs, et al., 1973). Synthetized glutamine diffuses readily out of the nervous system. The detoxication of $NH_4^+$ ions excess will be incomplete in the nervous system of hepatic encephalopathy, although the enzymatic activity of glutamate dehydrogenase is increased (Norenberg, 1976). As a consequence, it causes the disturbance of intracellular cation concentrations, especially $K^+$ ions, and of resting membrane potential in astroglia. The astrocytic swelling might reflect this disturbance induced by excess of ammonia.

Administration of methionine sulfoximine, an inhibitor of glutamine synthetase,

produced enlargement of astrocytic cytoplasm and its processes, proliferation of mitochondria and endoplsmic reticulum and accumulation of glycogen granules in rats (Rizzuto, et al., 1974; Gutierrez, et al., 1977), rabbits (Harris, 1964; Ule, 1968) and dogs (Harris,
1964). After sustained or severe convulsion, swelling of presynaptic ending was observed,
in addition to swelling of astrocytes (DeRobertis, et al., 1967; Rizzuto, et al., 1974).

When 6-aminonicotinamide (6-AN) was injected at a single or several repeated times
to suckling rats, all levels of cerebellar cortex exhibited a spongy state with numerous
vacuoles of various sizes. The spongy state was composed of progressive swelling of the
endoplasmic reticulum in astrocytes and less frequently in oligodendrocytes and swelling
of astrocytic processes including enlarged endoplasmic reticulum. Most of the neurons
remained unaffected, but in older rats 6-AN affected also cells of neuronal populations
(Schaarschmidt, 1975; Schaarschmidt, et al., 1975; Sotelo, et al., 1980). Administration of
6-AN to young adult rats (3-5 month old) produced acute pathologic change in the spinal
gray matter and several brainstem nuclei. The change was composed of swelling of
neuroglial cytoplasm, spongy state of the neuropil and, further damaged, petechial
hemorrhage, neuronal degeneration and dilatation of the extracellular space (Schneider, et
al., 1974; Horita, et al., 1978). Fifteen-, 20- and 25-month-old rats showed the spongy state
in the limbic structures, striatum and temporal cortex, becoming more prominent with
aging (Fig. 9) and increasing intervals after administration (Horita, et al., 1980 & 1981a).
Many neurons in the region of spongy change showed chromatolytic change in 25-month-
old rats (Fig. 9d). The spongy state was composed of swelling of astrocytic cytoplasm
and processes (Figs. 10 & 11). They contained membranous structures probably derived
from endoplasmic reticulum and glycogen granules. Astrocytic cytoplasm showed also
swelling filled with enlarged endoplasmic reticula (Fig. 12) and rarely proceeded to
degenerative change with pyknotic nucleus. With increasing intervals after administration of 6-AN, astrocytes exhibited hypertrophic change prominent in cytoplasmic
organella, enpecially gliofilaments (Figs. 13 & 14) and frequently proliferative change, such
as daughter cells with apposing cytoplasmic membrane (Fig. 15). Distended cytoplasm of
astrocyte was rarely packed with proliferation of smooth endoplasmic reticulum and
mitochondria (Fig. 16).

3-acetylpyridine (3-AP) produced patchy edema in hippocampal formation of mice 20
days and 1 year after administration (Lierse, 1965), while others reported neuronal
necrosis in the inferior olive (Denk, et al., 1968). The electronmicrograph exhibited
swelling of astroglial cytoplasm and process, and also of oligodendroglial ones (Lierse,
1965).

6-AN and 3-AP are synthetized to NAD(P)-anaglogues in the brain tissue because of
nonspecificity of synthetic enzymes (Coper, et al., 1963). These NAD(P)-analogues act
competitively as inhibitors of NAD(P)-dependent enzymes such as glutamate dehydrogenase (Fisher, 1973; Bielicki, et al., 1976). On the other hand, many authors reported also
6-phosphogluconate dehydrogenase as a most sensitive enzyme against the administration
of 6-AN (Coper, et al., 1963; Lange, et al., 1970). But, the suppression of hexose monophosphate shunt induced by 6-AN will not be a responsible factor for the pathologic
change as well as that of glycolysis pathway and hexose monophosphate shunt in cerebral
thiamine deficiency (Dreyfus, 1976). Glutamine synthetase and glutamate dehydrogenase
are key enzymes in ammonium detoxication and the latter is exclusively included in

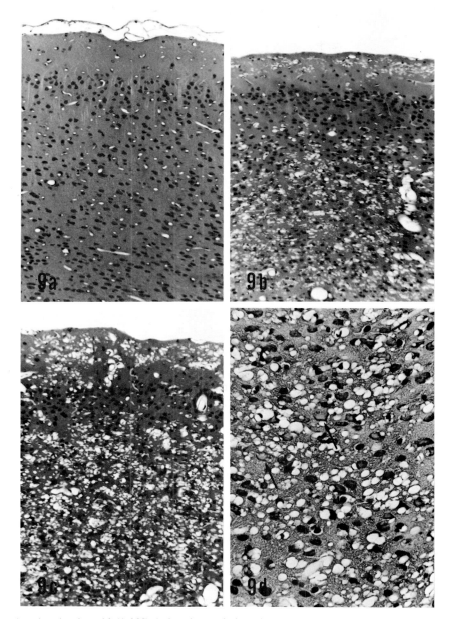

**Fig. 9.**  6-aminonicotinamide(6-AN) -induced encephalopathy.  **a:** Fourteen days after a single intraperitoneal injection of 6-AN 10 mg/kg.  Temporal lobe of 3-month-old rat.  No spongy state of the cortex. HE.  × 96.  **b:** Fourteen days after administration of 6-AN.  Temporal lobe of 15-month-old rat. Prominent multiple vacuoles in the cortex with tendency to coalesce.  Perivascular astrocytes were not always swollen.  HE.  × 96.  **c:** Fourteen days after administration of 6-AN.  Temporal lobe of 20-month-old rat.  Spongy state was more prominent and involved also superficial cortical layers.  HE. × 96.  **d:** Fourteen days after administration of 6-AN.  Temporal lobe of 25-month-old rat.  Neuronal chromatolysis (arrow) and the spongy state in the neuropil were present.  Nissl.  × 240.

236

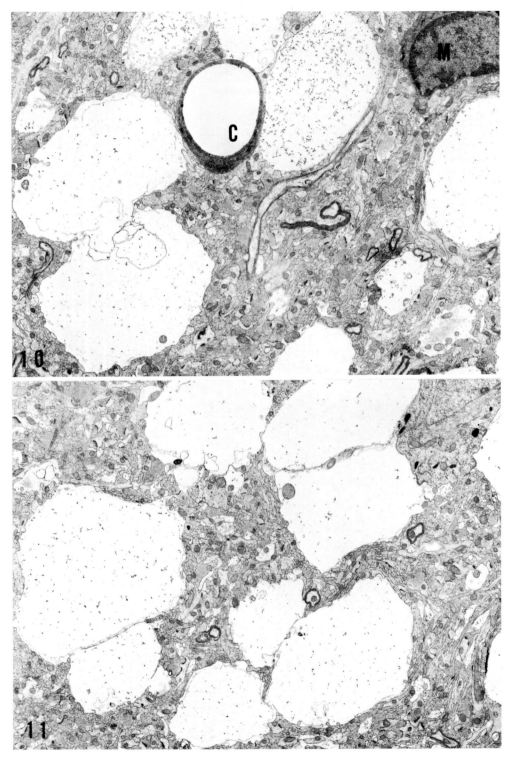

Fig. 10 and Fig. 11 (Legend in page 239)

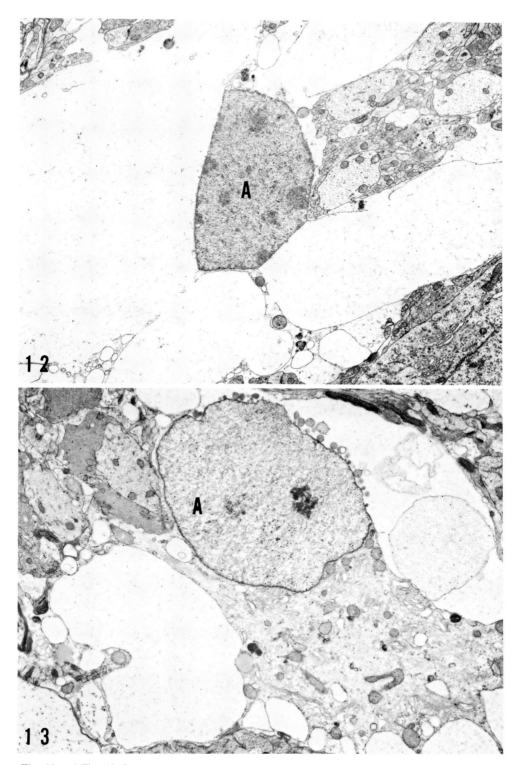

**Fig. 12** and **Fig. 13** (Legend in page 239)

238

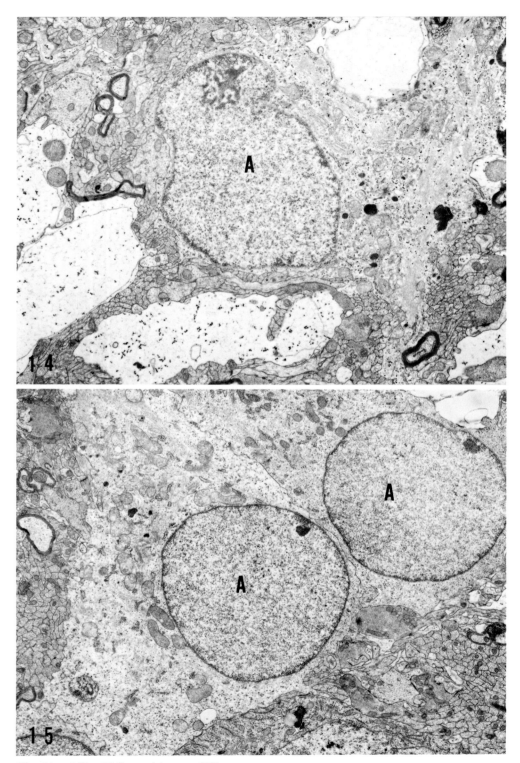

**Fig. 14** and **Fig. 15** (Legend in page 239)

astrocyte (Norenberg, et al., 1979).  The inhibition of these enzymes induced by methionine sulfoximine, 6-AN and 3-AP, might induce disturbance of ammonium detoxication and disequilibrium of the intra- and extra-cellular cation concentrations follwed by astrocytic swelling as well as hepatic encephalopathy.

In conclusion, substances producing status spongiosus in the gray matter will be divided roughly into the following 3 groups:

1: inhibitors of Na$^+$ , K$^+$-dependent ATPase on the excitable membrane.

2: neuroexcitatory substances such as aspartic acid, glutamic acid, L-cysteic acid and their analogues and inhibitors of enzymes associated with GABA biosynthesis and of GABA receptor.

3: substances disturbing the normal detoxication of ammonium ions associated with a small glutamate synthetic compartment.

The first is almost epileptogenic, and damages postsynaptic dendrites at the initial phase followed by swelling of astrocytes and dilatation of extracellular spaces.  The second induces initially astrocytic swelling followed by prominent distension and degene-

---

**Fig. 10.**  6-AN-induced encephaltpathy.  Temporal cortex of 25-month-old rat.  Fourteen days after administration of 6-AN.  Swollen cytoplasm or processes of astrocyte contained membranous structures and glycogen granules in various degree.  The perivascular foot processes were not always swollen.  This photograph exhibited a macrophage at the upper left corner, although it was generally rare.  C: capillary.  M: macrophage.  × 5,100.

**Fig. 11.**  6-AN-induced encephalopathy.  Temporal cortex of 25-month-old rat.  Fourteen days after administration of 6-AN.  The spongy state within the otherwise normal neuropil was composed of swelling of astrocytic cytoplasm or processes.  They contained glycogen granules and membranous structures probably derived from endoplasmic reticulum.  × 5,100.

**Fig. 12.**  6-AN-induced encephalopathy.  Temporal cortex of 25-month-old rat.  Five days after administration of 6-AN.  The cytoplasm of astrocyte was swollen and occupied with distended endoplasmic reticulum which were disrupted in some places.  In other photograph, astrocytes showed degenerative changes and the nucleus was pyknotic.  A: nucleus of astrocyte.  × 6,800.

**Fig. 13.**  6-AN-induced encephalopathy.  Hippocampus of 25-month-old rat.  Fourteen days after administration of 6-AN.  The astrocyte showed dilatation of endoplasmic reticulum and nuclear envelope with nuclear buddings.  The cytoplasm was prominent in organella such as mitochondria, endoplasmic reticulum and gliofilaments.  A: nucleus of astrocyte.  × 6,800.

**Fig. 14.**  6-AN-induced encephalopathy.  Temporal cortex of 25-month-old rat.  Fourteen days after administration of 6-AN.  The astrocyte was hypertrophic and prominent in organella, especially gliofilaments.  There ware swollen processes of astrocytes with enlarged endoplasmic reticulum, glycogen granules and mitochondria.  A: nucleus of astrocyte.  × 9,100.

**Fig, 15.**  6-AN-induced encephalopathy.  Hippocampus of 20-month-old rat.  Fourteen days after administration of 6-AN.  A pair of protoplasmic astrocytes.  Two daughter cells were separated by a set of apposing plasma membranes.  The cytoplasm was prominent in cytoplasmic organella such as mitochondria, glycogen granules, gliofilaments etc.  A: nucleus of astrocyte.  × 5,100.

ration of neuronal cells with some exceptions. The third exhibits principally swelling of astrocytic cytoplasm and processes at relatively long survivals after administration or surgical operation. These evidences suggest that each group showing the similar morphologic change may be produced by the disturbance of one specific metabolic pathway. The relationship between three groups remains to be solved.

## 3. Discussion

Status spongiosus in CJD and Inose type of hepatocerebral disease is mainly composed of swelling of astrocytic cytoplasm and processes and similar to that produced by substances belonging to third group of experimental encephalopathies. The characteristics of CJD are that status spongiosus is present in almost all layers of cerebral cortex, swollen cytoplasm contains often glycogen granules and disrupted or rounded membranous structures and enlarged vacuoles are frequently surrounded with cytoplasm containing gliofilaments and lipofuscin granules. These changes were similar to those induced

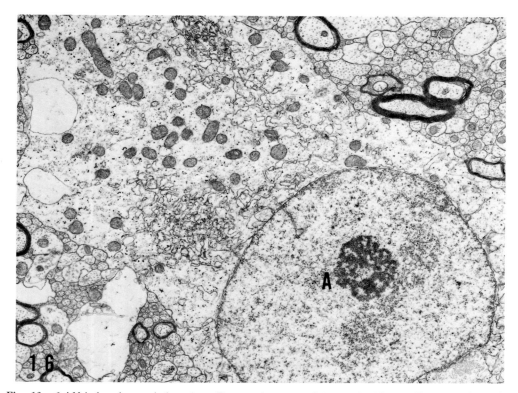

**Fig. 16.** 6-AN-induced encephalopathy. Temporal cortex of 25-month-old rat. Fourteen days after administration of 6-AN. The cytoplasm was plumped and packed with smooth endoplasmic reticulum, in addition to an increase of mitochondria, glycogen granules and gliofilaments. A: nucleus of astrocyte.- × 9,100.

by administration of 6-AN.   On the other hand, spongy state in Inose type is present in the laminar or pseudolaminar pattern and does not contain gliofilaments.   Alzheimer type II glia exhibits negative reaction for glial fibrillary acidic protein (GFAP) staining (Sobel, et al., 1981), although altered astrocytes in experimental hepatic encephalopathy includes gliofilaments at later stage (Cavanagh, et al., 1972).

CJD has been understood as a slow virus infection, since Gibbs et al. (1968) succeeded in its transmission to animals following the inoculation of brain homogenate into the CNS. However, the agent has not yet been isolated and the inflammatory response characteristic of virus encephalopathy is lacking.   On the other hand, the resemblance of CJD and pellagra encephalopathy probably caused by nicotinamide deficiency has been noted by some authors (Stadler, 1939; Jervis, et al., 1942).   Jacob (1960) examined neuropathological changes of seven autopsy cases, that showed initially endogenous psychotic symptoms and exogeneous or organic brain syndromes prior to death.   He concluded that the findings had something in common with those of CJD, Kraepelin's disease, unspecific cerebral atrophy and involutional pellagra, and were only differentiated from each other with some reservation.   Sluga et al. (1957) reported histochemically that the activity of TPN or DRN diaphorase was decreased in neuronal cells of CJD.   Lesions induced by 6-AN, an antimetabolite of nicotinamide showed spongy state in the limbic structures, striatum and cerebral cortex at the age corresponding to the involutional period in the human.   Neurons in damaged regions showed decreased activity of TPN and DPN diaphorase, although not always specific (Schotland, et al., 1965; Iglesias-Rozas, et al., 1974).

These evidences have lead to the hypothesis that CJD might be caused by dysfunction of NAD(H)- or NADP(H)-dependent enzymes and the affected exzymes in CJD and 6-AN-induced encephalopathy might be similar in metabolic pathways.   We postulate, therefore, that dysfunction of these enzymes in the CNS of the aged would be one possible pathoplastic factor for the formation of status spongiosus in CJD, even though it is not a primary pathogenetic factor.

## Acknowledgement

The author wishes to acknowledge the help of Drs. M. Suzuki and S. Fukunaga, Deperment of Pathology, Jikei University School of Medicine, and Dr. A. Okuno, Deperment of Pediatrics, Jikei University School of Medicine, in providing autopsy material for electron microscope and case notes of CJD.

# REFERENCES

**Atillo, A., Soederfeldt, B., Kalimo, H., Olsson, Y. and Siesjoe, B. K.:** Pathogenesis of brain lesions caused by experimental epilepsy. Light- and electronmicroncopic changes in the rat hippocampus following bicuculline-induced status epilepticus. Acta Neuropathol. (Berl.), 59: 11-24, 1983.

**Balázs, R., Patel, A. J. and Richter, D.:** Metabolic compartments in the brain: Their properties and relation to morphological structures. In: Balàzs, R. and Cremer, J. E. ed. Metabolic Compartmentation in the Brain, 1973: 167-184, London, McMillan.

**Barchi, R. L.:** The nonmetabolic role of thiamine in excitable membrane function. In: Gubler, C. J., Fujiwara, M. and Dreyfus, P. M. ed. Thiamine, 1976: 283-285, New York-London-Sydney-Tronto, John Wiley and Sons.

**Bielicki, L. and Krieglstein, J.:** Decreased GABA and glatumate concentration in rat brain after treatment with 6-aminonicotinamide. Naunyn-Schmiedeberg's Arch. Pharmacol., 294: 157-160, 1976.

**Bignami, A. and Forno, L. S.:** Status spongiosus in Jakob-Creutzfeldt disease: Electron microscopic study of a cortical biopsy. Brain, 93: 89-94, 1970.

**Brion, S., Mikol, J., Raverdy, P. and Isidor, P.:** Étude anatomo-clinique d'un cas de maladie de Creutzfeldt-Jakob. Aspects ultra-structuraux. Rev. Neurol. (Paris), 121: 165-179, 1969.

**Butler A. B., Willmore, L. J., Fuller, P. M. and Bass, N. H.:** Focal alteration of dendrites and astrocytes in rat cerebral cortex during initiation of cobalt-induced epileptiform activity. Exp. Neurol., 51: 216-228, 1976.

**Cavanagh, J. B. Lewis, P. D. Blakemore, W. F. and Kyu, M. H.:** Changes in the cerebellar cortex in rats after portocaval anastomosis. J. Neurol. Sci., 15: 13-26, 1972.

**Coper, H. and Herken, H.:** Schaedigung des Zentralnervensystems durch Antimetaboliten des Nicotinsaeureamids. Dtsch. Med. Wochenschr., 88: 2025-2036, 1963.

**Cornog, G. L. Gonatas, N. K. and Feierman, J. R.:** Effects of intracerebral injection of ouabain on the fine structure of rat cerebral cortex. Am. J. Pathol., 51: 573-590, 1967.

**Denk, H., Halder, M., Kovac, W. and Studynka, C.:** Verhaltensaenderung und Neuropathologie bei der 3-Acetylpyridinvergiftung der Ratte. Acta Neuropathol. (Berl.), 10: 34-44, 1968.

**DeRobertis, E., Sellinger, O. Z. DeLores Armaiz, G. R., Alberici, M. and Zieher, L. M.:** Nerve endings in methionine sulfoximine convulsant rats. A neurochemical and ultrastructure study. J. Neurochem., 14: 81-89, 1967.

**DeRobertis, E., Alberici, M. and DeLores Arnaiz, G. R.:** Astroglial swelling and phosphohydrolases in cerebral cortex of Metrazol convulsant rats. Brain Res., 12: 461-466, 1969.

**Dingledine, R. and Gjerstad, L.:** Reduced inhibition during epileptiform activity in the in vivo hippocampal slice. J. Physiol., 305: 297-313, 1980.

**Dreyfus, P. M.:** Thiamine-deficiency encephalopathy: Thoughts on its pathogenesis. In: Gubler, C., Fujiwara, M. and Dreyfus, P. M. ed. Thiamine, 1976: 229-239, New York-London-Sydney-Toronto, John Wiley and Sons.

**Ficher, J.:** Electron microscopic alterations in the vicinity of epileptogenic cobalt-gelatine necrosis in the cerebral cortex of the rat. A contribution to the ultrastructure of "plasmatic infiltration" of the central nervous system. Acta Neuropathol. (Berl.), 14: 201-214, 1969.

**Fisher, H. F.:** Glutamate dehydrogenase ---ligand complexes and their relationship to the mechanism of the reaction. In: Advances in enzymology and related areas of molecular biology, Vol. 39, 1973: 369-417, New York-London-Sydney-Toronto, John Wiley and Sons.

**Foncin, J. F.:** Étude ultrastructurale de la maladie Creutzfeldt-Jakob. Acta Neuropathol.

(Berl.), Suppl. 3: 127-130, 1967.

**Gibbs, C. J. Jr., Gajdusek, D. C., Asher, D. M., Alpers, M. P. Beck, E., Daniel, P. M. and Matthews, W. B.:**   Creutzfeldt-Jakob disease (spongiform encephalopathy): Transmission to the chimpanzee.   Science, 161: 388-389, 1968.

**Gonatas, N. K., Terry, R. D. and Weiss, M.:**   Electron microscopy study in two cases of Jakob-Creutzfeldt-disease.   J. Neuropathol. Exp. Neurol., 24: 575-598, 1965.

**Gonatas, N. K.:**   Comparative study of status spongiosus in human and experimental toxic encephalopathies.   In: VIe Congrés internat. Neuropathol., 1970: 49-59, Paris, Masson.

**Griffiths, T., Evans, M. C. and Meldrum, B. S.:**   Early hippocampal changes in the rat following bicuculline and L-allylglycine-induced seizures: a light and electron microscope study.   Neuropathol. Appl. Neurobiol., 8: 246, 1982.

**Grunnet, M. L.:**   Nuclear bodies in Creutzfeldt-Jakob and Alzheimer's disease. Neurology, 25: 1091-1093, 1975.

**Gutierrez, J. A. and Norenberg, M. D.:**   Ultrastructural study of methionine sulfoximine-induced Alzheimer type II astrocytosis.   Am. J. Pathol., 86: 285-300, 1977.

**Harris, B.:**   Cortical alterations due to methionine sulfoximine.   Arch. Neurol., 11: 388-406, 1964.

**Hirano, A., Ghatak, N. R., Johnson, A. B. Partnow, M. J. and Gomori, A. J.:**   Argentophilic plaques in Creutzfeldt-Jakob disease.   Arch. Neurol., 26: 530-542, 1972.

**Horita, N., Oyanagi, S., Ishii, T. and Izumiyama, Y.:**   Ultrastructure of 6-aminonicotinamide (6-AN)-induced lesions in the central nervous system of rats.   I. Chromatolysis and other lesions in the cervical cord.   Acta Neuropathol. (Berl.), 44: 111-119, 1978.

**Horita, N., Matsushita, M., Ishii, T., Oyanagi, S., Takenaka, H., Sakamoto, K., Hanawa, S., Hirota, I., Kumagai, M., Hato, K., Suzuki, J. and Mizutani, Y.:**   The fine structure of Alzheimer type II glia and its related pathological changes.   Psychiat. Neurol. Jpn., 81: 435-444, 1979.

**Horita, N., Ishii, T. and Izumiyama, Y.:**   Ultrastructure of 6-aminonicotinamide (6-AN)-induced lesions in the central nervous system of rats.   II. Alterations of the nervous susceptibility with aging.   Acta Neuropathol. (Berl.), 49: 19-27 1980.

**Horita, N., Ishii, T. and Izumiyama, Y.:**   Ultrastructure of 6-aminonicotinamide (6-AN)-induced lesions in the central nervous system of rats.   III. Alterations of the spinal gray matter lesion with aging.   Acta Neuropathol. (Berl.), 53: 227-235, 1981a.

**Horita, N., Matsushita, M., Ishii, T., Oyanagi, S. and Sakamoto, K.:**   Ultrastructure of Alzheimer type II glia in hepatocerebral disease.   Neuropathol. Appl. Neurobiol., 7: 97-102, 1981b

**Horita, N., Okuno, A. and Izumiyama, Y.:**   Neuropathologic changes in suckling and weanling rats with pyrithiamine-induced thiamine deficiency.   Acta Neuropathol. (Berl.), 61: 27-35, 1983.

**Iglesias-Rozas, J. R. and DeIglesias, R. E.:**   Histochemical changes in the rat spinal cord after exposure to 6-aminonicotinamide.   Acta Neuropathol. (Berl.), 28: 223-232, 1974.

**Inose, T.:**   Hepatocerebral degeneration a special type.   J. Neuropathol. Exp. Neurol., 11: 401-408, 1952.

**Itokawa, Y. and Cooper, J. R.:**   Ion movements and thiamine.   II. The release of the vitamin from menbrane fragments.   Biochim. Biophys. Acta, 196: 274-284, 1970.

**Jacob, H.:**   Differentialdiagnose pernicioeser Involutionspsychosen, praeseniler Psychosen und Psychosen bei Involutionspellagra. Zur Frage endogen-exogener Mischbilder (Intermediaer-syndrome) im hoeheren Lebensalter.   Arch. Psychiatr. Nervenkr., 201: 17-52, 1960.

**Jervis, G. A. Hurdum, H. M. and O'Neill, F. J.:**   Presenile psychosis of the Jakob type. Clinico-pathologic study of one case with a review of the literature.   Am. J. Psychiatry, 99: 101-109, 1942.

**Kida, H.:**   Histopathological studies on Alzheimer glia type II in various liver diseases.   A study of Best's carmine positive intranuclear inclusion.   Brain & Nerves (Japan), 32: 393-401, 1980.

**Kidd, M.:**   Some electron microscopical observations on status spongiosus.   Acta Neuropathol.

(Berl.), Suppl. 3: 137-144, 1967.

**Krammer, E. B.**: Anterograde and transsynaptic degeneration 'en cascade' in basal ganglia induced by intrastriatal injection of kainic acid: An animal analogue of Huntington's disease. Brain Res., 196: 209-221, 1980.

**Kuffler, S. W. and Nicholls, J. G.** The physiology of neuroglial cells. Ergebn. Physiol., 57: 1-90, 1966.

**Lampert, P, W., Gajdusek, D. C. and Gibbs, C. J. Jr.**: Subacute spongiform virus excephalopathies. Scrapie, Kuru and Creutzfeldt-Jakob disease. Am. J. Pathol., 68: 626-646, 1972.

**Lange, K., Kolbe, H., Keller, K. and Herken, H.**: Der Kohlenhydratstoffwechsel des Gehirns nach Blockade des Pentose-Phosphat-Weges durch 6-Aminonikotinamid. Hoppe-Seylers Z. Physiol. Chem., 351: 1241-1252, 1970.

**Lemkey-Johnston, N. and Reynolds, W. A.**: Nature and extent of brain lesions in mice related to injestion of monosodium glutamate. A light and electron microscope study. J. Neuropathol. Exp. Neurol., 33: 74-97, 1974.

**Lierse, W.**: Ultrastruktuelle Hirnveraenderungen der Ratte nach Gaben von 3-Acetylpyridin. Z. Zellforsch., 67: 86-95, 1965.

**Lovell, K. L. and Jones, M. Z.**: Kainic acid neurotoxicity in the mouse cerebellum. Brain Res., 186: 245-249, 1980.

**Lowe, D. A.**: Morphological changes in th cat cerebral cortex produced by superfusion of ouabain. Brain Res., 148: 347-363, 1978.

**Marin, O. and Vial, J. D.**: Neuropathological and ultrastructural findings in two cases of subacute spongiform encephalopathy. Acta Neuropathol. (Berl.), 4: 218-229, 1964.

**McGeer, P. L., McGerr, E. C. and Nagai, T.**: GABAergic and choninergic indices in various regions of rat brain after intracerebral injections of folic acid. Brain Res., 260: 107-116, 1983.

**Meldrum, B. S., Vigouroux, R. A. and Brierley, J. B.**: Systemic factors and epileptic brain damage. Arch. Neurol., 29: 82-87, 1973.

**Miyakawa, T., Kuramoto, R., Shimoji, A. and Higuchi, Y.**: Fine structure of inclusion body in the nucleus of Alzheimer glia type II in the brain of hepatocerebral degeneration. Acta Neuropathol. (Berl.), 56: 315-319, 1982.

**Nakamura, I., Endo, M., Hosokawa, K., Isaki, K., Koyama, Y. and Katsukawa, K.**: Fine structure of experimental epileptogenic focus produced by intracerebral implantation of cobalt-gelatine stick in rabbits. Folia Psychiat. Neurol. Jpn., 35: 103-111, 1981.

**Norenberg, M. D. and Lapham, L. W.**: The astrocyte response in experimental portal-systemic encephalopathy. An electron microscopic study. J. Neuropathol. Exp. Neurol., 33: 422-435, 1974.

**Norenberg, M. D.**: Histochemical studies in experimental portal-systemic encephalopathy. I. Glutamic dehydrogenase. Arch. Neurol., 33: 265-269, 1976

**Norenberg, M. D. and Martinez-Hernandez, A.**: Fine structural localization of glutamine synthetase in astrocytes of rat brain. Brain Res., 161: 303-310, 1979.

**Okada, K., Ayala, G. F. and Sung, J. H.**: Ultrastructure of penicillin-induced epileptogenic lesion of the cerebral cortex in cats. J. Neuropathol. Exp. Neurol., 30: 337-353, 1972.

**Olney, J. W.**: Glutamate-induced retinal degeneration in neonatal mice. Electron microscopy of the acutely evolving lesion. J. Neuropathol. Exp. Neurol., 28: 455-474, 1969.

**Olney, J. W.**: Glutamate-induced neuronal necrosis in the infant mouse hypothalamus. An electron microscopic study. J. Neuropathol. Exp. Neurol., 30: 75-90, 1971.

**Olney, J. W., Ho, O. L. and Rhee, V.**: Cytotoxic effects of acidic and sulphur containing amino acids on the infant mouse central nervous system. Exp. Brain Res., 14: 61-76, 1971.

**Olney, J. W., Fuller, T. and DeGubareff, T.**: Acute dendrotoxic changes in the hippocampus of kainate treated rats. Brain Res., 176: 91-100, 1979.

**Olney, J. W. Fuller, T. A. and DeGubareff, T.**:   Kainate-like neurotoxicity of folates.   Nature, 292: 165-167, 1981.

**Payne, C. M. and Sibley, W. A.**:   Intranuclear inclusions in a case of Creutufeldt-Jakob disease. An ultrastructural study.   Acta Neuropathol. (Berl.), 31: 353-361, 1975.

**Rizzuto, N. and Gonatas, N. K.**:   Ultrastructural study of effect of methionine sulfoximine on developing and adult rat cerebral cortex.   J. Neuropathol. Exp. Neurol., 33: 237-250, 1974.

**Schaarschmidt, W.**:   Licht- und elektronenmikroskopische Untersuchung am Kleinhirn 12 Tage alter Ratten nach Behandlung mit 6-Aminonikotinamid (6-AN). Acta Anat., 91: 362-375, 1975.

**Schaarschmidt, W. and Lierse, W.**:   Ultrastruktuelle Reaktion der multipotenten Glia im Kleinhirn der Ratte nach Behandlung mit 6-Aminonikotinamid.   Acta Anat., 93: 184-193, 1975.

**Schneider, H. and Cervos-Navarro, J.**:   Acute gliopathy in spinal cord and brainstem induced by 6-aminonicotinamide.   Acta Neuropathol. (Berl.), 27: 11-23, 1974.

**Schotland, D. L., Cowen, D., Geller, L. M. and Wolf, A.**:   A histochemical study of the effects of an antimetabolite, 6-aminonicotinamide, on the lumbar spinal cord of the adult rat.   J. Neuropathol. Exp. Neurol., 24: 97-107, 1965.

**Schwob, J. E., Fuller, T., Price, J. L. and Olney, J. W.**:   Widespread patterns of neuronal damage following systemic or intracerebral injections of kainic acid: A histological study. Neuroscience, 5: 991-1014, 1980.

**Sluga, E. and Seitelberger, F.**:   Beitrag zur spongioesen Encephalopathie.   Acta Neuropathol. (Berl.), Suppl., 3: 60-72, 1967.

**Sobel, R. A., DeArmond, S. J., Forno, L. S. and Eng, L. F.**:   Glial fibrillary acidic protein in hepatic encephalopathy.   An immunohistochemical study.   J. Neuropathol. Exp. Neurol., 40: 625-632, 1981.

**Soederfeldt, B., Kalimo, H., Olsson, Y. and Sjesjoe, B.**:   Pathogenesis of brain lesions caused by experimental epilepsy.   Light- and electron-microscopic changes in the rat cerebral cortex following bicuculline-induced status epilepticus.   Acta Neuropathol. (Berl.), 54: 219-231, 1981.

**Sotelo, C. and Rio, J. P.**:   Cerebellar malformation obtained in rats by early postnatal treatment with 6-aminonicotinamide.   Role of neuron-glia interactions in cerebellar development.   Neuroscience, 5: 1737-1759, 1980.

**Sperk, G., Lassmann, H., Baran, H., Kish, S. J., Seitelberger, F. and Hornykiewicz, O.**: Kainic acid induced seizures: Neurochemical and histopathological changes.   Neuroscience, 10: 1301-1315, 1983.

**Stadler, H.**:   Ueber Beziehungen zwischen Creutzfeldt-Jakobscher Krankheit und Pellagra. Z. Neurol., 165; 326-332, 1939.

**Suzuki, K. and Kikkawa. Y.**:   Status spongiosus of CNS and hepatic cahnges induced by Cuprizone (biscyclohexanone oxalyldihydrazone).   Am. J Pathol., 54: 307-325, 1969.

**Tanaka, R., Tanimura, K. and Ueki, K.**:   Ultrastructural and biochemical studies on ouabain-induced oedematous brain.   Acta Neuropathol. (Berl.), 37: 95-100, 1977.

**Torack, R. M.**:   Ultrastructural and histochemical studies of cortical biopsies in subacute dementia.   Acta Neuropathol. (Berl.), 13: 43-55, 1969.

**Towfighi, J. and Bonatas, N. K.**:   Effect of intracerebral injection of ouabain in adult and developing rats.   An ultrastructural and autoradiographic study.   Lab. Invest., 28: 170-180, 1973.

**Ule, G.**:   Feinstruktur der skongioesen Dystrophie der grauen Substanz.   Verh. Dtsch. Ges. Pathol., 52: 142-155, 1968.

**Ule, G. and Kolkmann, F. W.**:   Experimentelle Untersuchungen zur Wernicken Encephalopathie.   Acta Neuropathol. (Berl.), 11: 361-367, 1968.

**Watanabe, I. and Kanabe, S.**:   Early edematous lesion of pyrithiamine induced acute thiamine deficient encephalopathy in the mouse.   J Neuropathol. Exp. Neurol., 37: 401-413, 1978.

**Watanabe, I., Tomita, T., Hung, K.-S. and Iwasaki, Y.**: Edematous necrosis in thiamine-deficient encephalopathy of the mouse. J. Neuropathol. Exp. Neurol., 40: 454-471, 1981.

**Wolff, J. R., Schieweck, Ch., Emmenegger, H. and Meier-Ruge, W.**: Cerebrovascular ultra-structural alterations after intra-arterial infusions of ouabain, scillaglycosides, heparin and histamine. Acta Neuorpathol. (Berl.), 31: 45-58, 1975.

**Zamora, A. J., Cavanagh, J. B. and Kyu, M. H.**: Ultrastructural renponses of the astrocytes to portocaval anastomosis in the rat. J. Neurol. Sci., 18: 25-43, 1973.

# Chapter VII

# Changes in Water-soluble Brain Proteins in Creutzfeldt-Jakob Disease

Tsuyoshi Nishimura, M. D., Shiro Hariguchi, M. D., Kunitoshi Tada, M. D. and Masatoshi Takeda, M. D.,

In Creutzfeldt-Jakob disease (CJD), characteristic neuropathological changes such as nerve cell loss, status spongiosus, and astrocytic proliferation are extensively observed in the central nervous system. These highly destructive changes are claimed to be induced by the unknuwn transmissible agent, though the nature of the agent is not yet thoroughly clarified. Regardless of the etiology, there should be specific biochemical changes in the CJD brain and the investigation of the biochemical changes appears to be helpful to elucidate the characteristics of the etiologic agent.

So far, the changes of DNA (Bass, et al., 1975; Manuelidis, et al., 1981), RNA (Bass, et al., 1974) gangliosides (Yu, et al., 1974; Tamai, et al., 1979), lipids (Tamai, et al., 1978) and proteins (Nishimura, et al., 1974; Federico, et al., 1980; Olsson, 1980) have been reported in the CJD brain. Above all, as proteins are the most closely related to the brain function, it is required to investigate the change of proteins in detail along with the pathologic process. In this study we focused our attention on the changes of water-soluble proteins and those of fibrous proteins in the CJD brain.

## Materials and Methods

### 1) Brain tissues

CJD brains were obtained at autopsy for pathological diagnosis and stored at $-80°C$ until the experiments. The brief description of the cases used in this study are shown in Table 1.

The control brains were obtained at forensic autopsy and stored at $-80°C$ before use.

**Table 1.** CJD cases studied in the present study.

| Case number | Sex | Age of onset | Duration of illness |
|---|---|---|---|
| 1 | male | 56 | 2 y. |
| 2 | male | 43 | 2 y 6 m. |
| 3 | male | 51 | 4 m. |
| 4 | male | 39 | 2 y. |

## 2) Polyacrylamide gel electrophresis (PAAE)

The brain tissue was homegenized with 4 volumes (v/w) of 0.01 M phosphate buffer (pH 7.2) with a teflon homogenizer. After centrifugation at 10,000 ×g for 30 minutes, the supernatant was subjected to electrophoretic analysis of the water-soluble proteins.

PAAE with 7.5% polyacrylamide gel without detergents was done according to the Davis and Orstein's method. For SDS gradient PAAE, 4-30% gradient acrylamide gel slabs supplied by Pharmacia were used. For the analyses of the protein components of neurofilaments and proliferated glial fibers in CJD brain, the samples were dissolved with 6 M urea and 1% SDS and electrophoresed in 0.1 M Tris buffer (pH 7.4) containing 0.2 M sodium acetate, 0.02 M EDTA, 6 M urea and 0.1 % SDS.

## 3) Two-dimensional electrophoresis

The protein bands separated in 7.5 % polyacrylamide gel were analysed by two-dimensional electrophoresis, a reversed modification of the O'Farrell's method (O'Farrell, 1975): 7.5% disc PAAE for the first separation and isoelectric focusing (IEF) for the second separation. After electrophoresis in a 7.5% polyacrylamide gel disc, the gel was sliced into two halves, one for amideblack B10 staining, the other for IEF. The half disc was immersed in Phalmalyte (pH range 3.0-10.0) and set onto 11.5cm×11.5cm IEF slab gel for the second run at 30W for 2 hours. After the second run the slab was fixed with 10% TCA, 5% sulfosalicylate for 1 hour and immersed in a 30% methanol containing 10% acetate solution and stained with 0.02% Coomasie brilliant blue G. The pH gradient was measured with PI marker proteins (pI: 10.6, 8.7, 7.6, 6.2, 5.6, 3.9) from Oriental Yeast Co., Ltd.

## 4) Separation of glial filaments from CJD brain

Morphologically severely affected cortices of CJD brains (parietal cortex) were loosely homogenized by a teflon homogenizer with 4 volumes of 0.01 M phosphate buffer. After centrifugation at 100,000 ×g for 30 minutes, the precipitaed pellet was suspended in the same buffer containing 0.32 M sucrose. The suspension was layered on 1.6 M sucrose and centrifuged at 100,000 xg for 1 hour. The pellet obtained at the bottom was again suspended in 0.32 M sucrose, grained in half-frozen state, sonicated at 20W for 30 seconds, then centrifuged on the top of 2.0 M and 1.6 M sucrose layer. The interface between 2.0 M and 1.6 M sucrose was collected as a glial filament preparation. This fraction was mostly composed of fine fibrous aggregate and the fibrous structure with 10 nm in diameter was confirmed with electron microscopy.

## 5) Preparation of antisera for fibrous proteins

Astisera against purified neurofilament proteins, microtubule proteins, tubulin and actin were prepared. For neurofilament proteins, the triplet proteins were extracted from SDS-urea PAAE gels, 0.3-1.0 mg of the proteins were emulsified with 2 ml Freund's complete adjavent, and injected into rabbits subcutaneously. After 4 weeks, 0.5 mg of the booster proteins were intraperitoneally injected with incomplete adjavent. Out of 5 major bands derived from the neurofilament fraction, antisera against 200K, 160K, 68K and 50K were raised.

Microtubule proteins were purified by three cycles of temperature dependent cyclic polymerization, and tubulin was purified from microtuble preparation through phosphocellulose column chromatography. Actin was purified from chicken skeletal muscle. The antisera against these proteins were raised in rabbits in the same procedure as antineurofilament sera.

Anti-GFA rabbit serum was generously presented from Prof. Mori (Department of Surgery, Osaka University Medical School).

# Results

## 1) PAAE pattern of soluble proteins from the control brain

Soluble protein from healthy adult (16-50 years old) human brains showed 11 major bands and at least 7 minor bands, named from the anodal end B-1, B-2, B-2 and so on,

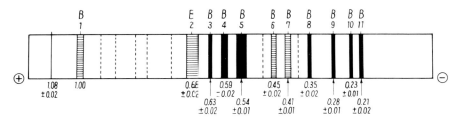

**Fig. 1.** Separation of human brain water-soluble proteins in normal adults by polyacrylamide gel (7.5%) electrophoresis. The figures below the band indicate the migration rate of each band relative to the migration distance of B-1.

**Table 2.** Age-related changes of B-2 and B-4 proteins. The figures indicate percent of B-2 and B-4 proteins in the total soluble protein.

| Age | B-2 | B-4 |
|-----|-----|-----|
| 7M | 2.0 | trace |
| 4Y | 3.5 | 2.4 |
| 16Y | 7.4 | 5.3 |
| 20Y | 7.1 | 1.1 |
| 27Y | 4.7 | 5.8 |
| 39Y | 5.7 | 5.4 |
| 53Y | 5.3 | 4.5 |
| 66Y | 5.1 | 1.5 |
| 68Y | 5.4 | 3.4 |
| 80Y | 3.0 | 1.7 |

consecutively (Fig. 1). The figures below the band are the calculated mobility of each band relative to that of band B-1. Band B-5 corresponds to serum albumin. In the brain tissue, more proteins are electrophoresed farther than B-5 band compared with other organ tissue. Especially the quantities of B-2 and B-4 proteins are much higher in the brain tissue than in other organs.

The age-relating changes of B-2 and B-4 proteins are expressed in percent to total soluble proteins in Table 2. Band B-4 is observed in trace amount in the new born and its amount increases with aging to the maximum level at 20 years of age, and it again declines in senescence. The change of band B-2 shows more or less the similar tendency with that of band B-4, but it is relatively moderate.

## 2) PAAE pattern of soluble proteins from CJD brain

Soluble proteins from CJD autopsied brains were electrophoresed in 7.5% polyacrylamide gel. The densitographic pattern is shown in Figure 2, with those of control and Alzheimer brains. In CJD, band B-2 decreases to 25-30% of the age-matched control brain and band B-4 nearly disappears. The more characteristic feature of CJD pattern is an intense band CJ-X located between B-10 and B-11. The density of CJ-X band is 43.7% of the whole density of the protein bands electrophoresed in the gel.

The PAAE pattern of the CJD brain was compared with those of Alzheimer's disease, senile dementia of Alzheimer type, Pick's disease, and amyotrophic lateral sclerosis. Disappearance of band B-2 and band B-4 is the common feature all through Alzheimer's disease, senile dementia of Alzheimer type, and Pick's disease. The increase of the density is noticed in the area around B-9 and B-10, slightly anodal side of CJ-X. In amyotrophic lateral sclerosis, decrease of B-2 and B-4 is observed in the precentral cortex and the occipital pole, but no clear change was observed in other cortical areas.

### 3) Analysis of CJ-X

Band CJ-X, specific to the CJD brain, is located between B-10 and B-11.   Since in this region no band is found in the control gel, CJ-X band is not likely to be formed by simple increment of the normal constituent proteins.   This suggests the possibility that CJ-X band could be the aggregate of the complex of smaller proteins existing in the control brain, or it could be the new protein specifically produced in the CJD brain.

Brain homogenate was electrophoresed in 4-30% gradient PAAE system with 0.2% SDS and 2mM EDTA after treating the brain homogenate with 1% 2-mercaptoethanol, and 1mM EDTA.   Soluble proteins of the CJD brain and the control brain were separated into about 40 protein bands and no difference was observed between the two groups.

Then, CJ-X band was cut off from the disc gel and extracted in 10mM Tris-HCl buffer (pH 8.0) with 1% SDS, 1% 2-mercaptoethanol and 1mM EDTA, and the extract was subjected to 4-30% gradient SDS PAAE.   The PAAE revealed that CJ-X is separated into 28 protein bands distributed between 20,000 and 100,000 of molecular weight (Fig. 3).

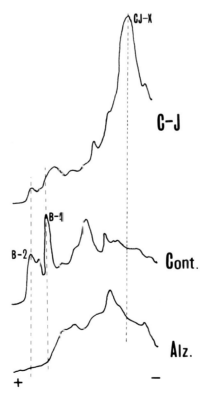

**Fig. 2.**   Densitometric representation of separation of water-soluble brain proteins by 7.5% PAAE. Cont.: Control. C-J: CJD.   Alz: Alzheimer's disease.

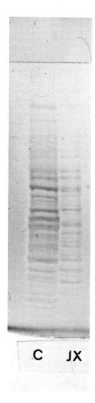

**Fig. 3.** Analysis of CJ-X protein by 4-30% gradient SDS-PAAE. C: Water-soluble proteins of the control brain. JX: CJ-X protein are separated into 28 protein bands distributed between 20,000 and 200,000 of molecular weight. To the most of the bands separated from CJ-X, corresponding bands are demonstrated in the control (C).

## 4) Two-dimensional electrophoresis of soluble proteins from CJD brain

Two dimensional electrophoretic patterns of the control and CJD proteins are shown in Fig. 4. In the control pattern, about 40 to 50 major spots are identified, the most intense spot in the central area is albumin, corresponding to B-5 in one-dimensional electrophoresis. The separation pattern of the CJD brain is clearly different from that of the control brain.

In the CJD brain, pI 5.5 protein derived from B-11 band is lost, and protein spots which normally migrate farther than albumin in both the first and the second run reduce their intensities and the relationship of the intensities among the spots is changed from the normal pattern.

## 5) Immunoelectrophoresis

CJD brain homegenate in 0.01 M phosphate buffer (pH 7.2) was centrifuged at

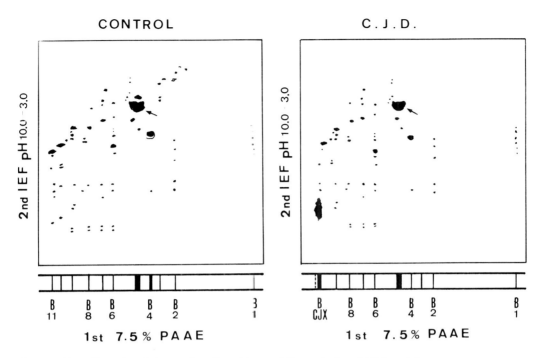

**Fig. 4.**   Two-dimensional electrophoretic patterns of the control and CJD proteins.
In the CJD brain, protein spots which migrate farther than albumin (indicated by an arrow) in both the first and the second run reduce their intensities.

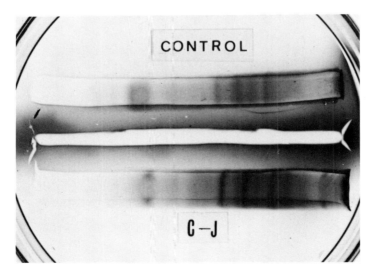

**Fig. 5.**   Immunoelectrophoretic demonstration of GFA in the water-soluble fraction.   In the CJD case (C-J), a definite precipion line is not formed, which is clearly demonstrated in the normal case.

100,000 ×g for 30 minutes.   The supernatant was electrophoresed in 7.5% polyacrylamide gel, and the gel slice was sujected to immunoelectrophoresis against anti-GFA serum. Soluble proteins from the control brain and also from astrocytoma formed precipitate lines just beside band B-11 against anti-GFA serun. (Fig. 5).   Soluble proteins from the CJD brain, however, did not show any precipitate line against anti-GFA serum, although the increase of GFA is expected from the marked astrocytosis in the CJD brain.

## 6) Immunodiffusion

The insoluble proteins from the CJD brain, which was obtained after centrifugation at 100,000 ×g for 30 minutes of the CJD brain homogenate, was suspended in 20 volumes of 10mM Tris-HCl buffer (pH 8.0) containing 1% SDS, 1% 2-mercaptoethanol and 1mM EDTA, and was heated at 100°C for 3 minutes.   Ouchterlony double immunodiffusion was studied by a modification by Yen, et al. (Yen, et al., 1976) in 1% agar containing 0.1% SDS and 0.5% Triton X-100.   The result is shown in Figure 6.   As suggested from the result of immunodiffusion, the soluble proteins from the control brain reacted with anti-GFA serum, forming definite precipitate lines, but the soluble proteins from the CJD brain did not show any precipitate lines.   On the other hand, insoluble proteins from the CJD brain showed precipitation with anti-GFA serum.   The brain proteins in Alzheimer's disease and senile dementia of Alzheimer type reacted against the anti-GFA serum in the same manner as the CJD brain proteins.

Anti-human tubulin serum reacted with insoluble proteins of the CJD brain and soluble proteins of the contral brain, but did not react with the soluble proteins of the CJD brain and with the insoluble proteins of the contral brain.   These results suggest that in the CJD brain GFA and tubulin are insolubilized to form abnormal fibrous structures.

## 7) Analysis of glial filaments from CJD brain

The component proteins of the glial filaments in the CJD brain were analysed by 4 –30% gradient SDS PAAE.   The glial filaments were separated into five major bands with molecular weights of a: 54000, b: 41000, c: 36000, d: 32000 and e: 3000, respectively.

These five bands were cut off from the gel and the proteins were extracted for immunological examinations.   Band-a reacted with anti-tubulin serum, bands-b and -c with anti-neurofilament serum and bands-d and -e with anti-GFA serum, respectively.

## Discussion

The separation pattern of SDS-PAAE of soluble proteins in the CJD brain has been reported not to be different from that of the healthy control brain.   Our results with SDS-PAAE is the same as in the previous report (Federict, et al., 1980), showing no noticeable difference between the CJD brain and the normal control brain.   Electrophoresis in 7.5%

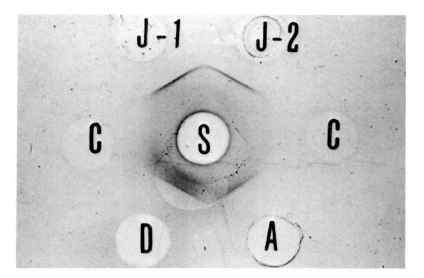

**Fig. 6.** Ouchterlony plate showing reaction between anti-GFA serum (S) and water-insoluble brain protein fractions from CJD (J-1 and J-2), Alzheimer's disease (A), senile dementia of Alzheimer type (D) and control cases (C).
Water-insoluble fractions from CJD, Alzheimer's disease and senile dementia of Alzheimer type show definite reaction with anti-GFA, while the fractions from control brains do not react.

PAAE without denaturants nor detergents, however, revealed the marked difference in soluble proteins between the CJD brain and the control brain. In PAAE with soluble proteins from the CJD brain, band B-2 and band B-4 decrease to the trace amounts and the new band CJ-X appears. The components of this CJ-X band are proteins with molecular weights of 20,000-100,000 which exist in the normal control brain. These findings seem to be explained by some mechanisms in the CJD brain which precipitate polymerization of lower molecular weight proteins to form highly polymerized molecules than in the control brain. The two-dimensional electrophoresis of CJD soluble proteins revealed the disappearance of pI 5.5 protein, however, we could not demonstrate the loss of pI 8.8 band in the the CJD brain which was reported by Olsson, et al. (Olsson, et al., 1980).

Due to marked proliferation of astrocytes in the CJD brain, the increase of glial fibrillary acidic protein (GFA) was expected, but the soluble protein fraction of the CJD brain did not show positive reaction against anti-GFA serum in immunoelectrophoresis. On the contrary, the increase of GFA was substantiated in the insoluble fraction of the CJD brain with positive immunologic reaction against anti-GFA serum. This finding suggests that the subunit protein of proliferating glail filaments in the CJD brain tends to polymerize to form the insoluble structure which is not observed in GFA of the normal brain.

Since the protein subunit of the purified glial filament from the CJD brain, as well as the protein from fibrous astrocytes of the control brain, showed positive immunologic reaction against anti-human glioma GFA serum, the immunogenecity of GFA in the CJD brain is not altered from that of the normal brain. The purified glial filaments from the

CJD brain were further analysed with SDS-PAAE and immunoelectrophoresis. The protein bands which showed positive precipitation against anti-GFA serum were those corresponding to the molecular weghts 32,000 and 30,000, lower than that of the normal GFA. It should wait for further study whether this is due to some modification of GFA subunit protein in the CJD brain or due to artifacts during the purification.

The same phenomenon was observed in the separation of proliferating neurofilaments of Alzheimer's disease by SDS-PAAE. In the separation by SDS-PAAE, it was demonstrated that the neurofilaments from Alzheimer cases are not composed of the normal triplet subnits, but of proteins with smaller molecular weights which do not exist in the control brain. These data suggest the possibility that in the pathological state where abnormal fibrous structures are accumulated, the composing protein subunits of these abnormal fibrous structure might be different from the normal subunits.

In SDS-PAAE pattern of the purified glial filaments from the CJD brain, there always found the band with molecular weight of 54,000 (band-a), which corresponds to tubulin. At present we can not conclude whether tubulin is the composing protein subunit of the proliferating filaments or it is only a contaminant in the purification process.

One of the present authors (Takeda, 1984) previously reported a possible mechanism of experimental neurofibrillary change formation in rabbits by aluminium or spindle inhibitors. In the process of the formation of experimental neurofibrillary change, proliferating neurofilaments attach to microtubule subunit proteins and insolubilize them, leading to the formation of insoluble fiber structures. It may be possible to postulate that a similar insolubilizing mechanism binds microtubule subunit proteins to proliferating glial filaments.

In immunological studies, sera from CJD patients reacted with anti-GFA serum, indicating the presence of GFA antigen in the sera of CJD patients. Sotelo, et al. (Sotelo, et al., 1980) reported the presence of autoantibodies against neurofilament proteins in sera from CJD patients, though we failed to verify the reported data. These findings arouse an interest for further investigation from diagnostic and pathophysiological points of view.

From the comprehensive understanding of the results presented in this paper, it is conceivable that in the CJD brain there are mechanisms and processes which form high degree polymers and insoluble structures of water-soluble proteins, especially of smaller sized proteins with molecular weights between 20,000 and 100,000.

We previously reported (Nishimura, et al., 1974; 1978) that a considerable part of the soluble proteins are insolubilized in the brains of patients with Alzheimer type dementia and Pick's disease as well as in the CJD brain. The insolubilization of GFA described in this paper is also observed in the Alzheimer's disease brain.

CJD has been shown to be caused by an unknown transmissible agent. So far, the demonstration of transmissible agents for Alzheimer type dementia and Pick's disease has been failed. However, the results of this paper and authors' other studies strongly suggest that there should be some common biochemical processes through CJD, Alzheimer type dementia and Pick's disease.

# REFERENCES

**Bass, N. H., Hess, H. H. and Pope, A.:** Altered cell membranes in Creutzfeldt-Jakob disease, Arch. Neurol., 31: 174-182, 1974.

**Federico, A., Annunziata, P. and Malantacchi, G.:** Neurochemical changes in Creutzfeldt-Jakob disease, J. Neurol., 223: 135-146, 1980.

**Manuelidis, L. and Manuelidis, E. E.:** Search for specific DNAs in Creutzfeldt-Jakob infectious brain fraction using "nick translation", Virology, 109: 435-443, 1981.

**Nishimura, T., Hariguchi, S., Tada, K. and Kaneko, Z.:** Changes in brain water-soluble proteins in presenile and senile dementia. In Környey, S. (ed): VII International Congress of Neuropathology (International Congress Series No. 362). Excerpta Medica, Amsterdam, pp. 139-142, 1975.

**Nishimura, T., Hariguchi, S., Tada, K. and Takeda, M.:** Changes in water-soluble brain protein in normal and abnormal aging. In Hirano, A. and Miyoshi, K (ed): Neuropsychiatric disorders in the elderly. Igaku-Shoin, Tokyo, pp. 79-84, 1983.

**O'Farrell, P. H.:** High resolution two-dimensional electrophoresis of proteins, J. Biol. Chem., 250: 4007-4021, 1975.

**Olsson, J. E.:** Brain and CSF proteins in Creutzfeldt-Jakob disease, Eur. Neurol., 19: 85-90, 1980.

**Sotelo, J., Gibbs, Jr. C. J. and Gajdusek, D. C.:** Autoantibodies against axonal neurofilaments in patients with kuru and Creutzfeldt-Jakob disease, Science, 210: 190-193, 1980.

**Takeda, M.:** Studies on mechanisms of experimental neurofibrillary change formation induced by aluminium and spindle inhibitors. Med. J. Osaka Univ. (Japan), 34: 145-161, 1984.

**Tamai, Y., Kojima, H., Ikuta, F. and Kuranishi, T.:** Alterations in the composition of brain lipids in patients with Creutzfeldt-Jakob disease, J. Neurol. Sci., 35: 59-76, 1978.

**Tamai, Y., Ohtani, Y., Miura, S., Narita, Y., Iwata, T., Kaiya, H. and Namba, M.:** Creutzfeldt-Jakob disease - Alteration in ganglioside sphingosine in the brain of a patient, Neurosci. Letters, 11: 81-86, 1979.

**Yen, S. C., Dahl, D., Schachner, M. and Shelanski, M. L.:** Biochemistry of the filaments of brain,. Proc. Nat. Acad. Sci. USA, 73: 529-533, 1976.

**Yu, R. K., Ledden, R. W., Gajdusek, D. C. and Gibbs, C. J.:** Brain Res., 70: 103-112, 1974.

# Chapter VIII

# Closing Remark

Hirotsugu Shiraki, M. D. and Toshio Mizutani, M. D.

In closing, the authors, particularly the editors, most sincerely hope that both the past history and present status of research on Creutzfeldt-Jakob disease, Creutzfeldt-Jakob disease group or allied disorders in the Japanese population have more or less been clarified. In this monograph a comparatively great emphasis has been paid to the clinicopathological classification of the disease and the interrelationship of each type of the disease.

The reasons are as follows: 1. The new types of the disease, such as the panencephalopathic type and/or chronic spongiform encephalopathy with plaques characterized by antecedent and longlasting cerebellar ataxia, which have rarely or never been reported in the western countries at least up to date, can be well documented in the Japanese population: 2. Among different approaches in an understanding of Creutzfeldt-Jakob disease it is true that epidemiological, clinical and etiological aspects have seriously been taken into consideration up to the present. Nevertheless, it is our opinion that in the previous current of research on the disease the pathogenetic aspect, particularly the morphopathogenetic aspect, has been neglected or paid little attention. For example, in the past there were only a few discussions in regard to the important findings in which single or multisystemic degeneration is most closely combined with the neuropathology of the disease, e.g., spongiform degeneration, astrocytosis and/or kuru or senile plaques.

Finally it should again be remembered that even when are different etiologic bases, the same pathogenetic mechanism can occur, whereas different pathogenetic mechanisms can in general be attributed to different etiologic bases.

# Appendix

# Creutzfeldt-Jakob Disease in Japan: Figures and Tables

Junichi Satoh, M. D. and Toshio Mizutani, M. D.

In this section the autopsy cases verified by postmortem examination, reported in Japan from 1961 to 1983, were listed, as completely as possible. Almost all cases were published in various Japanese journals, such as Clinical Neurology, Advances of Neurological Sciences, Psychiatrica et Neurologica Japonica, Neurological Medicine, Acta Pathologica Japonica, etc., while some cases were unpublished.

All the cases were numbered consecutively from No. 1 to No. 127. The number in italic type in the chapters corresponds to the number of Table 3 in this section. If either clinical or pathological findings of a case were not described in some chapter, you can find the information of its number in this table. The clinical and neuropathological findings in each case were translated to English with as much faithfulness as possible, but about one-third of all the cases were examined by us, and thus, some neuropathological findings not described originally by the authors were added in some such cases.

The number of the cases was 127. There were 74 males and 53 females. All the cases were classified into five clinicopathological subtypes as described in Chapter III: Simple poliodystrophic type of CJD ("SP", Nos. 1-16; M: F=12:4); Subacute spongiform encephalopathy ("SSE", Nos. 17-63, M:F=25:22); Ataxic form of CJD ("At", Nos. 64-72, M:F=8:1); Panencephalopathic type of CJD ("PE", Nos. 73-120, M:F=24:24); Chronic spongiform encephalopathy with plaques characterized by anteceded and longlasting cerebellar ataxia ("CSE", Nos. 121-127, M:F=5:2). Stern-Garcin syndrome was not included in this table (Chapter III-4).

SSE and PE accounted for 37% and 38% of all the cases respectively, while SP, At and CSE were a minor group. Thus, SSE and PE occupied an absolute majority of CJD in Japan. It was particularly remarked that the cases belonging to PE were prevailing in Japanese cases of CJD (sse Chapter III-6).

Frequency distribution of the age at death is shown in Fig. 1. The youngest case was

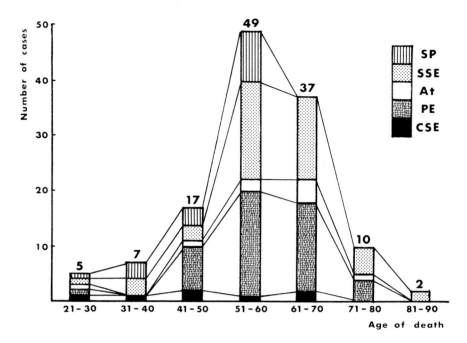

**Fig. 1.** Age at death of 127 cases with Creutzfeldt-Jakob disease. Abbreviations: SP: Simple poliodystrophic type of CJD; SSE: Subacute spongiform encephalopathy; At: Ataxic form of CJD; PE: Panencephalopathic type of CJD; CSE: Chronic spongiform encephalopathy with plaques characterized by antecedent and longlasting cerebellar ataxia.

24 years old with 43-months' duration (No. 19, SSE), while the oldest case was 88 years old with 5.5-months' duration (No.57, SSE). 68% of all cases died at the sixth and seventh decades of life. Each peak of age at death of SSE and PE existed in the sixth decade, while all the cases of SP died under the age of 60.

Fig. 2 indicates the distribution of the total duration of illness. The total duration of illness ranged from 2 months (No. 32, SSE) to 132 months (No. 121, CSE). 57% of all the cases died within 12 months of the duration, and 81.1% within 24 months. Average of the duration of each type was as follows: 7.4 months for At; 12.0 months for SP; 14.0 months for SSE; 18.6 months for PE; 73.9 months for CSE. The total duration of illness of CSE was statistically different from those of the other subtypes. Although the difference in the duration of illness was certainly important for each subtype of CJD, the evolution of clinical course could be much more significant in differentiation of clinicopathological subtypes (see Chapter III-6, Mizutani, et al., 1984).

Frequency distribution of brain weight of all cases is shown in Fig. 3. The brain weight ranged from 1560g (No. 4, SP) to 560g (No. 113, PE). Average was as follows: 1298g in SP; 1159g in SSE; 1092g in CSE; 1061g in At; 882g in PE. Thus, almost all cases of the subtypes except for PE showed more than 900g, and the atrophy remained slight to moderate in degree. The severest atrophy of the brain was found in PE, while SP showed the least atrophy.

Kirschbaum summarized the brain weight and the total duration of illness of 150 cases, and concluded that there was an inverse proportion between the brain weight and the total duration of illness (1968). However, our preliminary observation based on 88 cases showed that there was no evidence of such relationship (Mizutani, 1981). In this

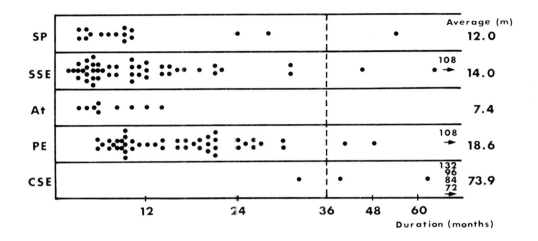

**Fig. 2.** Total duration of illness of each subtype of Creutzfeldt-Jakob disease. Each dot indicates one case. The average duration of each subtype is described at the left of the diagram. The arrows indicate the extremely protracted cases and each number indicates the total duration of illness (months). Abbreviations same as those in Fig. 1.

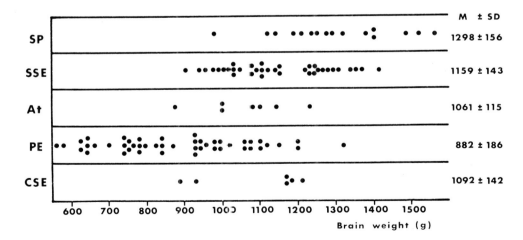

**Fig. 3.** Brain weight of each subtype of Creutzfeldt-Jakob disease. Each dot indicates one case. The average brain weight in each subtype is described at the left side of the diagram. Abbreviations same as those in Fig. 1.

survey its relationship was examined for each subtype of CJD. As a result, there was no distinct correlation of the brain weight to the total duration of illness with exception of PE. In PE, as the clinical course was more protracted, the brain atrophy became more severe. It is well-known that the brain shrinks with aging. For elimination of the effect of aging, it was examined whether the difference of the brain weight between the case of CJD and the age-matched control (Table 1) correlates to the total duration of illness. This is shown in Fig. 4. The result was that while PE showed a considerably obvious correlation of the brain atrophy to the total duration of illness, the other subtypes disclosed no relationship between the two factors. The difference of PE from the other subtypes for the brain weight was discussed in Chapter III-6.

Table 2 shows frequency of each clinical symptom which was described in the reported cases in Table 3. Unfortunately all symptoms and signs found in the clinical course of each case were not described. In some cases the clinical features were described in detail, while in the others only the outline of the clinical features was found. Furthermore, usage of the terminology for a symptom or sign was variable from case to case. For these reasons, in this section, the term "apallic state" is used as a synonym of akinetic mutism, since difference of description in both terms was obscure in many reported cases. "Ataxia" means incoordination of movement and does not always indicate clinical involvement of cerebellum. Unfortunately there were several cases in which nature of ataxia was not precisely described. Therefore, "ataxia" in this section indicates that of all types of clinical nature.

In spite of this disadvantage, the characteristics of each subtype were found in a certain degree in regard to the neuropathological findings.

Dementia, akinetic mutism, myoclonus, rigidity of muscle, gait disturbance and periodic synchronous discharge (PSD) were found in more than 50% of all the cases.

In CJD, it is not too much to say that all of the symptoms and signs in neurology and psychiatry were found. Thus, an obvious difference in frequency of clinical symptom or sign among the subtypes was scarcely able to be pointed out. However, negative symptom or sign appeared to be significant. Focal signs, such as aphasia, apraxia and agnosia were not found in SP and CSE and convulsion was not described in At. The other negative findings seemed to be insignificant, since clinical description of these symptoms was obscure in some cases. Some positive findings, on the other hand, were remarked. Lower motor neuron sign was found in 31% of the SP cases. These cases could be compatible with amyotrophic type of CJD (see Chapter III-2). Cerebellar signs and

**Table 1.** The average brain weight of the normal brains

| Age | Number of Cases | Average Weight |
|-----|-----------------|----------------|
| 21–30 | 2 | 1355g |
| 31–40 | 4 | 1278g |
| 41–50 | 8 | 1329g |
| 51–60 | 17 | 1312g |
| 61–70 | 3 | 1277g |
| 71–80 | 7 | 1210g |
| 81–90 | 3 | 1105g |

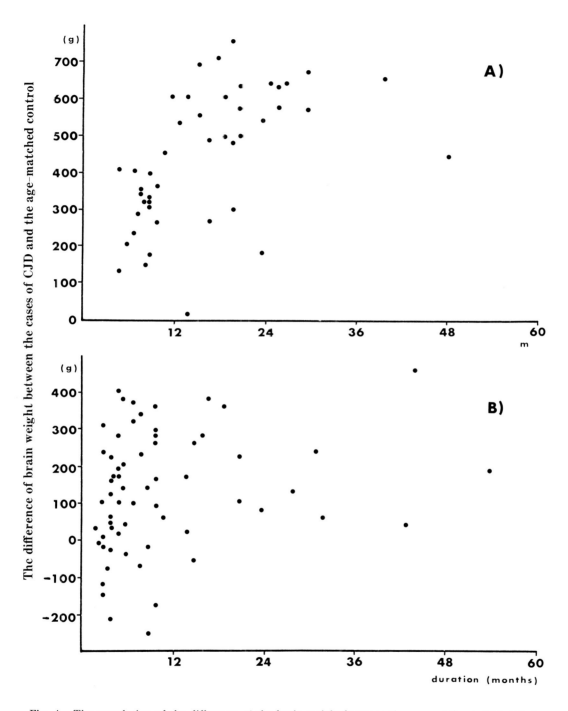

**Fig. 4.** The correlation of the difference of the brain weight between the case of Creutzfeldt-Jakob disease and the age-matched control to the total duration of illness. A) Panencephalopathic type of Creutzfeldt-Jakob disease, B) The other subtypes of Creutzfeldt-Jakob disease. Each dot indicates one case.

**Table 2.** Clinical Pictures in the Autopsy Cases of Creutzfeldt-Jakob disease

| Type of CJD | SP (n=16) | SSE (n=47) | At (n=9) | PE (n=48) | CSE (n=7) | Total (n=127) |
|---|---|---|---|---|---|---|
| **Mental** | | | | | | |
| Dementia | 100% | 87.4% | 55.6% | 87.5% | 85.7% | 86.6% |
| Akinetic mutism | 56.3 | 66.0 | 77.8 | 95.8 | 85.9 | 78.0 |
| Consciousness disturbance | 25.0 | 29.8 | 55.6 | 31.3 | 28.6 | 31.5 |
| Focal signs | 0.0 | 21.2 | 11.1 | 25.0 | 0.0 | 18.1 |
| Hallucination | 18.8 | 19.1 | 11.1 | 14.6 | 14.3 | 16.5 |
| Sleeplessness | 43.8 | 10.6 | 11.1 | 10.4 | 0.0 | 16.5 |
| Delusion | 18.8 | 10.6 | 0.0 | 12.5 | 14.3 | 11.8 |
| Perseveration | 0.0 | 12.8 | 11.1 | 6.3 | 0.0 | 7.9 |
| Psychomotor exicitement | 0.0 | 6.4 | 11.1 | 12.5 | 0.0 | 7.9 |
| **Neurological** | | | | | | |
| Myoclonus | 37.5 | 61.7 | 88.9 | 97.9 | 42.9 | 73.2 |
| Muscular rigidity | 62.5 | 74.5 | 44.4 | 60.4 | 42.9 | 63.8 |
| Gait disturbance | 93.8 | 44.7 | 44.4 | 60.4 | 100 | 59.8 |
| Para-, Tetraplegia in flexion | 18.8 | 34.0 | 22.2 | 41.7 | 14.3 | 33.1 |
| Visual disturbance (Diplopia) | 25.0 (12.5) | 31.9 (10.6) | 55.6 (22.2) | 27.1 (14.6) | 14.3 (0.0) | 33.1 (12.6) |
| Pyramidal sign | 37.5 | 25.5 | 44.4 | 31.6 | 14.3 | 29.1 |
| Dysarthria | 43.8 | 17.0 | 11.1 | 25.0 | 57.1 | 25.2 |
| Hand tremor | 43.8 | 25.5 | 11.1 | 18.6 | 42.9 | 25.2 |
| Ataxia | 37.5 | 17.0 | 22.2 | 18.6 | 71.4 | 23.6 |
| Convulsion | 18.8 | 14.9 | 0.0 | 27.1 | 14.3 | 18.9 |
| Cerebellar sign | 12.5 | 10.6 | 22.2 | 16.7 | 100 | 18.9 |
| Primitive reflex | 6.3 | 19.1 | 22.2 | 22.9 | 14.3 | 18.1 |
| Dysphagia | 18.8 | 8.5 | 11.1 | 16.7 | 28.6 | 14.2 |
| Choreo-athetoid movement | 12.5 | 6.4 | 0.0 | 16.7 | 0.0 | 10.2 |
| Lower motor neuron sign | 31.3 | 0.0 | 0.0 | 2.1 | 14.3 | 5.5 |
| Romberg's sign | 6.3 | 2.1 | 11.1 | 6.3 | 14.3 | 5.5 |
| Sensory disturbance | 0.0 | 4.2 | 11.1 | 2.1 | 28.6 | 4.7 |
| **Electroencephalographical** | | | | | | |
| Periodic synchronous discharge (PSD) (Abbreviations, see Fig. 1.) | 12.5 | 44.7 | 66.7 | 75.0 | 42.9 | 53.5 |

ataxia were found predominantly in CSE (see Chapter III-7). It was remarked that the frequencies of ataxia and/or cerebellar signs were surprisingly low in PE and At, since both subtypes had cerebello-cortical degeneration of granule cell type (see Chapter III-5 & 6). SP and SSE, on the other hand, showed ataxia and/or cerebellar signs, although their frequencies were low. In both subtypes there occurred no degeneration of the cerebellar cortex. Thus, there appears to exist clinicopathological dissociation of cerebellar signs and/or ataxia (Mizutani, et al., 1984).

Electroencephalographically, PSD was reported in 53.5% of all the cases. The SP cases showed a low rate (12.5%) as compared with the other subtypes. This may be related to the fact that almost all cases of SP were reported in the 1960s and the early

1970s, when the conception of CJD, particularly PSD was not widely recognized.

Finally, as mentioned above, it should be emphasized that the clinical characteristic of each subtype of CJD was represented more in the evolution of the clinical course than in the frequency of each symptom.

# REFERENCES

**Kirschbaum, W. R.**:  Jakob-Creutzfeldt Disease, American Elsevier, 1968.

**Mizutani, T.**:  Neuropathology of Creutzfeldt-Jakob disease in Japan.  With special reference to the panencephalopathic type, Acta Path. Jpn., 31: 903-922, 1981.

**Mizutani, T., Morimatsu, Y. and Shiraki, H.**:  Clinical pictures of Creutzfeldt-Jakob disease based on 97 autopsy cases in Japan - With special reference to clinicopathological correlation of cerebellar symptoms, Clin. Neurol. (Japan), 24: 23-32, 1984

**Table 3. Autopsy Cases of Creutzfeldt-Jakob Disease in Japan**

Simple poliodystrophic Type of Creutzfeldt-Jakob Disease

| No. | Age/Sex /Duration (months) | Authors, Year | Family History | Clinical Features | Macroscopic Findings | Microscopic Findings | |
|-----|------------|---------------|----------------|-------------------|----------------------|----------------------|---|
| 1 | 32/M/24 | Omaru, et al., 1961. | No. | Forgetfulness, slowness, unsteady gait, difficulty in articulation, emotional instability →Fasciculation in the palpebrae, tremor in the tongue, dysarthria, hyperreflexia, ataxic gait, childish behaviors→ Dirtiness, sleeplessness, nocturnal wandering→Lobotomy →Bizarre behaviors | 1190g. No gross atrophy of the brain. | Neuronal degeneration in the cerebral cortex, hippocampus, amygdaloid nucleus, dorsomedial nucleus of the thalamus, putamen and dentate nucleus; "primäre Reitzung" in Betz's giant cells. | |
| 2 | 54/M/9 | Same as No.1 | No. | Loss of activity, sleeplessness, wandering, forgetfulness, difficulty of speech→Fasciculation in the tongue, hypertonia, muscle weakness, hyperreflexia, tremor of the hand, ataxic and spastic gait, Wassermann's reaction (+) →Hallucination, increased hypertonia →Athetoid involuntary movement, dysphagia | 1400g. No gross atrophy of the brain. | Neuronal degeneration and loss in the cerebral cortex, caudate nucleus and thalamus; "primäre Reitzung" in the precentral cortex, striatum, thalamus, pallidum, dentate nucleus, oculomotor and pontine nuclei; Neuronophagia in the striatum; Mild astrocytosis; Calcification of blood vessel walls in the striatum, pallidum, thalamus, dentate nucleus, cerebral and cerebellar cortex, and white matter. | Some pathological findings comparable with Fahr's disease. |
| 3 | 53/M/4 | Same as No.1 | No. | Unsteadiness of gait and stance→tremor of the hand→ Emotional instability, sleeplessness, depressive state→ | 1320g. No gross atrophy. | Neuronal degeneration in the cerebral cortex; "primäre Reitzung" in the cerebral cortex, striatum, thalamus, den- | Authors considered as a presenile dementia of Kraepelin type. |

| No. | Age/Sex/Duration | Author | Family history | Clinical course | Brain | Neuropathology | Remarks |
|---|---|---|---|---|---|---|---|
| | | | | Ataxic gait, depression, delusion · Electric shock therapy → Wandering, incontinence, dirtiness | | ...tate nucleus and oculomotor nucleus; Mild astrcytosis. | |
| 4 | 59/M/10 | Ichikawa, et al., 1961. | No. | Forgetfulness, emotional instability → Hand tremor, sleeplessness→Euphoria, perseveration, dysarthria→Nocturnal wandering → Apathy, disorientation, gait disturbance, rigidity→Foreced grasping, adiadochokinesia, propulsion→Intention tremor, hyporeflexia→Incontinence | 1560g. No gross atrophy. | Severe neuronal degeneration and loss in the frontal, parietal and temporal cortex and striatum; "primäre Reitzung" of Betz's giant cells; Mild loss of Purkinje cells; Increased lipofuscin deposits in the striatum, dentate nucleus and brainstem nuclei; Marked hypertrophy and proliferation of astrocytes in the cerebral cortex, subcortical white matter, striatum and brainstem. | |
| 5 | 41/M/8 | Ishino, 1963. | No. | Diplopia, gait disturbance, difficulty to write→Hyperreflexia, adiadochokinesia, Romberg's sign→Amnesia→Rigidity, dysarthria, bedridden→Forced laughing, hallucination, psychomotor excitement→Ataxia in the upper limb, hyperreflexia, ankle clonus, fasciculation in the face and tongue, neurogenic EMG, paralysis of the lower limbs→Muscle atrophy, dysphagia, incontinence, fluctuation in psychic symptoms→Perforation of gastric ulcer | 1400g. No gross atrophy. | Diffuse neuronal degeneration and loss of the posterior frontal cortex; Marked astrocytosis in the frontal, hippocampal and insular cortex; "primäre Reitzung" in the precentral cortex, thalamus, oculomotor, pontine and gracile nuclei, and anterior horm; Corticospinal tract degeneration; Degeneration of Purkinje cells, loss of the granule cells in the cerebellum, degeneration of the dentate nucleus and demyelination of its hilus. | This case could be compatible with amyotrophic form of CJD. |
| 6 | 29/A/7 | Matsuoka, et al., 1964. | No. | Fever, pharyngitis→Dysphagia, mutism→Incontinence→Apallic syndrome, quadriple- | 980g. Diffuse cerebral atrophy. | Diffuse neuronal degeneration with proliferation of astrocytes, neuronophagia and glial | |

| No. | Age/Sex/Duration | Author | Heredity | Clinical course | Brain | Pathology | Characteristics |
|---|---|---|---|---|---|---|---|
| (continued) | | | | gia in flexion, choreo-athetoid movement in the extremities, hyperreflexia, ankle clonus → Fever → Fluctuation in the level of consciousness → Myclonus, rigidity →Convulsion | | rosettes in the parietal, frontal, occipital, temporal and insular cortex; "primäre Reitzung" in the precentral cortex; Neuronal degeneration with neuronophagia and glial rosettes in the striatum and thalamus; Neuronal degeneration of the dentate nucleus. | |
| 7 | 31/M/4 | Matsuoka, et al., 1968. | No. | Visual disturbance, unsteady gait →Remission for 2 years→ Reappearance→Car accident and transient unconsciousness →Bizarre behaviors, talkative, sleeplessness → Amnesia, disorientation, Gerstman's syndrome, decreased visual acuity, dysarthria, ataxic gait →Catatonic stupor→Hallucination, delusion → Stupor → Erythema in the face→Convulsion in the face and arm→ Hypertonia → High fever → Convulsion →Apallic syndrome, myclonus | 1485g. No gross atrophy. | Diffuse neuronal degeneration with focal loss, diffuse proliferation of astrocytes, neuronophagia in the frontal, superior temporal and occipital cortex; Status spongiosus in the cingulate, lateral occipital, hippocampal, middle and inferior temporal cortex; Severe neuronal changes in the thalamus (lateral, medial and ventral nuclei in decreasing order); Mild change in the striatum; Neuronal loss in the substantia nigra; "primäre Reitzung" in the precentral cortex, dentate nucleus, reticular formation, oculomotor and trigeminal sensory nuclei, and anterior horn; Diffuse myelin loss in the centrum semiovale. | |
| 8 | 51/M/10 | Yuasa, et al., 1969. | No. | Difficulty of gait →Bizarre behavior→Amnesia, disorientation, incontinence, emaciation→Fluctuation of mental disturbance→ Hyperreflexia, Babinski's sign →Amnesia→ Paraplegia in flexion→Apal- | 1120g. Mild atrophy of the frtnto-parietal lobe. | Diffuse neuronal loss and degeneration and astrocytic proliferation in the frontal, parietal and temporal cortex; Neuronal degeneration in the striatum and thalamus; "primäre Reitzung" in the cereb- | Fluctuation of mental disturbance, and lower motor neuron involvement. |

| No. | Age/Sex/Duration | Author, Year | Family history | Clinical course | Brain weight | Neuropathology | Conclusion |
|---|---|---|---|---|---|---|---|
|  |  |  |  | ...lic state→Marked muscle atrophy, fasciculation in the limbs→Tetraplegia in flexion, rigidity, coarse tremor in the upper limbs→Paralytic ileus |  | ...ral cortex, hypoglossal nucleus and anterior horn; No corticospinal tract degeneration. |  |
| 9 | 56/M/9 | Katayama, et al., 1969. | No. | Brief loss of consciousness after car accident→Gait disturbance→Bizarre behaviors, depressive, sleeplessness→Forgetfulness, confabulation, unsteady gait→Anxiety, confusion, dysarthria→Slowness, decreased activity, delusion→Disorientation→Hyporeflexia myoclonus-like movement of the trunk→Rigidity, coarse tremor of the trunk→Severe dementia, muscle atrophy of the hands, fasciculation→Dysarthria→Pneumonia | 1240g. No gross atrophy. | Diffuse neuronal loss, degeneration, and inflation in the orbital area of the frontal, insular and temporal cortex; Marked proliferation of astrocytes, spongy state in the temporal cortex; Inflated neurons and mild spongy state in the striatum; Slight loss of the granule cells of the cerebellum; Spinal cord not examined. |  |
| 10 | 46/F/6 | Mitsuyama, et al., 1970. | No. | Weakness of the lower limbs→Hypocalculia, difficulty of daily tasks→Gait disturbance, incontinence→Fasciculation, disorientation, decreased comprehension, decreased spontaneous speech→Akinetic mutism, Babinski's sign→Paralytic ileus→Startle reaction, muscle weakness of the hands and feet→Somnolence, rigidity→Pneumonia | 1290g. No obvious atrophy. | Senile plaques in the cerebral cortex, lenticular nucleus and thalamus; Mild neuronal degeneration, tissue loosening and astrocytosis in the cortex; Astrocytosis in the striatum; Severe neuronal loss and astrocytosis in the thalamus (medial and lateral nuclei); Mild loss of Purkinje cell, moderate neuronal loss in the dentate nucleus; Moderate neuronal loss in the inferior olive; "primäre Reitzung" in the cerebral cortex and anterior horn; Corticospinal tract degeneration and anterior horn cell depletion. | Senile changes in the cerebrum. Involvement of both upper and lower motor neurons |

| No. | | | | | | |
|---|---|---|---|---|---|---|
| 11 | 51/M/3 | Ishizaki, et al., 1971. | No. | Headache, diplopia, decreased visual field→Personality change→Forgetfulness, decreased comprehesion, unsteady gait→Disorientation, slowness, dysarthria, spastic gait →Forced grasp→Astasia -abasia→Paraplegia in flexion, Gegenhalten, Babinski's sign, athetoid movement of the hand→Dysphagia, startle reaction, PSD | 1380g. No gross atrophy. | Diffuse neuronal degeneration with focal loss in the frontal, parietal and occipital cortex; Inflated Betz's giant cells; Diffuse proliferation of astrocytes, coarse spongy state in the insular cortex; Astrocytosis in the striatum. | Authors considered as an intermediate case between CJD and SSE. |
| 12 | 51/F/3 | Uda, et al., 1972. | Similar clinical picture seen in one of her sisters. | Forgetfulness, disorientation →Convulsion→Decreased daily activity, apathy→Severe dementia→Rigidity→Coarse tremor of the hands→Gait disturbance→Convulsive seizures→Akinetic mutism | 1280g. Slight atrophy of the cerebrum. | Diffuse neuronal loss, degeneration and inflation in the cerebral cortex, diffuse proliferation of astrocytes; Widespread distribution of senile plaques and Alzheimer's neurofibrillary tangles; Neuronal loss and astrocytosis in the medial nucleus of the thalamus, hypoglossal nucleus, Purkinje cells, dentate nucleus and anterior horn of the spinal cord. | Senile changes in the cerebrum. |
| 13 | 47/M/54 | Ohta, et al., 1972. | No. | Spoke to himself, disturbance of thinking, hyperkinesia, wandering→Dementia, ataxic gait, dysarthria, Parkinsonism→Muscle atrophy→Akinetic mutism | 1140g. | Neuronal degeneration and loss, astrocytosis, neuronophagia in the cerebral cortex. | |
| 14 | 53/M/28 | Nakazima, et al., 1976. | No. | Gait disturbance, dementia → Pyramidal and extrapyramidal signs→PSD, myoclonus → Marked muscle atrophy → Apallic state | 1250g. | Neuronal loss, tissue loosening and proliferation of hypertrophic astrocytes in the temporal and insular cortex, slight spongy state in the tem- | |

| No. | Age/Sex/Duration | Author | | Clinical course | Gross | Microscopic | Remarks |
|---|---|---|---|---|---|---|---|
| 15 | 57/F/4.5 | Sugita, et al., 1977. | No. | Visual disturbance→Hypocalculia, forgetfulness, depressive state, gait disturbance→Delirium, emotional incontinence→Stupor→Akinetic mutism→Wernicke-Mann's posture→G.I. tract bleeding→Shock | 1210g. Mild and diffuse cerebral atrophy. | Diffuse neuronal degeneration of the cerebral cortex, focal loss of neurons, neuronophagia, astrocytic proliferation, and slight spongy state, particularly predominant in the parieto-occipital lobe, Similar changes in the striatum and thalamus; Increased glia in the cerebellar molecular layer; Inflated neurons in the cerebral cortex, dentate nucleus and dentate horn. | poral cortex; Pyramidal tract and posterior column degeneration. |
| 16 | 38/M/9 | Unpublished | No. | Depressive state→Sleeplessness, appetite loss→Gait disturbance→Remission of gait disturbance→Nocturnal excitement, wandering→Apathy, disorientation→Gait disturbance, dysarthria→Akinetic mutism, hyperreflexia, myoclonus→Rigidity→Clonic convulsion | 1520g. No gross atrophy. | Inflated neurons in the cerebral cortex including the precentral cortex, thalamus, brainstem reticular formation, and anterior horn of the spinal cord; Slight neuronal loss in the frontal, parietal and insular cortex; Proliferation of astrocytes and neuronophagia; Gliosis in the inferior olive and dentate nucleus. | |

**Subacute Spongiform Encephalopathy**

| No. | Age/Sex/Duration | Author | | Clinical course | Gross | Microscopic | Remarks |
|---|---|---|---|---|---|---|---|
| 17 | 59/M/11 | Shiraki, et al., 1963. | No. | Amnesia→Amnestic aphasia, paraphasia, iterative speech→High fever→Erythema, Wassermann's reaction (+)→Gait disturbance→Dementia→Apallic state→Emaciation | | Coarse and fine spongy state in the cerebral cortex except for the hippocampus, particularly predominant in the occipital, temporal and frontal lobes; Slight neuronal de- | The first case of SSE see Chapter III -3. |

| No. | Age/Sex/Duration | Author | Autopsy | Clinical course | Brain weight / Gross findings | Histological findings | Remarks |
|---|---|---|---|---|---|---|---|
| | | | | | | ...generation and slight proliferation of astrocytes; Mild spongy state in the striatum; No findings compatible with syphilis. | |
| 18 | 70/M/15 | Same as No. 17. | No. | Slight mental disturbance→Decreased daily activity, disorientation, anxiety, speech disturbance, tremor of the tongue→Restlessness, amnesia, perseveration, agraphia, aphasia, dysarthria, intention tremor→Dementia→Emaciation | Brain weight? | Coarse spongy state in the striate, temporal, frontal, precentral and insular cortex and striatum; Acute change more predominated in the depths of the sulci of the entire cortex; Senile plaques, neurofibrillary tangles and granulovacuolar degeneration in the Ammon's horn and frontal lobes. | Senile change and SSE. The first case of SSE. |
| 19 | 24/M/43 | Tsujiyama, et al., 1965. | No. | Delusion→Excitement→Remission→Delusion, hallucination→Electric shock therapy→Remission→Acute onset of numbness, weakness of the legs, unsteady gait, ataxia, dysarthria→Dysphagia, rigidity, hyperreflexia→Disturbance of consciousness | 1310g. Slight swelling of the brain. Laminar lesion in the striate cortex. | Spongy state in the entire cortex, particularly predominant in the striate cortex; Neuronal loss, particularly of the large size in the striate cortex; Marked proliferation of astrocytes; Severe neuronal loss and astrocytosis in the striatum; Moderate astrocytosis in the medial nucleus of the thalamus. | Authors considered as Heidenhain's syndrome. |
| 20 | 68/F/5 | Shinfuku, et al., 1965. | No. | Amnesia→Disorientation, perseveration, hyperreflexia, Romberg's sign→Gait disturbance→Dementia, visual loss, paralysis of the right arm→Forced laughing→Clonic convulsion, paraplegia in flexion→Myoclonus, rigidity, dysphagia→Apallic state | 1080g. Small brain. | Spongy state and astrocytic proliferation in the cerebral cortex, particularly of the occipital lobe; Neuronal loss in the occipital lobe; Spongy state in the striatum; Marked neuronal loss in the anterior and medial nuclei of the thalamus. | Thalamic degeneration. |

| | | | | | | | |
|---|---|---|---|---|---|---|---|
| 21 | 55/F/8 | Nishimura, 1965. | No. | Furuncles in the chest and abdomen→Vomiting, numbness in the ankles→Motor disturbance of the limbes, coarse tremor of the upper limbs→Incontinence→Visual loss→Disturbed consciousness →Tetraplegia in flexion→Hyperreflexia, primitive reflexes, Babinski's sign→Myoclonus, PSD → Delirium → Akinetic mutism | 1150g. No gross atrophy. | Status spongiosus in the cerebral cortex, particularly of the occipital lobe; Marked astrocytic proliferation and slight neuronal loss in the cortex; Slight loss of neurons in the striatum. | |
| 22 | 41/F/21 | Iwase, et al., 1967. | No. | Fatigability, appetite loss, weight loss→Slowness→Disorientation, amnesia → Delusion, personality change→Disorder of thinking, hallucination, delusion, ataxic gait, Babinski's sign → Dementia, stereotypy | 1230g. Diffuse atrophy. | Diffuse spongy state, astrocytosis and neuronal loss in the cerebral cortex including the precentral cortex; Similar changes in the caudate; Pyramidal tract degeneration. | Pyramidal tract degeneration. |
| 23 | 59/M/3 | Shirabe, et al., 1967. | No. | Gait disturbance→Speech disturbance→Intention tremor, poor coordination, hyperreflexia → Generalized convulsion →Mental deterioration→Decerebrate rigidity→Myoclonus | 1140g. | Spongy state and astrocytosis, acute changes and loss of neurons in the cerebral cortex; Slight loss of Purkinje cells. | |
| 24 | 59/M/4 | Unpublished | No. | Optic agnosia → Amnesia, disorientation, hypocalculia, agraphia→Mutism, unable to walk, incontinence→Dysphagia, perseveration→Myoclonus, convulsion→Akinetic mutism, Gegenhalten, paraplegia in flexion | 1410g. Atrophy of the cerebrum, particularly of the occipital lobes. | Severe spongy state, astrocytic proliferation, neuronal loss and inflation in the cerebral cortex, particularly predominant in the occipital cortex; Similar changes in the caudate; Astrocytosis in the putamen. | |

| No. | | | | | | | |
|---|---|---|---|---|---|---|---|
| 25 | 56/M/17 | Oikawa, et al., 1969. | Two members in this family suffered from CJD (Nos. 93 & 120). | Amnesia, slowness→Hand tremor→Rigidity, akinesia→Apathetic, athetoid movement, myoclonic jerk→Primitive reflexes→Incontinence, dementia→Blindness→Apallic state→Emaciation→Pneumonia | 1000g. Diffuse atrophy. | Spongy state, astrocytic proliferation and relatively well preserved neurons in the temporal, parietal, occipital and insular cortex; Slight spongy state in the striatum and thalamus; Swelling of oligodendroglia and ameboid change of astrocytes in the cerebral white matter. | Familial case of CJD. See Chapter IV, case 1 in Family H. |
| 26 | 57/M/5.5 | Matsuoka, et al., 1970. | No. | Common cold→Visual disturbance→Diplopia, gait disturbance, tinnitis→Clonic convulsion after cerebral angiography, constriction of the visual field→Unable to walk, unreasonable conversation, anxiety→Marked cerebellar ataxia, myoclonus→Disorientation, perseveration, decreased spontaneity, incontinence→Paraplegia in flexion, marked rigidity, cerebellar dysarthria, dysphagia→High fever→Cloudiness of conciousness→Apallic state, PSD | 1240g. Slight atrophy of the frontal and occipital lobes. Marked atrophy of the cerebellar vermis. | Coarse spongy state with relatively well preservation of neurons and slight astrocytic proliferation in the one-third of the cortex, and fine spongy state with marked astrocytic proliferation and disturbed cortical cytoarchitecture in the two-third of the cortex; Neuronophagia in the precentral cortex; Slight changes in the striatum; Marked loss of the granule cells with proliferation of Bergmann's glia in the Purkinje cell layer of the cerebellar vermis; Diffuse proliferation of astrocytes in the dentate nucleus; Neuronal degeneration and vacuolation in the anterior horn of the spinal cord. | Some findings compatible with those in the ataxic form of CJD. |
| 27 | 35/M/21 | Same as No. 26. | No. | Weakness of the left lower limb→Unsteady gait, amnesia, disorientation→Decreased activity, bradyphrenia, perseveration, dysarthria, gait ataxia, slight adiadochokine- | 1045g. Atrophy of the frtntal and occipital lobes. | Spongy state and proliferation of astrocytes with relatively well preservation of neurons in the cerebral cortex; Inflated neurons in the temporal and parietal cortex; | see Chapter III -3, case 3. |

| No. | Age/Sex/Duration | Author | Transmission | Clinical course | Brain weight | Pathology | Remark |
|---|---|---|---|---|---|---|---|
| | | | | sia, poor performance of finger-to-nose test, Gegenhalten →Coarse tremor, rigidity, marked ataxia, Babinski's sign→Apallic state, paraplegia in flexion→Myoclonus, PSD→Clonic convulsion→Recurrent high fever | | Senile plaques in the cerebral cortex; Tissue loosening and astrocytosis in the striatum and thalamus; Senile plaques in the cerebellar cortex; Well preserved Purkinje and granule cells, and proliferation of Bergmann's glia; Neuronal loss in the inferior olive and inflation of the remaining neurons; Spongy state with a few spheroids in both the lateral and posterior columns of the spinal cord. | SSE with senile change. |
| 28 | 66/M/4 | Ishida, et al., 1971 | No. | Visual loss→Hallucination→ Disorientation→Paraplegia of the legs→Delirium→Dementia →Rigidity, convulsion→ Dysarthria→Disturbance of consciousness→Fever | 1240g. Diffuse cerebral atrophy. | Diffuse neuronal loss and degeneration, senile plaques, spongy state, neuronophagia and astrocytic proliferation in the cortex, particularly of the occipital and frontal lobes; Neuronal degeneration and spongy state in the striatum; Microglia with fat droplets in the cerebellum; Slight loss of Purkinje cells; Widespread distribution of arteriosclerosis, particularly in the meninges. | |
| 29 | 62/M/8 | Rikimaru, et al., 1972. | No. | Visual loss→Disorientation, amnesia→Dementia→Rigidity, myoclonus, PSD | Brain weight? | Diffuse neuronal degeneration and spongy state with astrocytosis in the cerebral cortex, particularly pronounced in the occipital lobe; Neuronal degeneration in the basal ganglia, cerebellum, pons and medulla. | |

276

| No. | Age/Sex/Duration | Author | | Clinical course | | Histopathology | Remarks |
|---|---|---|---|---|---|---|---|
| 30 | 59/M/10 | Taniguchi, et al., 1972. | No. | Hand tremor, gait disturbance→General emaciation, amnesia→Dementia, hallucination→Myoclonus→Spasticity→Decerebrate posture | 1020g. Diffuse atrophy. | Marked spongy state in the cerebral cortex and subcortical white matter. | |
| 31 | 53/F/19 | Isaki, et al., 1972. | No. | Hypochondria → Amnesia, mutism→Amentia, rigidity→Akinetic mutism, convulsion, decerebrate rigidity | 1020g. Fronto-temporal atrophy, particularly marked in the left hemisphere. | Spongy state astrocytosis, and neuronal loss and degeneration, and inflation in the frontal, temporal, infraparietal and insular cortex; Astrocytic proliferation in the thalamus, hippocampus, pontine tegmentum in inferior olive. | Predominant change in the left cerebral hemisphere. |
| 32 | 64/M/2 | Hamaguchi, et al., 1972. | No. | Surgical operation for hemorrhoid under lumber anesthesia →2 days later, disorientation →Involuntary movement in the face and arm→Appetite loss, decreased spontaneity, incontinence→Astasia-abasia →High fever→Somnolence→ Rigidity→Myoclonus, rigidity, primitive reflexes, paraplegia in flexion, PSD→High fever | 1250g. Slight atrophy of the frntal lobes. | Marked spongy state, slight neuronal loss and astrocytosis in the frontal, supraparietal, temporal, insular and occipital cortex; Primitive plaques in the frontal cortex; Marked spongy state in the medial nucleus of the thalamus and less severe in the striatum; Slight neuronal loss in the inferior olive. | |
| 33 | 59/M/4 | Suetsugu, et al., 1973. | No. | Amnesia, sleeplessness, visual loss, diplopia→Gait disturbance→Ataxic gait→Limb ataxia, nystagmus→Chorea-like movement, myoclonus, PSD, paraplegia in flexion→Gegenhalten→Akinetic mutism | 1220g. No gross atrophy. | Marked spongy state and astrocytic proliferation predominant in the occipital cortex; Diffuse neuronal loss and degeneration in the temporal and frontal cortex; Inflated neurons in the superior frontal cortex; No remarkable findings in the striatum, globus pallidus and thalamus. | |

| | Reference | | Age/Sex | Clinical course | Brain | Histological findings | Remarks |
|---|---|---|---|---|---|---|---|
| 34 | Suetsugu, et al., 1973. | No. | 57/F/15 | Mutism, forgetfulness→Personality change→Amnesia, hypocalculia, hyperreflexia, rigidity→Babinski's sign, incontinence, forced grasp→Apallic state, quadriplegia in flexion→Myoclonus | 1120g. Slight atrophy of the frontal lobes. | Spongy state and astrocytic proliferation with slight neuronal degeneration in the frontal and parietal cortex; Primitive senile plaques in the frontal, temporal and parietal cortex; Moderate astrtocytosis in the pallidum, thalamus, striatum and claustrum. | Primitive plaques in the cerebral corrtex. |
| 35 | Same as No. 34. | No. | 65/M/3 | Sleeplessness→Disorientation→Amnesia→Delirium, unsteady gait→Nausea, vomiting→Perseveration→Incontinence→Marked ataxia, rigidity→Limb ataxia→Akinetic mutism→Myoclonus, PSD | 1410g. Slight swelling. | Moderate proliferation of astrocytes and slight neuronal changes particularly in the occipital cortex; Slight astrocytosis in the thalamus; No obvious changes in the striatum, brainstem and spinal cord. | No obvious anatomical substrate for marked ataxia. |
| 36 | Ogasawara, et al., 1973. | No. | 61/M/11 | Amnesia, hallucination, disorientation→Dementia→Rigidity | Brain weight? | Severe neuronal loss in the frontal and temporal cortex and mild astrocytosis; Spongy state in the cerebral cortex and white matter; Slight change in the striatum, thalamus and red nucleus. | The histological nature of the spongy state in the white matter was unclear. |
| 37 | Same as No. 36 | No. | 36/M/31 | Headache, tinnitus→Forgetfulness→Dysarthria, gait disturbance, hyperreflexia, ataxia→Dementia→Psychomotor excitement | Brain weight? | Severe neuronal loss and degeneration, spongy state and astrocytic proliferation in the cerebral cortex, striatum and thalamus; Spongy state in the cerebral white matter; Neuronal loss in the inferior olive. | The histological nature of the spongy state in the white matter was obscure. |
| 38 | Naito, et al., 1974. | No. | 60/M/11 | Forgetfulness, visual hallucination, strange behaviours→Disorientation, hypocalculia, apathy, hyporeflexia in the | 1320g. Slight atrophy of the frontal lobes. | Spongy state, neuronal loss and astrocytic proliferation in the cerebral cortex, particularly predominant in the tem- | |

| | | | | | | |
|---|---|---|---|---|---|---|
| 39 | 59/F/22 | Hirai, et al., 1974. | No. | right lower limb→Marked dementia→Mutism, incontinence→High fever→Tremor, rigidity→Akinetic mutism, decorticate rigidity | poral cortex; Slight to moderate spongy state in the striatum and thalamus; Inflated neurons in the pontine reticular formation. | |
| | | | | Dressing apraxia→Dementia, pyramidal sign, extrapyramidal symptoms, primitive reflexes myoclonus, PSD,→Intracerebral hemorrhage of the left hemisphere, and surgical removal→Decerebrate rigidity | Brain weight? Intracerebral hemorrhage in the striatum. | Spongy state, neuronal loss and astrocytosis in the cerebral cortex of the right hemisphere. |
| 40 | 42/M/2.5 | Hoshino, et al., 1974. | No. | Hand trauma→Complete recovery after surgical intervention→4 years later, speech disturbance. extrapyramidal signs→Pyramidal sign→Dementia, incontinence→Apallic state | 1340g. Adhesion of the dura matter, old scar and atrophy of the orbital area of the frontal and temporal lobes of the right hemisphere, old hemorrhage in the in the right frontal lobe. | Ulegyria in the superior temporal, middle and inferior frontal, insular and precentral cortex of the right side; Spongy state and proliferation of hypertrophic astrocytes in the cortex, particularly pronounced in the right occipital lobe; Spongy state, neuronal loss and astrocytosis in the striatum and thalamus; Pyramidal tract degeneration. | see Chapter III -3, case 5. Marked spongy state predominated in the right hemisphere damaged by head trauma. |
| 41 | 65/M/14 | Tadokoro, et al., 1975, Case 2. | No. | Amnesia→Apraxia, agnosia, agraphia, incontinence → Echolalia, pyramidal sign, tremor, rigidity→Apallic state | 1225g. Moderate atrophy. | Spongy state, neuronal degeneration and inflation of neurons in the cerebral cortex; Marked astrocytic proliferation in the corticomedullary junction; Inflated neurons and slight proliferation of astrocytes in the striatum and thalamus. | Widespread distribution of inflated neurons in the cerebral cortex, striatum and thalamus. |

| | | | | Clinical course | Brain weight / findings | Neuropathology | Comments |
|---|---|---|---|---|---|---|---|
| 42 | 60/F/5.5 | Suetsugu, et al., 1975. | No. | Common cold→Decreased visual acuity→Mutism, slowness → Right hemiparesis, cloudiness of consciousness, rigidity→Myoclonus, PSD→Apallic state, paraplegia in flexion | Brain weight? | Marked spongy state, neuronal loss and astrocytic proliferation in the cortex, particularly predominant in the occipital lobe; Proliferation of astrocytes in the striatum and thalamus. | |
| 43 | 48/F/6 | Narita, et al., 1976. | No. | Personality change → Optic agnosia→Sleeplessness, confusion → Rigidity → Stupor → Apallic state →Myoclonus | 1370g. | Spongy state, astrocytic proliferation, neuronal degeneration and loss in the cerebral cortex, particularly in the striate cortex; Fat granule cells in the cerebral cortex; Similar but less severe changes in the striatum, thalamus and cerebellar cortex. | The change in the cerebral cortex similar to case 8 in the Nevin's series (1960). |
| 44 | 34/M/108 | Ishii, et al., 1977. | No. | 25 yrs., Unsteady gait→29 yrs., Spastic gait, difficulty to write his name→30 yrs., Speech disturbance, apraxia → Constriction of visual field, spastic gait, hypertonia, poor coordination, tremor, Gerstmann's syndrome → Apallic state | 980g. Markedly diffuse atrophy of the cerebrum, particularly in the parieto-occipital lobe. | Spongy state, neuronal degeneration and loss, and proliferation of astrocytes in the cortex, particularly pronounced in the parieto-occipital lobe; Mild pallor of myelin in the subcortical white matter of the occipital lobe with fibrillary gliosis; Astrocytic proliferation in the striatum; Glial nodules in the inferior olive; Pyramidal tract degeneration; No remarkable changes in the cerebellum. | Strikingly long duration of the illness, typical changes of SSE in the cerebral cortex, and no obvious degeneration in the cerebral white matter. |
| 45 | 62/F/12 | Umezaki, et al., 1977. | No. | Appetite loss, vomiting→Gait disturbance → Hallucination, delusion → Myoclonus, PSD, Gegenhalten→Akinetic mutism | Brain weight? | Tissue loosening and spongy state, neuronal degeneration and loss, and marked proliferation of astrocytes in the cerebral cortex and basal ganglia. | |

| | | | | | | |
|---|---|---|---|---|---|---|
| 46 | 58/F/16 | Mukai, et al., 1978. | No. | Difficulty to speech→Involuntary movement in the right upper limb→Marked gait disturbance, paraplegia in flexion, hypertonia, mutism→Amnesia, distorientation, bizarre behaviours, hallucination, incontinence→Rigidity, tetraplegia in flexion→Apallic state | 1100g. No gross atrophy. | Marked spongy state, and less severe neuronal loss and astrocytosis in the cerebral cortex, particularly of the occipital lobe; Similar but far less severe changes in the thalamus and striatum; Spongy state in the substantia nigra, cerebellar cortex and dentate nucleus; Slight loss of Purkinje cells. |
| 47 | 73/F/4 | Teramoto, et al., 1978. | No. | Visual disturbance of color→Diplopia, headache, disorientation→Visual loss, cerebellar signs, hyperreflexia→Rigidity →Akinetic mutism | 1020g. Atrophy of the occipital lobes. | Neuronal loss, astrocytosis and spongy state in the cerebral cortex, particularly predominant in the occipital lobes; Similar changes in the thalamus and cerebellum. |
| 48 | 67/F/7 | Mizushima, 1978. | No. | Hypokinesia, amnesia, unaimed behaviors→Sleeplessness, nocturnal delirium, tremor of the trunk, gait disturbance, incontinence→Tremor of the hand, rigidity, myoclonus of the upper limbs, PSD→Akinetic mutism, paraplegia in flexion, hyperreflexia, pathological reflexes, primitive reflexes, myoclonus of the right upper and lower limbs→Fever, emaciation | 950g. More marked atrophy of the right hemisphere, moderate dilatation of the ventricular systems, moderate atrophy of the striatum. | Marked neuronal loss, spongy state and proliferation of astrocytes in the cerebral cortex, particularly in the frontal, rectal, cingular, insular, temporal and occipitotemporal cortex; Similar changes in the striatum, claustrum and thalamus (VL & A); Astrocytic proliferation and slight spongy state in the external pallidum, amygdaloid nucleus, superior colliculus, central gray of the midbrain and pontine reticular formation; Neuronal loss in the cerebellar vermis. |